Symbol	How it is read	What it means
s_p	s sub *p*	Pooled standard deviation
$s_{\bar{x}}$	s sub x-bar	Sample standard error of the mean; standard deviation of sampling distribution
SE(b)	standard error of *b*	Standard error of the regression coefficient
SE($\bar{x}$)	standard error of *x*-bar	Standard error of the mean (same as $s_{\bar{x}}$ or $\sigma_{\bar{x}}$)
SE($\hat{p}_1 - \hat{p}_2$)	standard error of *p*-one-hat minus *p*-two-hat	Standard error of the difference of two proportions
SE($\bar{x}_1 - \bar{x}_2$)	standard error of x-one-bar minus x-two-bar	Standard error of the difference of the two means
t	*t* value	*t* value from Student's *t* distribution
t_α	*t* sub alpha	*t* value corresponding to a specified tail area α
$\overline{X}$	*X*-bar	Sample mean; mean of *x* values
$\overline{Y}$	*Y*-bar	Mean of *y* values
Z	*Z* score	Standard normal deviate

II. Symbols taken from letters of the Greek alphabet

Symbol	How it is read	What it means
α	alpha	Significance level
α_0	alpha sub zero	Baseline value of α
α error	alpha error	Type I error in hypothesis testing
β error	beta error	Type II error in hypothesis testing
α	alpha	*y* intercept of population regression line
β	beta	Slope of population regression line
χ^2	chi-square (pronounced "ki-square")	Test statistic for contingency table
δ	delta	Mean difference of population observations
Δ	delta (capital delta)	Δx means change in x
μ	mu	Population mean
μ_0	mu sub zero	Baseline value of μ
$\mu_{\bar{x}}$	mu sub x-bar	Mean of sampling distribution
σ	sigma	Population standard deviation
σ^2	sigma squared	Population variance
$\sigma_{\hat{p}}$	sigma sub *p* hat	Standard error of $\hat{p}$

continued on inside back cover

Basic Statistics for the Health Sciences

Jan W. Kuzma

LOMA LINDA UNIVERSITY

Mayfield Publishing Company

To my mother, Elizabeth, my wife, Kay, and my children, Kim, Kari and Kevin, who have given me faith, love, and joy.

First edition

Library of Congress Catalog Card Number: 83-062835
International Standard Book Number: 0-87484-587-4

Manufactured in the United States of America
Mayfield Publishing Company
285 Hamilton Avenue
Palo Alto, California 94301

Sponsoring editor: C. Lansing Hays
Manuscript editor: Lieselotte Hofmann
Managing editor: Pat Herbst
Art director: Nancy Sears
Designer: Albert Burkhardt
Cover designer: Albert Burkhardt
Illustrator: Mary Burkhardt
Production manager: Cathy Willkie
Compositor: Jonathan Peck Typographers, Ltd.
Printer and binder: Lehigh Press/R. R. Donnelley

Credits

Contents

Preface xiii

Chapter 1

Statistics and How They Are Used 1

1.1 The Meaning of Statistics 2

What Does "Statistics" Mean? 2

What Do Statisticians Do? 2

1.2 The Uses of Statistics 3

1.3 Why Study Statistics? 4

1.4 Sources of Data 5

Surveys and Experiments 5

Retrospective Studies 6

Prospective Studies 7

Comparison of Ratios 8

Descriptive and Analytical Surveys 8

1.5 Clinical Trials 8

1.6 Planning of Surveys 10

Exercises 10

Chapter 2

Populations and Samples 12

2.1 Selecting Appropriate Samples 13

2.2 Why Sample? 14

2.3 How Samples Are Selected 14

2.4 How to Select a Random Sample 15
2.5 Effectiveness of a Random Sample 18
Exercises 19

Chapter **3**

Organizing and Displaying Data **20**

3.1 The Use of Numbers in Organizing Data 21
3.2 Quantitative and Qualitative Data 21
3.3 The Frequency Table 24
3.4 Graphing Data 26
Histograms 27
Frequency Polygons 28
Cumulative Frequency Polygons 29
Stem-and-Leaf Displays 29
Bar Charts 30
Pie Charts 32
Exercises 34

Chapter **4**

Summarizing Data **36**

4.1 Measures of Central Tendency 37
The Mean 37
The Median 38
The Mode 38
Which Average Should You Use? 38
4.2 Measures of Variation 39
Range 39
Mean Deviation 39
Standard Deviation 40
4.3 Coefficient of Variation 42
4.4 Means and Standard Deviations from Grouped Data 42
4.5 Means and Standard Deviations of a Population 44
Exercises 46

Chapter 5

Probability 48

5.1 What Is Probability? 49

5.2 Probability Rules 51

Multiplication Rule 51

Addition Rule 52

5.3 Counting Rules 54

Rule 1: Number of Ways 54

Rule 2: Permutations 55

Rule 3: Combinations 56

5.4 Probability Distributions 56

5.5 Binomial Distribution 57

Exercises 61

Chapter 6

The Normal Distribution 65

6.1 The Importance of Normal Distributions 66

6.2 Properties of the Normal Distribution 67

6.3 Areas Under the Normal Curve 68

Exercises 75

Chapter 7

Sampling Distribution of Means 77

7.1 The Distribution of a Population and the Distribution of Its Sample Means 78

7.2 Central Limit Theorem 80

7.3 Standard Error of the Mean 81

7.4 Student's *t* Distribution 83

7.5 Application 86

Exercises 87

Chapter **8**

Estimation of Population Means 89

8.1 Estimation 90
8.2 Point Estimates and Confidence Intervals 90
8.3 Two Independent Samples 93
8.4 Confidence Intervals for the Difference Between Two Means 94
8.5 The Before-and-After Experiment 97
8.6 Determination of Sample Size 99
Exercises 101

Chapter **9**

Tests of Significance 103

9.1 Definitions 104
9.2 Basis for a Test of Significance 105
9.3 Procedure for a Test of Significance 106
9.4 One-Tailed Versus Two-Tailed Tests 108
9.5 Meaning of "Statistically Significant" 110
9.6 Type I and Type II Errors 111
9.7 Test of Significance of Two Independent Sample Means 113
9.8 Relationship of Tests of Significance to Confidence Intervals 115
Exercises 116

Chapter **10**

Analysis of Variance 121

10.1 Function of ANOVA 122
10.2 Rationale for ANOVA 122
10.3 ANOVA Calculations 123
10.4 Assumptions 126
10.5 Application 126
Exercises 129

Chapter 11

Inferences Regarding Proportions 131

11.1 Introduction 132
11.2 Mean and Standard Deviation of the Binomial Distribution 132
11.3 Approximation of the Normal to the Binomial Distribution 133
11.4 Test of Significance of a Binomial Proportion 134
11.5 Test of Significance of the Difference Between Two Proportions 135
11.6 Confidence Intervals 137
Confidence Interval for p 137
Confidence Interval for the Difference of $p_1 - p_2$ 138
Exercises 139

Chapter 12

The Chi-Square Test 141

12.1 Rationale for the Chi-Square Test 142
12.2 The Basics of a Chi-Square Test 142
12.3 Types of Chi-Square Tests 145
12.4 Test of Association Between Two Variables 146
12.5 Test of Homogeneity 148
12.6 Test of Significance of the Difference Between Two Proportions 150
12.7 Test of Goodness of Fit 151
12.8 Two-by-Two Contingency Tables 152
12.9 Measures of Strength of Association 153
12.10 Limitations in the Use of Chi-Square 155
Exercises 156

Chapter 13

Correlation and Linear Regression 158

13.1 Relationship Between Two Variables 159
13.2 Differences Between Correlation and Regression 161
13.3 The Scatter Diagram 162

13.4 The Correlation Coefficient 164
13.5 Tests of Hypotheses and Confidence Belts for a Population Correlation Coefficient 166
13.6 Limitations of the Correlation Coefficient 167
13.7 Regression Analysis 169
13.8 Inferences Regarding the Slope of the Regression Line 174
Exercises 176

Chapter **14**

Nonparametric Methods **178**
14.1 Rationale for Nonparametric Methods 179
14.2 Advantages and Disadvantages 179
14.3 Wilcoxon Rank-Sum Test 180
14.4 Wilcoxon Signed-Rank Test 182
14.5 Spearman Rank-Order Correlation Coefficient 184
Exercises 186

Chapter **15**

Vital Statistics and Demographic Methods **189**
15.1 Introduction 190
15.2 Sources of Vital Statistics and Demographic Data 190
The Census 190
Annual Registration of Vital Events 191
Morbidity Surveys 192
15.3 Vital Statistics Rates, Ratios, and Proportions 194
15.4 Measures of Mortality 195
Annual Crude Death Rate 195
Age-Specific Death Rate 195
Cause-Specific Death Rate 196
Cause-Race–Specific Death Rate 196
Proportional Mortality 197

Maternal Mortality Ratio 198
Infant Mortality Rate 198
Neonatal Mortality Proportion 199
Fetal Death Ratio 199
Perinatal Mortality Proportion 200
15.5 Measures of Fertility 200
Crude Birthrate 200
General Fertility Rate 201
15.6 Measures of Morbidity 201
Incidence Rate 201
Prevalence Proportion 202
Case-Fatality Proportion 202
15.7 Adjustment of Rates 202
The Direct Method 203
The Indirect Method 205
Exercises 206

Chapter 16

Life Tables **207**

16.1 Introduction 207
16.2 Current Life Tables 208
Age Interval 210
Age-Specific Death Rate 210
Correction Term 210
Corrected Death Rate 210
Number Living at Beginning of Age Interval 210
Number Dying During Age Interval 211
Person-Years Lived in Interval 211
Total Number of Person-Years 211
Expectation of Life 211
16.3 Follow-up Life Tables 214
Construction of a Follow-up Life Table 214
Exercises 217

Chapter 17

The Health Survey and the Research Report 219

17.1 Planning a Health Survey 210

Step 1: Making a Written Statement of the Purpose 220

Step 2: Formulating Objectives and Hypotheses 221

Step 3: Specifying the Target Population 221

Step 4: Listing the Variables 221

Step 5: Reviewing Existing Data 221

Step 6: Deciding How to Collect Data 222

Step 7: Establishing the Time Frame 222

Step 8: Designing the Questionnaire 222

Step 9: Pretesting the Questionnaire 223

Step 10: Selecting the Sample 223

Step 11: Collecting the Data 223

Step 12: Editing and Coding the Data 223

Step 13: Analyzing the Data 224

Step 14: Reporting the Findings 224

17.2 Evaluation of a Research Report 224

Observer Bias 225

Sampling Bias 225

Selection Bias 225

Response Bias 225

Dropout Bias 226

Memory Bias 226

Participant Bias 226

Lead-Time Bias 226

Keys to a Systematic Approach 226

Exercises 228

Chapter 18

Computers: An Introduction 229

18.1 Introduction 230

18.2 Hardware 230

18.3 Software 231
18.4 Computer Programs 232
18.5 Computerized Data Entry: An Example 233
18.6 Computerized Data Output: An Example 237
18.7 Microcomputers 238
Exercises 240

Appendix A: Binomial Probability Table 241
Appendix B: Percentiles of the F Distribution 244

Bibliography 248
Answers to Selected Exercises 251
Index 269

Preface

Statistics is a peculiar subject. Unaccountably, many students who handle their toughest studies with aplomb view statistics as a nearly insurmountable barrier. Perhaps this derives from the inherent difficulty of viewing the world in probabilistic terms, or from the underlying mathematics, or from the often abstruse mode of presentation. I hope that *Basic Statistics for the Health Sciences* is a step in the direction of overcoming these problems.

The purpose of this book is to present some of the concepts, principles, and methods of statistics in as clear and understandable a manner as possible. The level is appropriate to students with a limited mathematical background but for whom a working knowledge of statistics is indispensable. In my own teaching I have found this approach to be particularly effective with students of medicine, nursing, public health, and the allied health sciences. The underlying objective is to introduce concepts intuitively rather than via rigorous mathematics.

Certain features of this book's organization have proven to be especially effective. These include in each chapter an outline, learning objectives (which may easily be used as review questions), a highlighting of important terms, a concluding statement, and a list of newly introduced vocabulary. My colleagues and I have found these to be simple but effective aids for any student striving for mastery of the material. Since nearly all the examples and exercises are adapted from actual data in health research, students are quite likely to appreciate the relevance of the material to their chosen field. My own extended research is reflected in the steady theme of these pages—the effect our life-style choices have on our health.

This text goes somewhat beyond the coverage of most elementary statistics books by including a number of special topics for students of different disciplines and interests. Some key principles of epidemiology are introduced; the topics of age-adjustment and relative risk are covered. A chapter on probability, often reserved for more sophisticated treatments, is included. By understanding probability, the student gains a better insight into several of the subsequent topics. There are chapters devoted to correlation, regression, and analysis of variance, as well as to distribution-free methods, a subject that appears to be gaining rapidly in favor. Chapters on vital statistics and life tables are included to meet the special needs of medical and public health students. Two important subjects, how to perform a health survey and how to evaluate a research report, should be of real benefit to persons who will carry out or use the results of research projects. And, with the explosive impact of computers on data analysis, an introduction to computers and their use could not be overlooked.

This text can be used for a course of three quarter units or three semester units, depending on the topics the instructor chooses to emphasize. It contains the material I have found to be uncommonly effective in motivating students' interest in statistics, so that they begin to see it as a very satisfying form of detective work. The book should be especially useful for the student who enters the course with some lingering doubts about his or her ability to master statistics or for the student who initially questions the relevance of studying the subject. My experience with the prepublication version of the text has been gratifying. May your experience be even more so.

Writing a textbook is a labor of love—filled with pleasure and agony. Its completion follows the convergence of a number of factors: the idea, the encouragement of friends and colleagues, and the cooperation of assistants. I wish especially to acknowledge the inspiring influence of my teachers—John W. Fertig, Chin Long Ching, and Richard D. Remington—and my mentor, Wilfred J. Dixon. They demonstrated to me that statistics, an often abstruse subject, can indeed be taught in a clear and understandable fashion. Special thanks go to my colleague Gerald Shavlik, who assisted in preparing the initial manuscript; to the countless students who have provided me with constructive criticism and valuable feedback; to Burton Brin for his brilliant editorial input; and to Marcella Harrom for her always precise secretarial assistance. The manuscript benefited from the professional insights of Paul S. Anderson Jr. of the University of Oklahoma at Oklahoma City, Gary R. Cutter and Richard A. Windsor of the University of Alabama at Birmingham, and Patricia W. Wahl of the University of Washington. I wish also to acknowledge the cooperation of the various publishers who generously granted permission to reproduce tables from their books.

J.W.K.

Basic Statistics for the Health Sciences

Chapter **1**

Statistics and How They Are Used

Chapter Outline

1.1 The Meaning of Statistics
The term "statistics" is formally defined and illustrated by describing what a statistician does.

1.2 The Uses of Statistics
It is shown how descriptive statistics are used to describe data and how inferential statistics are used to reach conclusions from the analysis of the data.

1.3 Why Study Statistics?
It is shown how the study of statistics is important for research, for writing publishable reports, for understanding scientific journals, and for discriminating between appropriate and inappropriate uses of statistics.

1.4 Sources of Data
Surveys and experiments, two main sources of data, are discussed, and surveys are further classified as retrospective or prospective, and descriptive or analytical.

1.5 Clinical Trials
The use of a clinical trial to determine the value of a new drug or procedure is described.

1.6 Planning of Surveys
Some hints are given on how to make survey data be of maximum value.

Learning Objectives

After studying this chapter, you should be able to

1. Define "statistics"
2. List several reasons for studying statistics
3. Distinguish clearly between
   (a) descriptive and inferential statistics
   (b) surveys and experiments
   (c) retrospective and prospective studies
   (d) descriptive and analytical surveys
4. Define "bias"
5. Describe the purpose and components of a clinical trial

1.1 The Meaning of Statistics

One way to understand statistics is to consider two basic questions: What does the term "statistics" mean? What do statisticians do? Once we have the answers to these questions, we can delve into how statistics are used.

What Does "Statistics" Mean?

The word **"statistics"** has several meanings. It is frequently used in referring to recorded data such as the number of traffic accidents, the size of enrollment, or the number of patients visiting a clinic. Statistics also denotes characteristics calculated for a set of data: for example, mean, standard deviation, correlation coefficient. In another context, statistics refers to statistical methodology and theory.

In short, statistics is a body of techniques and procedures dealing with the collection, organization, analysis, interpretation, and presentation of information that can be stated numerically.

What Do Statisticians Do?

A statistician is usually a member of a group that works on challenging scientific tasks. Frequently engaged in projects that explore the frontiers of human knowledge, the statistician is primarily concerned with developing and applying methods that can be used in collecting and analyzing data. He or she may select a well-established technique or develop a new one that may provide a unique approach to a particular study, thus leading to valid conclusions. Specifically, the statistician's tasks are as follows:

1. *To guide the design of an experiment or survey.* A statistician ought to be consulted in the early planning stages of an investigation so that it can be carried out efficiently with a minimum of bias. Once data are collected, it is too late to plan ahead. By then, it is impossible to impose an appropriate statistical design or compensate for the lack of a randomly selected sample.
2. *To analyze data.* Data analysis may take many forms, such as examining the relationships among several variables, describing and analyzing the variation of certain characteristics (e.g., blood pressure, temperature, height, weight), or determining whether a difference in some response is significant.
3. *To present and interpret results.* Results are best evaluated in terms of probability statements that will facilitate the decision-making process. Mainland (1963:3) defines statistics as the "science and art of dealing with variation in such a way as to obtain reliable results." The art of statistics is especially pertinent to this task and involves skills that are usually acquired through experience.

As the interpretation of statistics is more of an art than a science, it is all too easy to emphasize some inappropriate aspect of the results and consequently misuse statistics. An interesting little book, *How to Lie with Statistics* by Darrell Huff (1954), provides an enlightening and entertaining view of the problems involved in presenting statistics.

1.2 The Uses of Statistics

It is helpful to distinguish between the two major categories of statistics. **Descriptive statistics** deal with the enumeration, organization, and graphical representation of data. **Inferential statistics** are concerned with reaching conclusions from incomplete information, that is, generalizing from the specific. Inferential statistics use information obtained from a sample to say something about an entire population.

An example of *descriptive* statistics is the decennial **census** of the United States in which all the residents are requested to provide such information as age, sex, race, and marital status. The data obtained in such a census can then be compiled and prepared into tables and graphs that describe the characteristics of the population at a given time. An example of *inferential* statistics is an opinion poll, such as the Gallup Poll, which attempts to draw inferences as to the outcome of an election. In such a poll, a sample of individuals (frequently less than 2000) is selected; their preferences are tabulated and inferences made as to how more than 80 million persons will vote on election day.

Statistical methods provide a logical basis for making decisions in a variety of areas when incomplete information is available. Here are some examples of scientific questions to which the application of statistical methodology has been useful:

1. How can researchers test the effectiveness of a new vaccine against the common cold?
2. How effective is a trial that seeks to reduce the risk of coronary heart disease?
3. How effective have several family planning programs been?
4. How much, if at all, does use of oral contraceptives increase a woman's chances of developing a thromboembolism?

The three specific studies described next further amplify the application of statistics.

Smoking During Pregnancy. A pioneering study of the effects of smoking during pregnancy on the newborn infant was reported by Simpson (1957). She examined the data of 7499 patients in three hospitals in and near Loma Linda University and found from the records that prematurity rates increased with the number of cigarettes smoked per day. A more recent review of the various studies on this topic is given by the Surgeon General's Report on Smoking and Health (1979). The principal conclusion of that report is: "Maternal smoking during pregnancy has a significant adverse effect upon the well-being of the fetus and the health of the newborn baby."

Health Practices and Mortality. Belloc (1973) reported on a very interesting study done by the Human Population Laboratory of the California State Health Department on a representative sample of 6928 Alameda County residents. She concluded that there was a striking inverse relationship between the *number* of personal health practices (not smoking, not being obese, not drinking, being physically active, eating regularly, etc.) and mortality.

The Multiple Risk Factor Intervention Trial (MRFIT). Paul (1976) reported on a national study of the primary prevention of coronary heart disease. Its approach was to determine whether the risk of coronary disease in middle-aged men can be significantly reduced through intervention. This intervention entailed simultaneously reducing their serum cholesterol levels, treating any high blood pressure, and encouraging the men to stop smoking. The six-year trial involved 20 clinical centers and 11,000 subjects, all initially healthy but at high risk for coronary disease. At random, half the men were assigned to be followed through the intervention program and the other half through their usual medical care, augmented only by annual physicals and lab tests.

Since skills, facilities, and funds are never unlimited, the problem arises as how to extract the maximum amount of information in the most efficient manner. With the aid of statistics it is usually possible to achieve greater precision at minimum cost by effectively using the available resources.

1.3 Why Study Statistics?

Many students ask: "Why should I study statistics?" or "How useful will statistics be in my future career?" There are answers to these questions; the appropriateness of each depends on one's career objectives.

A knowledge of statistics is essential for people going into research management or graduate study in a specialized area. Persons active in research will find that a basic understanding of statistics is useful not only in the conduct of their investigations, but also in the effective presentation of their findings in papers, in reports for publication, and at professional meetings. Some proficiency in statistics is helpful to those who are preparing, or may be called upon to evaluate, research proposals. Further, a person with an understanding of statistics is better able to decide whether his or her professional colleagues use their statistics for illumination or merely for support of their personal biases. That is, it helps one to decide whether the claims are valid or otherwise.

A knowledge of statistics is essential for persons who wish to keep their education up-to-date. To keep abreast of current developments in one's field, it is important to review and understand the writings in scientific journals, many of which use statistical terminology and methodology.

An understanding of statistics can help anyone discriminate between fact and fancy in everyday life—in newspapers and on television and in making daily comparisons and evaluations.

Finally, a course in statistics should help one know when, and for what purpose, a statistician should be consulted.

1.4 Sources of Data

In observing various phenomona, we are usually interested in obtaining observations on specific characteristics: for instance, age, weight, height, marital status, or smoking habits. These characteristics are referred to as **variables**; the values of the observations recorded for them are referred to as **data.** Data are the raw materials of statistics. They are derived from incredibly diverse sources. Knowing our sources provides clues to our data—their reliability, their validity, and the inferences we might draw.

Surveys and Experiments

Data may come from anywhere: observational surveys, planned surveys, or experiments. The two fundamental kinds of investigations are **surveys** and **experiments.** Data from a survey may represent observations of events or phenomena over which few, if any, controls are imposed. The study of the effects of the explosion of the atomic bomb on the inhabitants of Hiroshima and Nagasaki is an example of a survey. In this case, the radiation to which the survivors were exposed (referred to as "treatment" in statistics) was in no way controlled or assigned. By contrast, in an experiment we design a research plan purposely to impose controls over the amount of exposure (treatment) to a phenomenon such as radiation. The distinction between them is that an experiment imposes controls on the methods, treatment, or conditions under which it is performed, whereas in a survey such controls are seldom possible.

A classic example of an experiment is the Veterans Administration Cooperative Study. It began in 1963 and involved 523 hypertensive men, patients in 16 Veterans Administration hospitals (Veterans Administration, 1970, 1972). The study demonstrated that oral hypertensive medications, judiciously administered, could significantly reduce blood pressure levels, whereas placebos (substances or treatments that have no therapeutic value) had no effect on blood pressure.

Although experimental investigations are preferable to surveys, in some cases there are reasons for not conducting them: for instance, ethical reasons, as when a beneficial treatment may be withheld from one of the groups; or administrative reasons, as when an experiment may seriously disrupt an established routine of the patients' care.

A variety of surveys on human populations are always being conducted by health researchers. These may be categorized as retrospective or prospective.

Retrospective Studies

Retrospective studies gather past data from selected cases and controls to determine differences, if any, in the exposure to a suspected factor. They are commonly referred to as **case-control studies.** The purpose of the comparison is to determine if the two groups differ as to their exposure to some specific factor. In retrospective studies, the researcher identifies individuals with a specific disease or condition (cases) and also identifies a comparable sample without that disease or condition (controls). An example: comparing the smoking habits of women who bore premature babies to those of others who carried their pregnancies to term. Given the comparative data, the researcher then seeks to determine whether there is a statistical relation between the possible **stimulus variable,** or causative factor (smoking), and the **outcome variable** (prematurity).

A disadvantage of retrospective studies is that the data were usually collected for other purposes and may be incomplete. Surveys frequently fail to include relevant variables that may be essential to determine whether the two groups studied are comparable. This absence of demonstrated comparability between cases and controls may envelop the results in a cloud of doubt.

Because of the historical nature of such records or the necessity of relying on memory, serious difficulties may attend the selection of appropriate controls. Unknown biases frequently hinder such studies. The major advantages of a retrospective study are that it is economical and is particularly applicable to the study of rare diseases. Such a study also makes it possible to obtain answers relatively quickly because the cases are usually easily identified.

In retrospective studies, sample selection begins with the outcome variable (disease). The researcher looks back in time to identify the stimulus variable (factor). In prospective studies (discussed next), the stimulus variable is known in advance and the study population is followed through time, while occurrences of the outcome are noted. A generalized **2 × 2 table** may be used to illustrate the study design (Table 1.1). This table is applicable to both retrospective and prospective studies and is called a fourfold table because it consists of four elements, a, b, c, and d:

Element a represents persons without the stimulus variable who developed the disease anyway.

Table 1.1 Generalized 2 × 2 Table

Stimulus variable	Outcome variable: With disease	Outcome variable: Without disease
Absent	*a*	*b*
Present	*c*	*d*

Element *b* represents persons without the stimulus variable who did not contract the disease.
Element *c* represents persons with the stimulus variable who developed the disease.
Element *d* represents persons with the stimulus variable who did not contract the disease.

Prospective Studies

Prospective studies are usually **cohort studies** in which one enrolls a group of healthy persons and follows them over a certain period to determine the frequency with which a disease develops. The group is divided statistically according to the presence or absence of a stimulus variable (e.g., smoking history). This is done because the group cannot, of course, be divided according to a disease that has not yet occurred (e.g., the presence or absence of lung cancer). The prospective study then compares the proportion of smokers (exposed cohort) who developed lung cancer to the proportion of nonsmokers (nonexposed cohort) who developed the same disease.

The prime advantage of prospective studies is that they permit the accurate estimation of disease incidence in a population. They make it possible to include relevant variables, such as age, sex, and occupation, that may be related to the outcome variable. Furthermore, they permit data collection under uniform conditions. Data are obtained for specified reasons; there are better opportunities for making appropriate comparisons and limiting or controlling the amount of **bias,** which may be considered *systematic error*. The *disadvantages* of prospective studies are that they take considerable time, are expensive, and are not useful in studying diseases of low incidence.

A good example of a prospective study is one that seeks to determine if there are long-term health effects on women who take oral contraceptives. Prospective studies do not prove a causal relationship with the factor under study because the characteristics (such as smoking or not smoking) are not randomly assigned and persons with an inherent tendency to lung cancer are arguably more likely to be included in the smoking group. Nevertheless, such studies provide the best mechanism for providing "causal" evidence. The results should be taken as important, though less than perfect, scientific evidence. In some studies, such as those of smoking and lung cancer, the relationship, although not proven, may well be established beyond a reasonable doubt. On this point, MacMahon and Pugh (1970:22) aptly state, "When the derivation of experiential evidence is either impracticable or unethical, there comes a point in the accumulation of evidence when it is more prudent to act on the basis that the association is causal rather than to await further evidence."

Comparison of Ratios

For each type of study, it is instructive to note the different ratios that can be constructed and the questions that can be answered. For *retrospective* studies the ratios to be compared (using the notation of Table 1.1) are

$$\frac{a}{a+c} \quad \text{and} \quad \frac{b}{b+d}$$

By comparing them we can answer the question: Were mothers of premature infants more likely to have been smokers than mothers of normal infants?

For *prospective* studies the ratios to be compared are

$$\frac{a}{a+b} \quad \text{and} \quad \frac{c}{c+d}$$

This comparison answers the question: Which group has the higher frequency of premature infants—mothers who smoke or mothers who don't smoke?

Descriptive and Analytical Surveys

Retrospective surveys are usually *descriptive.* Such surveys provide estimates of a population's characteristics, such as the proportion of individuals who had a physical examination during the last 12 months. Prospective surveys may be descriptive or *analytical.* In an analytical survey one seeks to determine the degree of association between a variable and a factor in the population. An example is the relationship between having (or not having) regular physical examinations and some measure of health status.

1.5 Clinical Trials

A **clinical trial** is a carefully designed experiment that seeks to determine, under controlled conditions, the effectiveness of a new drug or treatment method. Clinical trials are used extensively today by investigators seeking to determine the effectiveness of newly proposed drugs such as cancer chemotherapeutic agents. One of the pioneer clinical trials evaluated the effectiveness of streptomycin in the treatment of tuberculosis (Medical Research Council, 1948). Other clinical trials have been used in evaluating polio vaccine, ACTH for multiple sclerosis, tolbutamide for the control of diabetes, and hundreds of new cancer chemotherapeutic agents.

In short, a clinical trial involves a comparison of two or more comparable groups of patients. The **treatment group,** which receives a potentially therapeutic agent, is compared with a similar **control group,** which instead receives a placebo or the standard therapeutic treatment. It is important that the two groups of patients be comparable. To assure that they are, **random allocation** is ordinarily used. That is, each patient is given an equal chance of being assigned to the treatment or the control group.

The investigator is interested not only in establishing comparable groups, but also in limiting the amount of bias entering a trial. One way to do this is in **single-blind** fashion: the patient does not know whether he or she is in the treatment or the control group. An even better way is **double blind;** that is, neither the patient nor the experimenter knows to which group the patient is assigned. A neutral party keeps the code as to who's who and discloses it only at the end of data-gathering. Numerous clinical trials have failed because bias was not adequately controlled. Bias falls into a number of categories, and is discussed further in Chapter 17.

A clinical trial demands an appropriate control group. One such group is a *concurrent* control group, which is selected at the same time and from the same pool of individuals as the treatment group. Since the use of controls usually doubles the size of the experiment, some investigators have tried alternatives such as historical controls. But historical controls present problems because of changes in the population over time and no means to control selection bias. Volunteer groups have also been used as controls. As such a group is self-selected, it is usually atypical of the rest of the population, thus limiting the inferences that may be drawn. Some investigators have chosen controls from patients in certain hospital wards. This method presents problems of selection for a particular kind of disease or condition. It may overrepresent patients hospitalized for a long time or those recently admitted. Since a clinical trial is, in actuality, an experiment on human beings, a number of ethical issues arise. For instance, is it ethical to withhold a probably effective mode of treatment from a control group? For further discussion of such problems see Hill (1963) and Colton (1974). For a step-by-step procedure of preparing a protocol for a clinical trial, see Kuzma (1970).

Clinical trials as used today have developed since World War II and are of considerable worth in distinguishing between effective and ineffective agents. Had clinical trials been used more commonly in the early days of medicine, the futility of such drastic and dangerous methods as blood letting and purging would have been exposed early on.

In summary, then, the salient features of a clinical trial are

1. Simultaneous treatment and control groups
2. Subjects who are randomly allocated to the two groups
3. A double-blind technique used when feasible

1.6 Planning of Surveys

The previous section discussed several types of medical surveys that may give rise to data. Before starting a survey it is essential to formulate a clear plan of action. An outline of such a plan, including the major steps that should be followed in pursuing the investigation, is given in Chapter 17.

Conclusion

A statistician is involved in designing efficient and unbiased investigations that provide data that he or she then analyzes, interprets, and presents to others so that decisions can be made. To do this work the statistician uses techniques that are collectively called statistics. The student of statistics learns these techniques and how they may relate to his or her work and everyday life. Students need to know not only how to understand the scientific literature of their field but also how to select from various kinds of investigations the one that best fits their research purpose.

Vocabulary List

analytical survey
bias
case-control study
census
clinical trial
cohort study
control group
data
descriptive statistics
descriptive survey
double blind
experiment
inferential statistics
outcome variable
prospective studies
random allocation
retrospective studies
single blind
statistics
stimulus variable
survey
treatment group
two-by-two table (2 × 2 table)
variable

Exercises

1.1 (a) Suggest and describe briefly a survey and its objectives.
(b) Is it a descriptive or an analytical survey?
(c) List some potential sources of bias.

1.2 (a) Suggest and describe an experiment.
(b) What research question are you testing?
(c) What is the "treatment" in this experiment?
(d) List some potential sources of bias.

1.3 (a) Suggest a clinical trial for some phenomenon of interest to you, such as drug use or exercise.
(b) Describe how you would select and allocate cases.
(c) What would the treatment be?
(d) What would be the outcome variable for determining the effectiveness of the treatment?
(e) What double-blind feature would you include, if any?

1.4 (a) Find a newspaper or magazine article that uses data or statistics.
(b) Were the data obtained from a survey or an experiment?
(c) Is the study descriptive or inferential?
(d) What research question was the author trying to answer?
(e) How did he or she select the cases? What population do the cases represent?
(f) Was there a control group? How were the control subjects selected?
(g) Are possible sources of bias mentioned?
(h) If conclusions are stated, are they warranted?
(i) Make a copy of the article to turn in with your answers to these questions.

Chapter **2**

Populations and Samples

Chapter Outline

2.1 Selecting Appropriate Samples
It is explained why the selection of an appropriate sample has an important bearing on the reliability of inferences made about a population.

2.2 Why Sample?
A number of reasons are given as to why sampling is often preferable to census-taking.

2.3 How Samples Are Selected
Explanations are given of several ways in which samples are selected.

2.4 How to Select a Random Sample
The method of selecting a sample by the use of a random number table is illustrated with a specific example.

2.5 Effectiveness of a Random Sample
A demonstration is presented of the credibility of the random sampling process.

Learning Objectives

After studying this chapter, you should be able to

1. Distinguish between
   (a) population and sample
   (b) parameter and statistic
   (c) the various methods of sampling
2. Explain why the method of selecting a sample is important
3. State the reasons why samples are used
4. Define a random sample
5. Explain why it is important to use random sampling
6. Select a sample using a random number table

2.1 Selecting Appropriate Samples

A **population** is a set of persons (or objects) having a common observable characteristic. A **sample** is a subset of a population.

The real challenge of statistics is how to come up with a reliable statement about a population on the basis of sample information. For example, if we want to know how many persons in a community have quit smoking or have health insurance or plan to vote for a certain candidate, we usually obtain information on an appropriate sample of the community and generalize from it to the entire population. How a subgroup is selected is of critical importance. Take this classic example: *Literary Digest Poll.* The Literary Digest Poll attained considerable prestige by successfully predicting the outcomes of four presidential elections before 1936. Using the same methods, the *Literary Digest* in 1936 mailed out some 10 million ballots asking persons to indicate their preference in the upcoming presidential election. About 2.3 million ballots were returned; on this basis the *Literary Digest* confidently predicted that Alfred M. Landon would win by a landslide. In fact, Franklin D. Roosevelt won with a 62% majority. Soon after this fiasco the *Literary Digest* ceased publication. A postmortem examination of its methods revealed that the sample of 10 million was selected primarily from telephone directories and motor vehicle registration lists, which then overrepresented persons with high incomes. Since in 1936 there was a strong relation between income and party preference, the poll's failure was virtually inevitable.

The moral of this incident is clear. The *way* the sample is selected, not its *size*, determines whether we may draw appropriate inferences about a population. Modern sampling techniques can quite reliably predict the winner of a presidential election from a nationwide sample of less than 2000 persons. This is remarkable, considering that the nation's population today is over 75% larger than it was in 1936.

Here are some examples of populations that one may wish to sample: veterans of foreign wars, marijuana users, persons convicted of driving while intoxicated, persons who have difficulty gaining access to medical care, gifted children, or residents of a certain city. The primary reason for selecting a sample from a population is to draw inferences about that population. Note that the population may consist of persons, objects, or the observations of a characteristic. The set of observations may be summarized by a descriptive characteristic, called a **parameter.** The same characteristic of a sample is called a **statistic.** Sample statistics help us draw inferences about population parameters.

The value of the population parameter is constant but usually unknown. The value of the statistic is known because it is computed from the sample.

Observations differ from one sample to the next; consequently, the value of the statistic varies from sample to sample.

2.2 Why Sample?

You may be wondering, "Why not study the entire population?" There are many reasons. It is *impossible* to obtain the weight of every tuna in the Pacific Ocean. It is too costly to inspect every manifold housing that comes off an assembly line. The Internal Revenue Service doesn't have the work force to review every income tax return. Some testing is inherently destructive: tensile strength of structural steel, flight of a solid propellant rocket, measurement of white blood count. We certainly can't launch all the rockets to learn the number of defective ones; we can't drain all the blood from a person and count every white cell. Often it is not justifiable to enumerate the entire population, because for most purposes we can obtain suitable accuracy quickly and inexpensively on the basis of the information gained from a sample.

2.3 How Samples Are Selected

How reliable are our inferences regarding a population? That depends on how well the population is specified and on the method of sample selection. Having a poorly specified or enumerated population or an inappropriately selected sample will surely introduce bias. But bias is controllable. The best way to limit bias is to use **random sampling,** a technique that is simple to apply (which is why it is sometimes called simple random sampling). We use a means of randomization such as a random number table (described in the next section) to ensure that each individual in the population has an equal chance of being selected. This technique meets some of the important assumptions underlying several statistical methods. It also makes possible the estimation of error.

There are several other ways in which samples can be selected. In **convenience sampling** a group is selected at will or in a particular program or clinic. These cases are often self-selected. Since the data obtained are seldom representative of the underlying population, problems arise in analysis and in drawing inferences.

Systematic sampling is frequently used when a **sampling frame** (a complete, nonoverlapping list of the persons or objects constituting the population) is available. We randomly select a first case and then proceed by selecting every nth (say $n = 30$) case, where n depends on the desired sample size. The symbol N is used to denote the size of the entire population.

Stratified sampling is used when we wish the sample proportionately to represent the various **strata** (subgroups) of the population. A random sample is taken from each stratum.

In **cluster sampling** we select a simple random sample of groups, such as city blocks, and then interview a person in each household of the selected blocks. This technique is more economical than the random selection of persons throughout the city.

For a complete discussion of the various kinds of sampling methods, you should consult a textbook on the subject. A good one is by Scheaffer and Mendenhall (1979).

2.4 How to Select a Random Sample

One of the easiest ways of selecting a random sample is to use a **random number table.** Such tables are easy to find; they are in many statistical texts and mathematical handbooks. A portion of one is reproduced in Table 2.1.

Table 2.1 Random Numbers

						col. 31 ↓				
00439	81846	45446	93971	84217	74968	62758	49813	13666	12981	
29676	37909	95673	66757	72420	40567	81119	87494	85471	81520	
69306	71708	88608	67251	22512	00169	58624	04059	05557	73345	
68381	61725	49122	75836	15368	52551	54604	61136	51990	19921	
69158	38683	41374	17028	09304	10834	61546	33503	84277	44800	
00858	04352	17833	41105	46569	90109	14713	15905	84555	92326	
86972	51707	58242	16035	94887	83510	56462	83759	68279	64873	
30606	45225	30161	07973	03034	82983	78242	06519	96345	53424	
93864	49044	57169	43125	11703	87009	76463	48263	99273	79449	
61937	90217	56708	35351	60820	90729	90472	68749	23171	67640	
94551	69538	52924	08530	79302	34981	12155	42714	39810	92772	
79385	49498	48569	57888	70564	17660	50411	19640	07597	34550	
14796	51195	69638	55111	06883	13761	53688	44212	71380	56294	
79793	05845	58100	24112	26866	26299	74127	63514	04218	07584	
98488	68394	65390	41384	52188	81868	74272	77608	34806	46529	
96773	24159	28290	31915	30365	06082	73440	16701	78019	49144	
18849	96248	46509	56863	27018	64818	40938	66102	65833	39169	
71447	27337	62158	25679	63325	98699	16926	28929	06692	05049	
97091	42397	08406	04213	52727	08328 →	24057	78695	91207	18451	← row 19
56644	52133	55069	57102	67821	54934	66318	35153	36755	88011	
60138	40435	75526	35949	84558	13211	29579	30084	47671	44720	
80089	48271	45519	64328	48167	14794	07440	53407	32341	30360	
54302	81734	15723	10921	20123	02787	97407	02481	69785	58025	
61763	77188	54997	28352	57192	22751	82470	92971	29091	35441	
25769	28265	26135	52688	11867	05398	43797	45228	28086	84568	
80142	64567	38915	40716	76797	37083	53872	30022	43767	60257	
69481	57748	93003	99900	25413	64661	17132	53464	52705	69602	
40431	28106	28655	84536	71208	47599	36136	46412	99748	76167	
16264	39564	37178	61382	51274	89407	11283	77207	90547	50981	
19618	87653	18682	22917	56801	81679	93285	68284	11203	47990	

Random number tables are prepared in such a way that each digit gets equal representation. Selecting a random sample involves three steps: define the population, enumerate it, and use a random number table to select the sample.

Here is an illustration of how to select 10 persons from a population of 83 cases in a hypertension study (Table 2.2). Observe that the population is clearly defined: 83 cases classified according to their dietary status. Also note that the cases have been numbered arbitrarily from 01 to 83. If the random number table covered four pages, you might flip a coin twice and arbitrarily agree to assign HH (two heads) to page 1, HT to page 2, TH to page 3, and TT to page 4. Suppose you flip heads on both tosses (HH); you then turn to page 1. To choose an arbitrary starting place, you could blindly stab at row 19 and column 31. The row–column intersection of the starting place should be recorded, just in case you wish later to verify your selection, hence your sample. Next, begin reading the two-digit numerals. Why use two digits? Because your sampling frame is identified by two-digit numerals. The first number selected is 24. By advance agreement, you could proceed by reading down the column: 66, 29, 7, 97, and so on. Alternatively, you could agree to read the table in some other reasonable way, say from left to right, but not changing the pattern during the selection process. Continuing the process, you would select the following individuals:

ID	Diastolic blood pressure
24	58
66	82
29	56
7	58
82	66
43	102
53	92
17	68
36	60
11	78

Why was number 97 excluded? The answer is simple: the sampling frame defines only numbers 01 through 83. Disregard all others. A corollary problem is the duplication of a number already selected; in practice the duplicate is simply ignored. It is important to remember that the selected numerals only identify the sample; the sample itself is the set of blood pressure values.

Occasionally it may be uneconomical or impractical to implement a random selection scheme that requires enumeration of the entire population. For example, it would be nearly impossible to obtain a list of all persons in a city who have VD or are obese. In such cases one might have to resort to whatever lists are conveniently available.

Table 2.2 Hypertension Study Cases
by Diastolic Blood Pressure, Diet Status, and Sex

ID	Diastolic blood pressure (mmHg)	Sex	Vegetarian status	ID	Diastolic blood pressure (mmHg)	Sex	Vegetarian status
01	88	M	V	42	70	M	NV
02	98	M	V	43	102	M	NV
03	64	M	V	44	84	M	NV
04	80	M	V	45	74	M	NV
05	60	M	V	46	76	M	NV
06	68	M	V	47	84	M	NV
07	58	M	V	48	84	M	NV
08	82	M	V	49	82	M	NV
09	74	M	V	50	82	M	NV
10	64	M	V	51	74	M	NV
11	78	M	V	52	70	M	NV
12	68	M	V	53	92	M	NV
13	60	M	V	54	68	M	NV
14	96	M	V	55	70	M	NV
15	64	M	V	56	70	M	NV
16	78	M	V	57	70	M	NV
17	68	M	V	58	40	M	NV
18	72	M	V	59	83	M	NV
19	76	F	V	60	74	M	NV
20	68	F	V	61	56	F	NV
21	70	F	V	62	89	F	NV
22	62	F	V	63	84	F	NV
23	82	F	V	64	58	F	NV
24	58	F	V	65	58	F	NV
25	72	F	V	66	82	F	NV
26	56	F	V	67	78	F	NV
27	84	F	V	68	82	F	NV
28	80	F	V	69	71	F	NV
29	56	F	V	70	56	F	NV
30	58	F	V	71	68	F	NV
31	82	F	V	72	58	F	NV
32	88	F	V	73	72	F	NV
33	100	F	V	74	80	F	NV
34	88	F	V	75	88	F	NV
35	74	F	V	76	72	F	NV
36	60	F	V	77	68	F	NV
37	74	F	V	78	66	F	NV
38	70	F	V	79	78	F	NV
39	70	F	V	80	74	F	NV
40	66	F	V	81	60	F	NV
41	76	M	NV	82	66	F	NV
				83	72	F	NV

NOTE: ID = identification; mmHg = millimeters of mercury; V = vegetarian; NV = nonvegetarian.

Simple random sampling is well named, for you can see how simple it is to apply. Yet it is one of the statistician's most vital tools and is used in countless applications. It is the basic building block for every method of sampling, no matter how sophisticated.

2.5 Effectiveness of a Random Sample

Students who encounter random sampling for the first time are somewhat skeptical about its effectiveness. The reliability of sampling is usually demonstrated by defining a fairly small population and then selecting from it all conceivable samples of a particular size, say three observations. Then, for each sample, the mean (average) is computed and the variation from the population mean is observed. A comparison of these sample means (statistics) with the population mean (parameter) neatly demonstrates the credibility of the sampling scheme.

In this chapter an attempt is made to establish credibility by a different approach. If you page ahead to Chapter 3 (p. 22), you will find a table listing characteristics of a representative sample of 100 individuals from the 7683 participants in the Honolulu Heart Study, which investigated heart disease among men ages 45 through 67. Five separate samples of 100 observations each were selected from this population, and the mean ages were compared with the population mean. The results of this comparison are shown in Table 2.3. It can be seen that the population parameter is 54.36 and that the five statistics representing this mean are all very close to it. The difference between the sample estimate and the population mean never exceeds 0.5 years, even though each sample represents only 1.3% of the entire population. This comparison underscores how much similarity you can expect among sample means.

Table 2.3 Effectiveness of a Random Sample

	Population (N = 7683)	Sample (n = 100 each)				
		1	2	3	4	5
Mean age	54.36	54.85	54.31	54.31	54.67	54.02

Conclusion

As assessing all individuals may be impossible, impractical, expensive, or inaccurate, it is usually advantageous to study a sample of the original population. To do this we must clearly identify the population, be able to list it in a sampling frame, and utilize an appropriate sampling technique.

Although several methods of selecting samples are possible, random sampling is the most practical, in that it is easy to apply, limits bias, provides estimates of error, and meets the assumptions of the statistical tests. The effectiveness of random sampling can easily be demonstrated by comparing sample statistics with population parameters. The statistics obtained from a sample are used as estimates of the unknown parameters of the population.

Vocabulary List

cluster sample	random number table	statistic
convenience sample	random sample	stratified sample
parameter	sample	systematic sample
population	sampling frame	

Exercises

2.1. Draw a sample of 10 from Table 2.2 by the use of the random number table (Table 2.1). Make note of
(a) the row and column where you started
(b) the direction in which you proceeded
(c) the 10 values you selected (show the ID and blood pressure for each)
What is this type of sample called?

2.2 Suppose in Exercise 2.1 you had selected the sample by taking two simple random samples of five from each of the two diet groups. What name would you apply to such a sample?

2.3 Select a sample of 10 from Table 2.2 by taking every eighth individual beginning with ID number 6.
(a) What is the name of such a sample?
(b) Do you see a possible source of bias in taking the sample in this way?

2.4 Look ahead to the blood glucose values listed in Table 3.1.
(a) Describe the population.
(b) Select a simple random sample of 10.
(c) What statistical term describes the characteristic for the sample?
(d) What statistical term describes the characteristic for the population?

Chapter **3**

Organizing and Displaying Data

Chapter Outline

3.1 The Use of Numbers in Organizing Data
The three types of numbers are discussed in relation to organizing data.
3.2 Quantitative and Qualitative Data
A distinction is drawn among qualitative data, discrete quantitative data, and continuous quantitative data.
3.3 The Frequency Table
Instructions are given on how to organize data in the form of a frequency table.
3.4 Graphing Data
Various methods of graphing are discussed and illustrated, with emphasis on those that apply specifically to frequency distributions.

Learning Objectives

After studying this chapter, you should be able to

1. Distinguish between
   (a) qualitative and quantitative variables
   (b) discrete and continuous variables
   (c) symmetrical, bimodal, and skewed distributions
   (d) positively and negatively skewed distributions
2. Construct a frequency table that includes class limits, class frequency, relative frequency, and cumulative frequency
3. Indicate the appropriate types of graphs that can be used for displaying quantitative and qualitative data
4. Distinguish which form of data presentation is appropriate for different situations
5. Construct a histogram, a frequency polygon, an ogive, and a bar chart
6. Interpret a frequency table
7. Distinguish among and interpret the various kinds of graphs
8. Determine and interpret percentiles from an ogive

3.1 The Use of Numbers in Organizing Data

Any survey or experiment yields a list of observations. These need to be organized and summarized in a logical fashion so that we may perceive the outcome clearly. There are three general ways of organizing and presenting data: tables, graphs, and numerical methods. Each of these ways will be illustrated by reference to a sample of 100 individuals, selected by systematic random sampling from a Honolulu Heart Study population of 7683. The data for this sample are presented in Table 3.1 (see p. 22).

We must take a few moments to discuss the subject of *numbers.* There are many different types of numbers. Those used most frequently in everyday life—telephone, zip code, social security, driver's license, and the like—do not represent an amount or quantity. Such numbers are used as names or identifiers of a person's status, category, or attribute and are referred to as **nominal** numerals. In Table 3.1 the nominal variables are the ID number and smoking status (smoker vs. nonsmoker).

An **ordinal** is another kind of number. Ordinals represent an ordered series of relationships. *First, second,* and *third* are ordinals. They may be applied, for example, to the rank order of causes of death by type of disease. Note that an ordinal indicates position in an ordered series but nothing at all about the magnitude of difference between any two successive entries. In Table 3.1 educational level and physical activity status are examples of ordinal variables.

The third kind of number is one measured on an **interval scale** having equal units but an arbitrary zero point. Temperature is an example of an interval scale data. Interval scale units may be added or subtracted but they may not be multiplied or divided. Common statistics such as the mean, standard deviation and t can be computed on interval scale data. For example, an average age or height is meaningful, whereas an average zip code (a nominal variable) is senseless. It is *not* appropriate to perform arithmetic operations on nominal data. Variables such as weight (or height) for which we can compare meaningfully one weight versus another (say, 50 kg is twice 25 kg), are said to be measured on a **ratio scale.**

3.2 Quantitative and Qualitative Data

As noted in Chapter 1, specific characteristics (e.g., age, height, and weight) that we may want to assess for a certain population are referred to as variables. Variables may further be categorized as qualitative or quantitative. Variables that yield observations on which individuals can be categorized according to some characteristic or quality are referred to as **qualitative**

Table 3.1 Data for a Sample of 100 Individuals of the Honolulu Heart Study Population of 7683 Persons, 1969

ID	Educational level	Weight (KG)	Height (CM)	Age	Smoking status	Physical activity at home	Blood glucose	Serum cholesterol	Systolic blood pressure	Ponderal index
1	2	70	165	61	1	1	107	199	102	40.0361
2	1	60	162	52	0	2	145	267	138	41.3808
3	1	62	150	52	1	1	237	272	190	37.8990
4	2	66	165	51	1	1	91	166	122	40.8291
5	2	70	162	51	0	1	185	239	128	39.3082
6	4	59	165	53	0	2	106	189	112	42.3838
7	1	47	160	61	0	1	177	238	128	44.3358
8	3	66	170	48	1	1	120	223	116	42.0663
9	5	56	155	54	0	2	116	279	134	40.5138
10	2	62	167	48	0	1	105	190	104	42.1942
11	4	68	165	49	1	2	109	240	116	40.4248
12	1	65	166	48	0	1	186	209	152	41.2862
13	1	56	157	55	0	2	257	210	134	41.0365
14	2	80	161	49	0	1	218	171	132	37.3648
15	3	66	160	50	0	2	164	255	130	39.5918
16	4	91	170	52	0	2	158	232	118	37.7951
17	3	71	170	48	1	1	117	147	136	41.0547
18	5	66	152	59	0	2	130	268	108	37.6123
19	1	73	159	59	0	2	132	231	108	38.0444
20	4	59	161	52	0	1	138	199	128	41.3563
21	1	64	162	52	1	1	131	255	118	40.5001
22	3	55	161	52	1	1	88	199	134	42.3356
23	2	78	175	50	1	1	161	228	178	40.9582
24	2	59	160	54	0	1	145	240	134	41.0995
25	3	51	167	48	1	2	128	184	162	45.0326
26	3	83	171	55	0	1	231	192	162	39.2016
27	2	66	157	49	1	2	78	211	120	38.8495
28	4	61	165	51	0	1	113	201	98	41.9155
29	2	65	160	53	0	1	134	203	144	39.7939
30	3	75	172	49	0	1	104	243	118	40.7858
31	4	61	164	49	0	2	122	181	118	41.6615
32	1	73	157	53	1	2	442	382	138	37.5658
33	2	66	157	52	0	1	237	186	134	38.8495
34	1	73	155	48	0	2	148	198	108	37.0873
35	2	61	160	53	0	1	231	165	96	40.6453
36	3	68	162	50	0	2	161	219	142	39.6898
37	2	52	157	50	0	2	119	196	122	42.0629
38	5	73	162	50	0	1	185	239	146	38.7622
39	1	52	165	61	1	2	118	259	126	44.2062
40	1	56	162	53	1	1	98	162	176	42.3434
41	3	67	170	48	1	2	218	178	104	41.8560
42	1	61	160	47	0	1	147	246	112	40.6453
43	3	52	166	62	1	2	176	176	140	44.4741
44	2	61	172	56	1	2	106	157	102	43.6937
45	3	62	164	55	1	2	109	179	142	41.4362
46	2	56	155	57	1	2	138	231	146	40.5138
47	1	55	157	50	0	2	84	183	92	41.2838
48	3	66	165	48	1	2	137	213	112	40.8291
49	1	59	159	51	0	2	139	230	152	40.8426
50	3	53	152	53	1	2	97	134	116	40.4655
51	5	71	173	52	0	2	169	181	118	41.7792
52	2	57	152	49	0	1	160	234	128	39.4959
53	2	73	165	50	1	1	123	161	116	39.4800
54	3	75	170	49	0	2	130	289	134	40.3115
55	3	80	171	50	1	2	198	186	108	39.6856

Table 3.1
Continued

ID	Educational level	Weight (KG)	Height (CM)	Age	Smoking status	Physical activity at home	Blood glucose	Serum cholesterol	Systolic blood pressure	Ponderal index
56	4	49	157	53	0	1	215	298	134	42.9044
57	4	65	162	52	0	1	177	211	124	40.2913
58	2	82	170	56	0	2	100	189	124	39.1302
59	3	55	155	52	0	2	91	164	114	40.7578
60	3	61	165	58	0	1	141	219	154	41.9155
61	2	50	155	54	1	2	139	287	114	42.0735
62	5	58	160	56	0	1	176	179	114	41.3343
63	1	55	166	50	1	2	218	216	98	43.6503
64	5	59	161	47	0	2	146	224	128	41.3564
65	2	68	165	53	1	1	128	212	130	40.4248
66	2	60	170	53	1	2	127	230	122	43.4243
67	1	77	160	47	1	1	76	231	112	37.6089
68	5	60	155	52	0	1	126	185	106	39.5927
69	3	70	164	54	0	1	184	180	128	39.7935
70	2	70	165	46	0	1	58	205	128	40.0361
71	3	77	160	58	1	1	95	219	116	37.6089
72	5	86	160	53	0	2	144	288	154	36.2483
73	2	67	152	49	1	2	124	261	126	37.4242
74	3	77	165	53	1	1	167	221	140	38.7841
75	3	75	169	57	0	2	150	194	122	40.0744
76	2	70	165	52	0	2	156	248	154	40.0361
77	2	70	165	49	1	1	193	216	140	40.0361
78	1	71	157	53	0	1	194	195	120	37.9153
79	1	55	162	49	0	2	73	217	140	42.5985
80	2	59	165	53	1	2	98	186	114	42.3838
81	3	64	159	50	0	2	127	218	122	39.7501
82	1	66	160	54	0	1	153	173	94	39.5918
83	4	59	165	60	0	2	161	221	122	42.3838
84	3	68	165	57	0	1	194	206	172	40.4248
85	5	58	160	52	0	1	87	215	100	41.3343
86	1	57	154	65	1	1	188	176	150	40.0156
87	2	60	160	65	0	2	149	240	154	40.5699
88	2	53	162	62	0	1	215	234	170	43.1277
89	2	61	159	62	1	2	163	190	140	40.3913
90	1	66	154	62	0	1	111	204	144	38.1072
91	1	61	152	67	0	2	198	256	156	38.6131
92	2	52	152	66	0	2	265	296	132	40.7233
93	1	59	155	62	0	2	143	223	140	39.8151
94	1	63	155	62	1	1	136	225	150	38.9540
95	2	61	165	63	0	2	298	217	130	41.9155
96	2	68	155	67	0	2	173	251	118	37.9749
97	1	58	170	62	0	1	148	187	162	43.9178
98	3	68	160	55	0	1	110	290	128	39.1998
99	5	60	159	50	0	2	188	238	130	40.6144
100	2	61	160	54	1	1	208	218	208	40.6453

Code for variables:

Education: 1 = none, 2 = primary, 3 = intermediate, 4 = senior high, 5 = technical school, 6 = university
Weight: in kilograms
Height: in centimeters
Smoking: 0 = no, 1 = yes
Physical activity: 1 = mostly sitting, 2 = moderate, 3 = much
Blood glucose: in milligrams percent
Serum cholesterol: in milligrams percent
Systolic blood pressure: in millimeters of mercury
Ponderal index: height $\div \sqrt[3]{\text{weight}}$

variables. Examples of qualitative variables are occupation, sex, marital status, and education level. Variables that yield observations that can be measured are considered to be **quantitative variables.** Examples of quantitative variables are weight, height, and serum cholesterol.

Quantitative variables can further be classified as **discrete** or **continuous.** The number of children in one's family, the number of times you visit a doctor, and the number of missing teeth are termed discrete variables; they must always be integers, that is, whole numbers (e.g., 0, 1, and 2). Variables such as age, height, and weight may take on fractional values (e.g., 37.8, 138.2, and 112.9). They are referred to as **continuous** variables.

Different types of variables are analyzed differently. Know what type of data you have. This will enable you quickly to select the appropriate method of analysis.

3.3 The Frequency Table

Perhaps the most convenient way of summarizing data is by means of a **frequency table.** Tables 3.2 and 3.3 are examples, constructed from the systolic blood pressure readings (by smoking status) of our Honolulu Heart Study sample, Table 3.1. The first step is to compute the interval spanned by the data. We can obtain this interval by arranging the data into an **array,** a listing of all observations from smallest to largest. We find that the overall blood pressure interval is 92–208 mm, a range of 116 mm.

The next step is to divide the range into a number of arbitrary but usually equal and nonoverlapping segments called **class intervals.** Intervals are traditionally equal in length, thereby aiding the comparisons between

Table 3.2 Frequency Table for Systolic Blood Pressure of *Nonsmokers* from Table 3.1

Class interval (systolic blood pressure*)	Tally	f (frequency)	Relative frequency (%)
90–109	𝍸 𝍸	10	16
110–129	𝍸 𝍸 𝍸 𝍸 𝍷𝍷𝍷𝍷	24	38
130–149	𝍸 𝍸 𝍸 𝍷𝍷𝍷	18	29
150–169	𝍸 𝍷𝍷𝍷𝍷	9	14
170–189	𝍷𝍷	2	3
190–209		0	0
Total		63	100

SOURCE: Honolulu Heart Study.
*In millimeters of mercury.

Table 3.3 Frequency Table for Systolic Blood Pressure of *Smokers* from Table 3.1

Class interval (systolic blood pressure*)	Tally	*f* (frequency)	Relative frequency (%)
90–109	||||/	5	14
110–129	||||/ ||||/ ||||/	15	41
130–149	||||/ ||||/	10	27
150–169	|||	3	8
170–189	||	2	5
190–209	||	2	5
Total		37	100

SOURCE: Honolulu Heart Study.
*In millimeters of mercury.

the frequencies of any two intervals. The beginning and length of the class intervals should be reasonably convenient and correspond, so far as possible, to meaningful stopping points. The number of intervals depends, of course, on the number of observations but in general should range from 5 to 15. With too many class intervals, the data are not summarized enough for a clear visualization of how they are distributed. With too few, the data are oversummarized and some of the details of the distribution may be lost. The first interval in Table 3.2 is 90–109 mm, where 90 and 109 are called **class limits.** The number of observations falling into any given interval is called the **class frequency,** usually symbolized by *f*. For the first interval, *f* is 10, obtained from the **tally.** The tally is a familiar and convenient way of keeping score of a set of observations.

A completed frequency table provides a frequency distribution. A frequency distribution is a table (or a graph or an equation) that includes a set of intervals and displays the number of measurements in each interval. From Tables 3.2 and 3.3 we can derive the range, the frequency in each of the intervals, and the total number of observations collected. Frequency tables should include an appropriate descriptive title, specify the *units of measurement,* and cite the source of data.

Frequency tables often include other features, for example, the **relative frequency,** which represents the relative percentage to total cases of any class interval. It is obtained by dividing the number of cases in the class interval by the total number of cases and multiplying by 100. For example, in Table 3.2, the relative frequency of the first class, 90–109 mm, is (10/63)100 =16%. It indicates that percentage of total cases that fall in a given class interval. The use of relative frequency is particularly helpful in making a comparison between two sets of data that have a different number of observations, like our 63 nonsmokers and 37 smokers. For example, in the blood

Table 3.4 Comparison of Systolic Blood Pressure Between Smokers and Nonsmokers from Table 3.1

Class interval (Systolic blood pressure*)	Relative frequency (%)		Cumulative relative frequency (%)	
	Nonsmokers	Smokers	Nonsmokers	Smokers
90–109	16	14	16	14
110–129	38	41	54	55
130–149	29	27	83	82
150–169	14	8	97	90
170–189	3	5	100	95
190–209	0	5	100	100

SOURCE: Honolulu Heart Study.
*In millimeters of mercury.

pressure range of 90–109 mm, 10 (16%) of the nonsmokers and 5 (14%) of the smokers were represented.

Class boundaries are points that demarcate the true upper limit of one class and the true lower limit of the next. For example, the class boundary between classes 90–109 and 110–129 is 109.5; it is the upper boundary for the former and the lower boundary for the latter. Class boundaries may be used in place of class limits.

Cumulative relative frequency, also known as **cumulative percentage,** gives that percentage of individuals having a measurement less than or equal to the upper boundary of the class interval. The cumulative percentage distribution is of value in obtaining such commonly used statistics as the median and percentile scores, which we will discuss later. It also makes possible a rapid comparison of entire frequency distributions, ruling out any need to compare individual class intervals. Cumulative relative frequency is easy to compute. You do it by successively cumulating the relative frequencies of each of the various class intervals. In our example, for nonsmokers the cumulative percentage for the first four intervals is 16 + 38 + 29 + 14 = 97% (Table 3.4). The interpretation: 97% of the nonsmokers in the sample have a systolic blood pressure below 169.5. By comparison, 90% of the smokers have a blood pressure below the same level. An alternate way of looking at this is to note that 3% of the nonsmokers and 10% of the smokers have a systolic blood pressure above 169.5.

3.4 Graphing Data

The second way of displaying data is by use of **graphs.** They give the user a nice overview of the essential features of the data. Although such visual aids are even easier to read than tables, they do not give the same detail.

Graphs are designed to help the user obtain an intuitive feeling for the data at a glance. So it is essential that each graph be self-explanatory—that is, with a descriptive title, labeled axes, and an indication of the units of observation. An effective graph is simple and clean. It should not attempt to present so much information that it is difficult to comprehend.

Histograms

Perhaps the most common graph is the **histogram.** A histogram is nothing more than a pictorial representation of the frequency table. It consists of an **abscissa** (horizontal axis), which depicts the class boundaries (not limits), and a perpendicular **ordinate** (vertical axis), which depicts the frequency (or relative frequency) of observations. The vertical scale should begin at zero. A general rule in laying out the two scales is to make the height of the vertical scale equal to approximately three-fourths the length of the horizontal scale. Otherwise, the histogram may appear to be out of proportion with reality. Once the scales have been laid out, a vertical bar is constructed above each class interval equal in height to its class frequency. For our Honolulu Heart Study example, the bar over the first class interval is 10 units high (Figure 3.1). Frequencies are represented not only by the height but also by the area of each bar. The total area represents 100%.

From Figure 3.1 it is possible to measure that 16% of the area corresponds to the 10 scores in the class interval 89.5–109.5 and that 38% of the area corresponds to the 24 observations in the second bar. Since area is proportional to the number of observations, you must be especially careful when constructing histograms from frequency tables that have unequal class intervals.

Figure 3.1 Histogram Illustrating the Data of Table 3.2: Systolic Blood Pressure of a Sample of 63 Nonsmokers from the Honolulu Heart Study

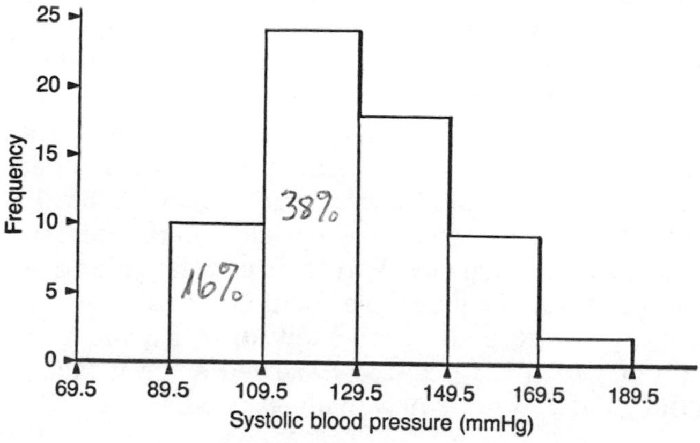

Figure 3.2 Frequency Polygon Illustrating the Data of Table 3.2: Systolic Blood Pressure of a Sample of 63 Nonsmokers from the Honolulu Heart Study

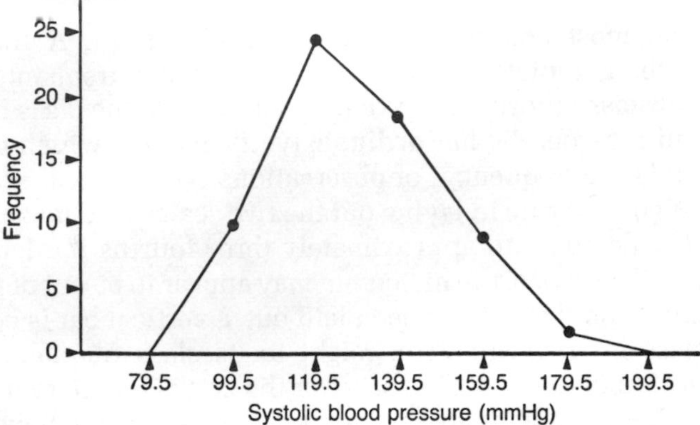

Frequency Polygons

Another commonly used graph is the **frequency polygon.** It uses the same axes as the histogram. It is constructed by marking a point (at the same height as the histogram's bar) at the **midpoint** of the class interval. These points are then connected with straight lines. At the ends, the points are connected to the midpoints of the previous (and succeeding) intervals of zero frequency (Figure 3.2). Frequency polygons, especially when superimposed, are superior to histograms in providing means of comparing two frequency distributions. In frequency polygons, the frequency of observations in a given class interval is represented by the area contained beneath the line segment and within the class interval. This area is proportional to the total number of observations in the frequency distribution. Frequency polygons should be used to graph only quantitative (numerical) data, never qualitative (i.e., nominal or ordinal) data.

Frequency polygons may take on a number of different shapes. Some of those most commonly encountered are shown in Figure 3.3. Part (a) of the figure is the classic "bell-shaped" **symmetrical** distribution. Part (b) is a **bimodal** (having two peaks) distribution that could represent an overlapping group of males and females. Part (c) is a **rectangular** distribution in which each class interval is equally represented. Parts (a) and (c) are symmetrical, whereas parts (d) and (e) are **skewed,** or asymmetrical. The frequency polygon of part (d) is positively skewed since it tapers off in the positive direction, and part (e) is negatively skewed.

Figure 3.3 Various Shapes of Frequency Polygons

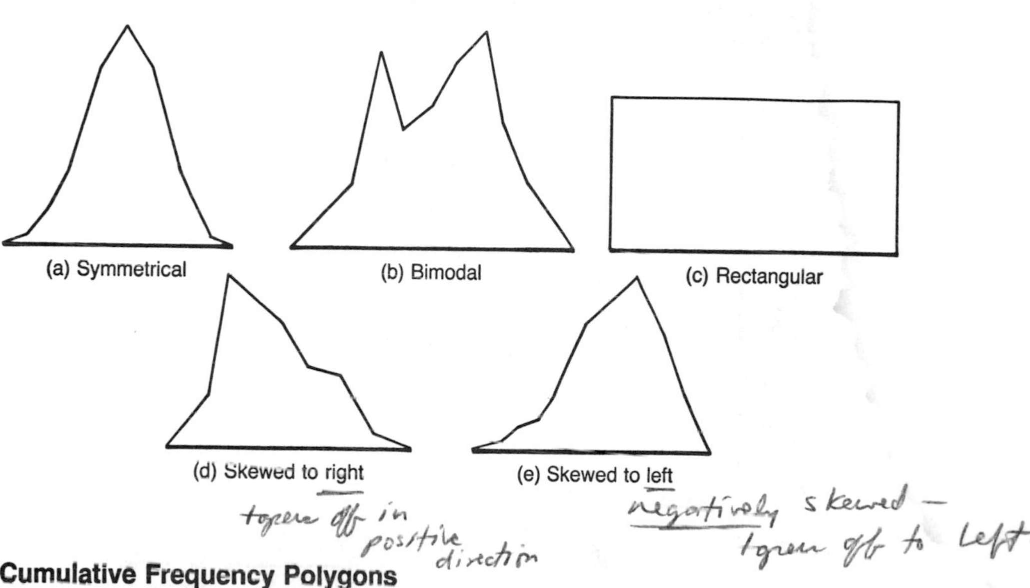

Cumulative Frequency Polygons

At times it is useful to construct a **cumulative frequency polygon,** also called an **ogive.** Although the horizontal scale is the same as that used for a histogram, the vertical scale indicates cumulative frequency or cumulative relative frequency. To construct the ogive, we place a point at the upper class boundary of each class interval. Each point represents the cumulative relative frequency for that class. Note that not until the upper class boundary has been reached have all the data of a class interval been accumulated. The ogive is completed by connecting the points (Figure 3.4). Ogives are useful in comparing two sets of data, as, for example, data on healthy and diseased individuals. In Figure 3.4 we can see that 90% of the nonsmokers and 86% of the smokers had systolic blood pressures below 160 mmHg. The ogive gives for each interval the cumulative relative frequency—that is, the percentage of cases having systolic blood pressures in that interval or a lower one.

Percentiles may be obtained from an ogive. The 90th **percentile** is that observation that exceeds 90% of the set of observations and is exceeded by only 10% of them. Percentiles are readily obtained, as in Figure 3.4. In our example, the 50th percentile, or median, for nonsmokers, is a blood pressure of 127.5 mmHg, and the 90th percentile is 159.5 mmHg.

Stem-and-Leaf Displays

Tukey (1977) has suggested an innovative technique for summarizing data that utilizes characteristics of the frequency distribution and the his-

Figure 3.4 Ogives Illustrating the Data of Table 3.4: Systolic Blood Pressure of a Sample of 63 Nonsmokers and 37 Smokers from the Honolulu Heart Study

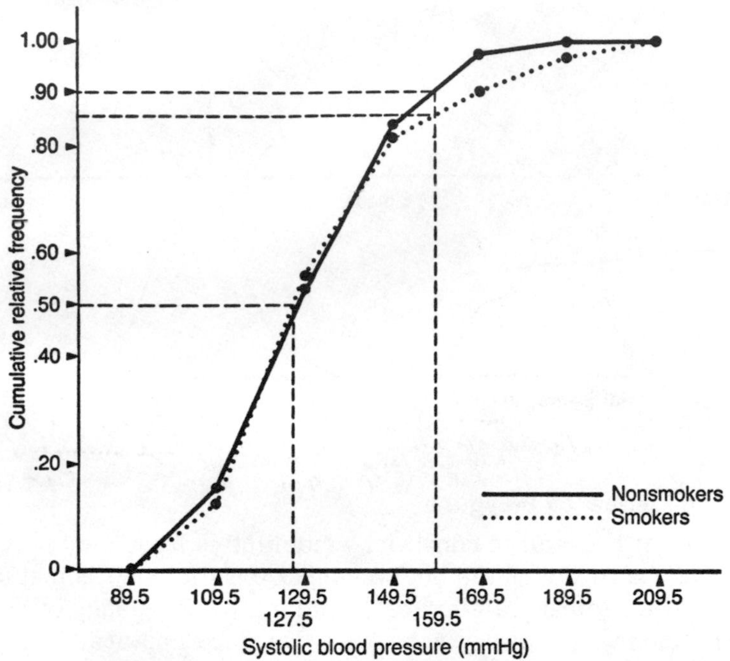

togram. It is referred to as the **stem-and-leaf display,** in which the "stems" represent the class intervals and the "leaves" are the strings of values within each class interval. Table 3.5 illustrates the usefulness of this technique in helping you develop a better feel for your data. The table is a stem-and-leaf display that utilizes the observations of systolic blood pressures of the 63 nonsmokers of Table 3.2. For each stem (interval) we arrange the last digits of the observations from the lowest to the highest. This arrangement is referred to as the leaf. The leaves (strings of observations) portray a histogram laid on its side; each leaf reflects the values of the observations from which it is easy to note their size and frequencies. Consequently, we have displayed all observations and provided a visual description of the shape of the distribution. It is often useful to present the stem-and-leaf display together with a conventional frequency distribution.

Bar Charts

The **bar chart** is a convenient graphical device that is particularly useful for displaying nominal or ordinal data—data like ethnicity, sex, and treat-

Table 3.5 Stem-and-Leaf Display of Systolic Blood Pressure of 63 *Nonsmokers* (Data from Table 3.2)

Stems (intervals)	Leaves (observations)	Frequency (*f*)
90–99	2 4 6 8	4
100–109	0 4 6 8 8 8	6
110–119	2 2 4 4 8 8 8 8 8	9
120–129	0 2 2 2 2 4 4 8 8 8 8 8 8 8 8	15
130–139	0 0 0 2 2 4 4 4 4 4 4 8	12
140–149	0 0 2 4 4 6	6
150–159	2 2 4 4 4 4 6	7
160–169	2 2	2
170–179	0 2	2
180–189		0
Total		63

ment category. The various categories are represented along the horizontal axis. They may be arranged alphabetically, by frequency within a category, or on some other rational basis. The height of each bar is equal to the frequency of items for that category. To prevent any impression of continuity, it is important that all the bars be of equal width and separate, as in Figure 3.5.

Figure 3.5 Bar Chart of Excess Mortality of Smokers over Nonsmokers According to Number of Cigarettes Smoked

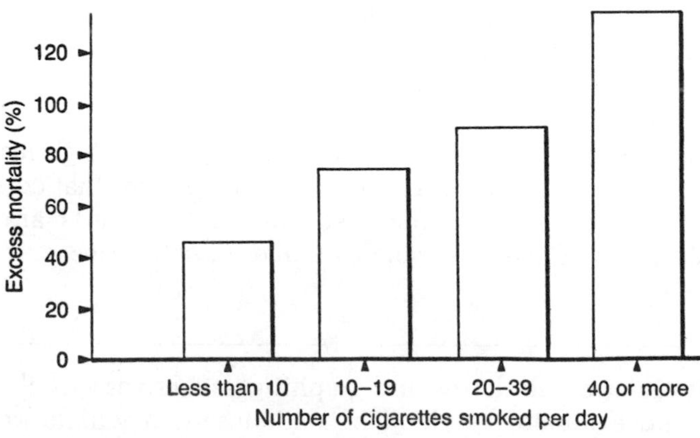

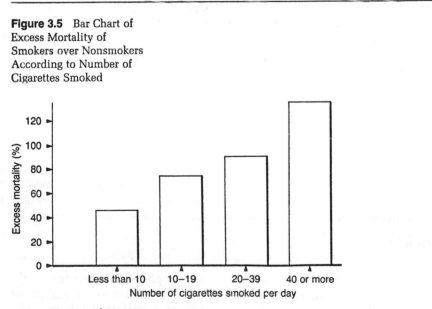

SOURCE: Hammond (1966).

Figure 3.6 Bars Broken to Show Vertical Scale Does Not Begin at Zero

SOURCE: Hammond (1966).

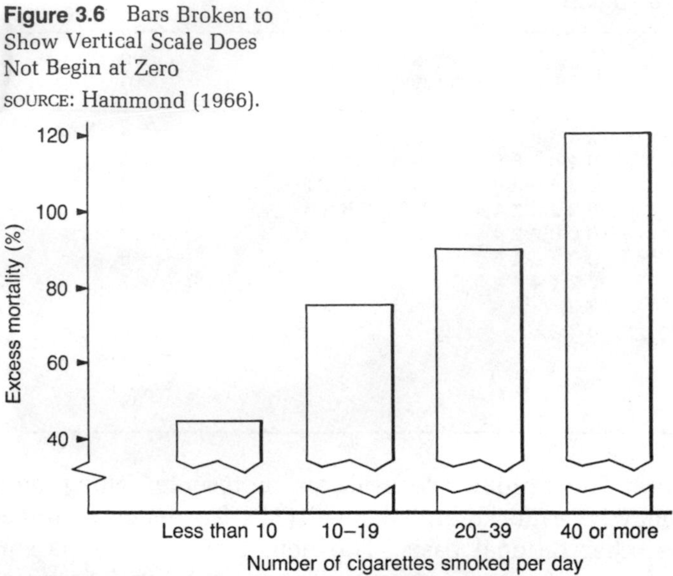

To avoid misleading a reader it is essential that the scale on the vertical axis begin at zero. If that is impractical, one should employ broken bars (or a similar device), as shown in Figure 3.6. Here is an example of what can happen if neither procedure is followed. The public relations department of a West Coast college recently circulated the graph shown in Figure 3.7a. It gives the clear impression that enrollment doubled between 1976 and 1982. The reason for this is that the bars begin not at zero but at 2000. Persons unskilled in interpreting graphical data may find themselves drawn into one of the many pitfalls that are so well documented in books on the misuse of statistics. Figure 3.7b illustrates the correct way of presenting the same enrollment statistics. This graph makes clear that the enrollment increased only about 50% over the seven years.

Pie Charts

A common device for displaying data arranged in categories is the **pie chart** (Figure 3.8; see p. 34), a circle divided into wedges that correspond to the percentage frequencies of the distribution. Pie charts are useful in conveying data that consist of a small number of categories.

Conclusion

The principles of tabulating and graphing data are essential if we are to understand and evaluate the flood of statistics with which we are bombarded. By proper use of these principles, the statistician is able to present

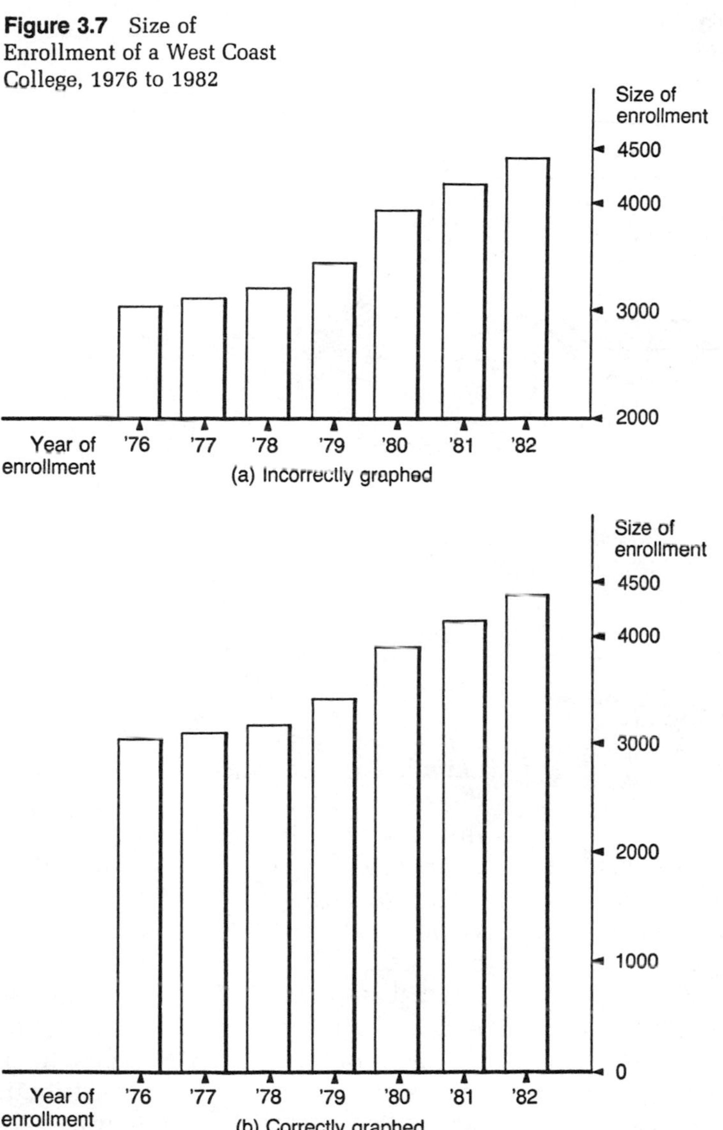

Figure 3.7 Size of Enrollment of a West Coast College, 1976 to 1982

data accurately and lucidly. It is also important to know which method of presentation to choose for each specific type of data. Tables are usually comprehensive but do not convey the information as quickly or as impressively as do graphs. Remember that graphs and tables must tell their own story. They should be complete in themselves and require little (if any) explanation in the text.

Figure 3.8 Pie Chart of Leading Causes of Death in the United States, 1979

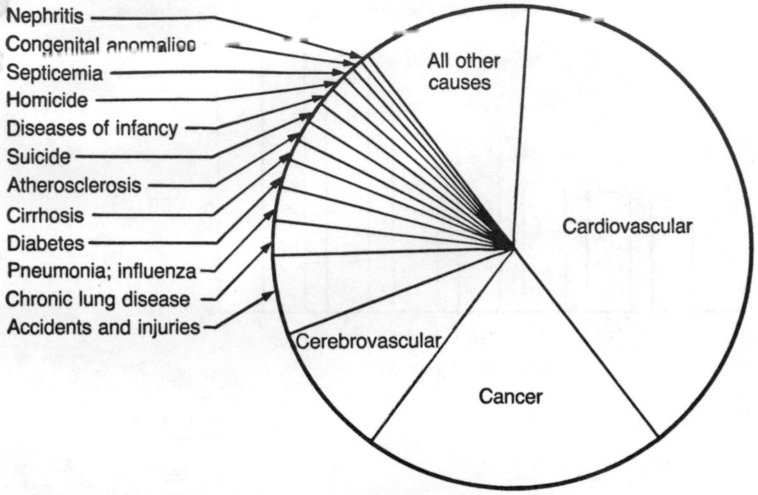

SOURCE: National Center for Health Statistics (1982).

Vocabulary List

abscissa
array
bar chart
bimodal distribution
class boundaries
class frequency
class interval
class limits
class midpoint
continuous variable
cumulative frequency polygon (ogive)
cumulative percentage
discrete variable
frequency distribution
frequency polygon
frequency table
graph
histogram
interval scale
nominal number
ordinal number
ordinate
percentile
pie chart
qualitative variable
quantitative variable
ratio scale
rectangular distribution
relative frequency
skewed distribution
stem-and-leaf display
symmetrical distribution
tally

Exercises

3.1 Refer to the variables of Table 3.1.
(a) Classify each variable as to whether it is qualitative or quantitative.
(b) Which of the quantitative variables are discrete? Which continuous?
(c) Name an appropriate type of graph for presenting each variable.
(d) Name a discrete variable that one might be interested in measuring for the Honolulu Heart Study group.

3.2 Name the variables represented in Table 2.2 and state which type each is.

3.3 How would you describe the shape of Figure 3.2? Refer to Table 3.4 and state whether the distribution of smokers' systolic blood pressures would be similar in shape to that of nonsmokers.

3.4 State the principal difference between a negatively skewed distribution and a positively skewed one.

3.5 (a) From the 83 observations of diastolic blood pressure in Table 2.2, prepare a frequency table like Table 3.2 that includes class interval, class frequency, relative frequency, cumulative relative frequency, and class midpoint.
(b) Using the same sheet of graph paper, draw a histogram and a frequency polygon for the same data.
(c) Construct an ogive for the same data.
(d) Find the following percentiles from the ogive: 20th, 50th (median), and 90th.
(e) What percentage of the observations are less than 70? 80? 90?

3.6 For the serum cholesterol values of Table 3.1, perform the same operations as suggested in (a) and (b) of Exercise 3.5. Do this by activity status; that is, for those who reported their physical activity as (a) mostly sitting (code #1) and (b) moderate (code #2), make separate frequency tables, histograms, and frequency polygons for the serum cholesterol values.

3.7 Make a bar graph of the educational levels of Table 3.1.

3.8 With each of the variables listed below, two graphical methods are mentioned. Indicate which method is more appropriate. State why one method is more appropriate than the other.
(a) Number of dental cavities per person
histogram, bar graph
(b) Triglyceride level
frequency polygon, bar graph
(c) Occupational classification
pie chart, histogram
(d) Birthrate by year
line graph, histogram

3.9 Prepare a stem-and-leaf display for the heights listed in Table 3.1.

Chapter 4

Summarizing Data

Chapter Outline

4.1 Measures of Central Tendency
Three common measures of central tendency—mean, median, and mode—are described, illustrated, and contrasted.

4.2 Measures of Variation
Several measures of variation or variability, including the standard deviation, are described.

4.3 Coefficient of Variation
The coefficient of variation, useful in comparing levels of variation, is defined.

4.4 Means and Standard Deviations from Grouped Data
The equations for computing means and standard deviations from grouped and ungrouped data are listed.

4.5 Means and Standard Deviations of a Population
The equations for the parameters of a population are contrasted with the statistics of a sample.

Learning Objectives

After studying this chapter, you should be able to

1. Compute and distinguish between the uses of measures of central tendency: mean, median, and mode
2. Compute and list some uses for measures of variation: range, variance, and standard deviation
3. Compare sets of data by computing and comparing their coefficients of variation
4. Select the correct equations for computing the mean and the standard deviation
5. Be able to compute the mean and the standard deviation for grouped and ungrouped data
6. Understand the distinction between the population mean and the sample mean

4.1 Measures of Central Tendency

Suppose you are considering accepting a new job with a well-known company. Salary is foremost in your mind, so you ask, "What is an employee's typical annual salary?" One person tells you, "$18,000"; another, "$10,000." You decide to check further into these inconsistent responses. Finally, you obtain some information you regard as reliable. Specifically, you are interested in knowing the lowest and the highest salary, the typical salary, and relative frequencies of the various annual salaries. A small but representative sample of salaries shows them to be $6000, $10,000, $10,000, $14,000, and $50,000. With this information at hand, you are now prepared to describe the salaries in the company. But to do this, you need to know how to compute statistics that characterize the center of the frequency distribution.

Given a set of data, one invariably wishes to find a value about which the observations tend to cluster. The three most common values are the mean, the median, and the mode. They are known as measures of **central tendency**—the tendency of a set of data to center around certain numerical values.

The Mean

The arithmetic mean (or, simply, **mean**) is computed by summing all the observations in the sample and dividing the sum by the number of observations. As there are other means, such as the harmonic and geometric means, it is essential to designate which type of mean one uses. In this textbook we will use only the arithmetic mean.

Symbolically, the mean is represented by

$$\bar{x} = \frac{x_1 + x_2 + x_3 \cdots + x_n}{n} \tag{4.1}$$

or

$$\bar{x} = \frac{\sum_{i=1}^{n} x_i}{n} \tag{4.2}$$

In these expressions the symbol $\bar{x}$, representing the sample mean, is read "x-bar"; x_1 is the first and x_i the ith in a series of observations. In this textbook we will use $\bar{X}$ (uppercase) to denote a random variable, and $\bar{x}$ (lowercase) to indicate a particular value of a function. The symbol Σ is the uppercase Greek letter sigma and denotes "the sum of." Thus $\Sigma_{i=1}^{n}$ indicates that the sum is to begin with $i = 1$ and increment by one up to and including the last observation n.

For the sample of the five salaries,

$$\bar{x} = \frac{\$6,000 + \$10,000 + \$10,000 + \$14,000 + \$50,000}{5} = \$18,000$$

The arithmetic mean may be considered the balance point, or fulcrum, in a distribution of observations. It considers the magnitude of each observation and is the point that balances the positive and negative deviations from the fulcrum.

The Median

In a list ranked according to size, the **median** is the observation that divides the distribution into equal halves. The median is considered the most typical observation in a distribution. It is that value above which there are the same number of observations as below. In short, it is the middlemost value. In our example of five salaries, the median is $10,000. For an even number of observations, the median is the average of the two middlemost values.

The Mode

The **mode** is the observation that occurs most frequently. In the salary example, the mode is equal to $10,000. It can be read from a graph as that value on the abscissa that corresponds to the peak of the distribution.

Which Average Should You Use?

With a bit of experience you can readily determine which measure of central tendency is appropriate to a given situation. The arithmetic mean is by far the most common. Since it considers, for example, the average amount of product consumed by a user, it is indispensable in business and commerce. If, for example, the average per capita consumption of sugar per year is 25 lb, then the amount of sugar to be sold in a town of 10,000 people would be 250,000 lb.

If you desire to know the typical observation in a distribution, particularly if it's skewed, the median proves to be a better measure. Income is the most common example of a distribution that is typically skewed. Because of the disproportionate weight of a few top-salary jobs, the arithmetic mean for income is nearly always artificially inflated.

Suppose an emergency stock clerk who handles different sizes of crutches wants to know which is the most popular size (the mode) so that he can order enough to meet his demand. By looking at the several measures of central tendency, he can obtain some idea of the shape of the frequency distribution. In a symmetrical distribution (Figure 4.1) the three measures of central tendency are identical. In an asymmetrical distribution (Figure 4.2) the mode remains located (by definition) at the peak; the mean is off to the right; and the median is in-between. Left-skewed distributions are the same, but in mirror-image.

The mode is used for nominal scores, the median for ordinal scores, and the mean for interval scores.

Figure 4.1 Symmetrical Frequency Distribution

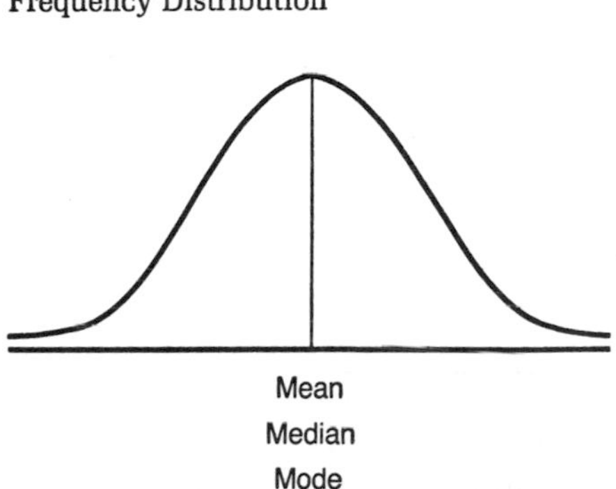

Figure 4.2 Asymmetrical Distribution, Skewed to the Right

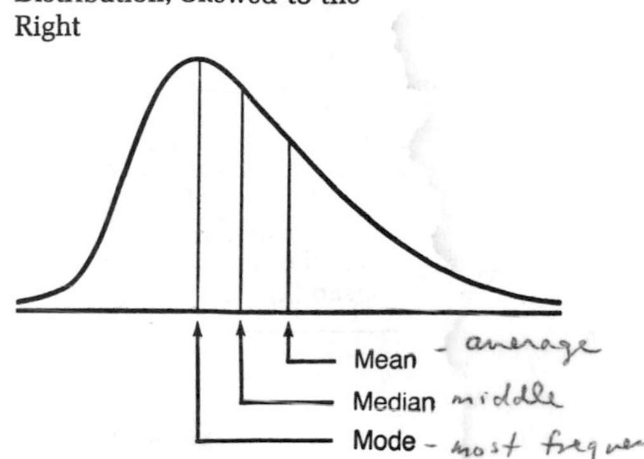

4.2 Measures of Variation

Knowing a distribution's central tendency is helpful, but it's not enough. It is also important to know whether the observations tend to be quite similar (homogeneous) or whether they vary considerably (heterogeneous). To describe variability, measures of **variation** have been devised. The most common of these are the **range,** the **mean deviation,** and the **standard deviation.**

Range

The **range** is defined as the difference in value between the highest (maximum) and lowest (minimum) observation:

$$\text{Range} = x_{max} - x_{min} \tag{4.3}$$

The range is quick to compute but fails to be very useful since it considers only the extremes and does not take into consideration the bulk of the observations. It is not widely used.

Mean Deviation

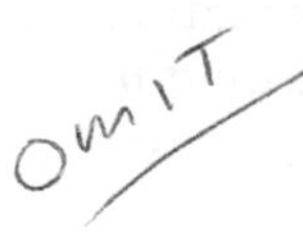

By knowing the range of a data set, we can gain some idea of the set's variability. The **mean deviation** is a bit more sophisticated than the range. It is defined as the average deviation of all observations from the mean. We can compute how far observations deviate from the mean by subtracting the mean from the value of each observation. The mean deviation is the sum of all of the **absolute values** of the deviations divided by the number of observations. That is,

$$\text{Mean deviation} = \frac{|x_1 - \bar{x}| + |x_2 - \bar{x}| + \cdots + |x_n - \bar{x}|}{n} \tag{4.4}$$

Table 4.1 Annual Percentage of Medical School National Board Honorees, 1978–1982

	Year of graduation				
	1978	1979	1980	1981	1982
Honors graduates (x_i)	4	6	5	8	7
Deviation from mean ($x_i - \bar{x}$)	−2	0	−1	+2	+1
Absolute value of deviation from mean ($\lvert x_i - \bar{x} \rvert$)	2	0	1	2	1
Squared deviation from mean $(x_i - \bar{x})^2$	4	0	1	4	1

where $|x_1 - \bar{x}|$ is read as "the absolute value of x sub one minus x-bar." Absolute value ignores the sign of the difference; that is, the mean deviation indicates how much, on average, the observations deviate from the arithmetic mean. The mean deviation is now mainly of historical interest; the measure was more commonly used before the age of electronic calculators and computers.

As an example, consider the percentage of graduates of a medical school who passed their National Boards with honors during a five-year period (Table 4.1). Note that some of the deviations are positive, some are negative, and one is zero. In sum, they add to zero, because $\bar{x}$ is the balance point of the observations. By using absolute values, we can eliminate the negatives and thus compute a mean deviation:

$$\text{Mean deviation} = \frac{\Sigma|x - \bar{x}|}{n} = \frac{6}{5} = 1.20$$

For the five-year period, the percentage of graduates earning honors differed, on average, by 1.2 percentage points from the mean of 6%.

Standard Deviation

By far the most useful measure of variation is the **standard deviation,** represented by the symbol s. It is the square root of the **variance** of the observations. The variance, or s^2, is computed by squaring each deviation from the mean, adding them up, and dividing their sum by one less than n, the sample size:

$$s^2 = \frac{\sum_{i=1}^{n}(x_i - \bar{x})^2}{n - 1} \tag{4.5}$$

The sample variance may thus be thought of as the mean squared deviation from the mean. Some old texts refer to standard deviation as "root-mean-squared deviation."

The variance is readily computed for the data of Table 4.1 as follows:

$$\bar{x} = \frac{30}{5} = 6$$

$$s^2 = \frac{\sum_{i=1}^{n} (x_i - \bar{x})^2}{n - 1}$$

$$s^2 = \frac{4 + 0 + 1 + 4 + 1}{4} = \frac{10}{4} = 2.5$$

The standard deviation is computed by extracting the square root of the variance. Or symbolically,

$$s = \sqrt{s^2} \tag{4.6}$$

For our example, $s = \sqrt{2.5} = 1.58$. (The square root of a number is best obtained with a calculator or from square root tables found as an appendix in many statistics books.)

Both the variance and the standard deviation are measures of variation in a set of data. The larger they are, the more heterogeneous the distribution. For example, if we were to compare the National Board scores of graduates of two medical schools, the school with the smaller standard deviation would have students who are more homogeneous in ability than the school with the larger. As a measure of variation, standard deviation is much preferred over all other choices. The units of the standard deviation turn out to be the same as the units of the raw data (e.g., inches, millimeters, kilograms), whereas the units of variance are squared. Standard deviation is arithmetically easy to handle and avoids the awkwardness of absolute values. Since the magnitude of the standard deviation depends on the phenomenon being observed, which may be represented by large or small numbers, the standard deviation itself can be large or small. What is a large deviation for one variable may be small for another.

Understanding the sources of variation may help you appreciate the meaning of standard deviation. For example, among subjects, one source of variation may be due to a personal characteristic like age or sex. Another source may be individual variation; still another, the varying condition of the subject (i.e., observations obtained before or after dinner, or before or after exercise, may differ). Yet another source of variation is measurement error. A certain amount is inherent in any observation; scientists strive mightily to keep it to a minimum.

4.3 Coefficient of Variation

One important application of the mean and the standard deviation is the **coefficient of variation.** It is defined as the ratio of the standard deviation to the mean, expressed as a percentage.

$$CV = \frac{100s}{\bar{x}}\% \tag{4.7}$$

The coefficient of variation depicts the size of the standard deviation relative to its mean. Since both standard deviation and the mean represent the same units, the units cancel out and the coefficient of variation becomes a pure number. That is, it is free of the measurement units of the original data. Therefore it is possible to use it to compare the relative variation of even unrelated quantities. For example, we may wish to know whether the variation of blood glucose readings is greater or less than the variation of serum cholesterol levels. From Table 3.1, we can compute the variation exactly. The coefficient of variation for blood glucose (in milligrams per deciliter) is = 54.72/152.14 × 100 = 36%; and for serum cholesterol it is 38.82/216.96 × 100 = 18%. From this we see that the variation in blood glucose is relatively greater than that for serum cholesterol.

4.4 Means and Standard Deviations from Grouped Data

More often than not, data are presented in *grouped* form. That is, the data are in part summarized and grouped in a frequency table. In actuality, this simplifies the handling of data—it's easier to work with 28 serum cholesterol readings of 130.5 than to list the value 130.5 separately 28 times. Means and standard deviations may be computed from grouped data, but the equations are a bit different. Table 4.2 presents both the definition equations and the calculating equations for obtaining these quantities. In the equations for grouped data, f_i denotes the number of observations in the ith class interval and c the number of classes. We can apply the equations of Table 4.2 to our Honolulu Heart Study subjects by using the data on heights from Table 4.3.

Table 4.2 Equations for Means and Standard Deviations

	Definition equation		Calculating equation	
	Ungrouped data			
Mean	$\bar{x} = \dfrac{\sum_{i=1}^{n} x_i}{n}$	(4.2)	same	
Standard deviation	$s = \sqrt{\dfrac{\sum_{i=1}^{n} (x_i - \bar{x})^2}{n-1}}$	(4.5)	$\sqrt{\dfrac{\sum_{i=1}^{n} x_i^2 - \dfrac{\left(\sum_{i=1}^{n} x_i\right)^2}{n}}{n-1}}$	(4.8)
	Grouped data			
Mean	$\bar{x} = \dfrac{\sum_{i=1}^{c} f_i x_i}{\sum_{i=1}^{c} f_i}$		$\dfrac{\sum_{i=1}^{c} f_i x_i}{n}$	(4.9)
Standard deviation	$s = \sqrt{\dfrac{\sum_{i=1}^{c} f_i (x_i - \bar{x})^2}{n-1}}$		$\sqrt{\dfrac{\sum_{i=1}^{c} f_i x_i^2 - \dfrac{\left(\sum_{i=1}^{c} f_i x_i\right)^2}{n}}{n-1}}$	(4.10)

Table 4.3 Frequency of Heights (in centimeters) of a Sample of 100 Males from the Honolulu Heart Study

Class interval	Class midpoint (x_i)	f_i	fx_i	fx_i^2
150–154	152	9	1,368	207,936
155–159	157	22	3,454	542,278
160–164	162	31	5,022	813,564
165–169	167	24	4,008	669,336
170–174	172	13	2,236	384,592
175–179	177	1	177	31,329
Total		100	16,265	2,649,035

For the grouped data, we obtain

$$\bar{x} = \frac{\sum_{i=1}^{c} f_i x_i}{\sum_{i=1}^{c} f_i} = \frac{16{,}265}{100} = 162.65 \text{ cm}$$

$$s = \sqrt{\frac{\sum_{i=1}^{c} f_i x_i^2 - \frac{\left(\sum_{i=1}^{c} f_i x_i\right)^2}{n}}{n-1}} = \sqrt{\frac{2{,}649{,}035 - 2{,}645{,}502.25}{99}}$$

$$= \sqrt{35.68}$$

$$= 5.97 \text{ cm}$$

Using Equations 4.2 and 4.8 for ungrouped data, we find $\bar{x} = 161.75$ cm, so that

$$s = \sqrt{\frac{\sum_{i=1}^{n} x_i^2 - \frac{\left(\sum_{i=1}^{n} x_i\right)^2}{n}}{n-1}} = \sqrt{\frac{2{,}619{,}407 - \frac{(16{,}175)^2}{100}}{99}}$$

$$= \sqrt{\frac{3100.75}{99}} = \sqrt{31.32}$$

$$= 5.60 \text{ cm}$$

Note that there is some difference between results from computations for ungrouped and grouped data. The size of the discrepancy depends on the width of the class interval and on the number of observations within an interval. With short class intervals and large samples, the discrepancy is negligible.

4.5 Means and Standard Deviations of a Population

The equations given for the mean and the standard deviation apply to the data of a sample selected from a population. When we have data for an *entire* population, we use similar equations but different symbols. Table 4.4 compares equations used for the two purposes. The **population mean, μ** (lowercase Greek mu), is defined as the sum of the values divided by N, the number of observations for the entire population. The sample mean, $\bar{x}$, is an estimate of μ and is the sum of the values in the sample divided by n, the

Table 4.4 Equations for Population and Sample Means and Standard Deviations

Quantity	Sample		Population	
Mean	$\bar{x} = \frac{\sum_{i=1}^{n} x_i}{n}$	(4.2)	$\mu = \frac{\sum_{i=1}^{N} x_i}{N}$	(4.11)
Variance	$s^2 = \frac{\sum_{i=1}^{n} (x_i - \bar{x})^2}{n - 1}$	(4.5)	$\sigma^2 = \frac{\sum_{i=1}^{N} (x_i - \mu)^2}{N}$	(4.12)
Standard deviation	$s = \sqrt{s^2}$	(4.6)	$\sigma = \sqrt{\sigma^2}$	(4.13)

number of observations in the sample alone. (Convention dictates the use of Greek letters for population parameters and Roman letters for sample statistics.) The population variance, σ^2, is the sum of the squared deviations from the population mean μ divided by N, whereas the sample variance s^2 (an estimation of σ^2) is the sum of the squared deviations from the sample mean $\bar{x}$ divided by $n - 1$. Dividing by $n - 1$ looks like a peculiarity, but it provides an equation that gives an unbiased sample variance. Therefore the use of $n - 1$, instead of n, gives a more accurate estimate of σ^2. Convention dictates the use of some shorthand to replace more awkward notation. Hence, in subsequent chapters, we will use x instead of x_i and Σ instead of $\Sigma_{i=1}^{n}$.

Conclusion

In describing data by use of a summary measure it is important to select that measure of central tendency that best represents the data and does not give a false impression. A better way of representing data is to use two summary measures—one to indicate central tendency and one to indicate variation. The most commonly used pair is the arithmetic mean and the standard deviation.

Vocabulary List

absolute values
central tendency
coefficient of variation
mean
mean deviation
median
mode
population mean
range
standard deviation
variance
variation

Exercises

4.1 Find the mean, median, mode, range, variance, and standard deviation for the data 8, 5, 3, 5, 2, 1. (For variance, use Equation 4.5.)

4.2 Using the sample 3, 1, 6, 4, 10, 6,
(a) Find the median, mean, and range.
(b) Compute the standard deviation using Equations 4.5 and 4.6.
(c) Compute the standard deviation using Equation 4.8.
(d) Compare the results of (b) and (c).
Why is the standard deviation of this example larger than that of Exercise 4.1?

4.3 Determine the range, median, and mode for the data of Table 2.2.

4.4 Assuming that Table 2.2 is a population of values, compute the mean, variance, and standard deviation. (Use the equation $\sigma^2 = \Sigma x^2/N - \mu^2$ for the calculation of variance.)

4.5 Compute $\bar{x}$, s^2, and s for the sample of ten that you took in Exercise 2.1. (Use Equation 4.8.) Compare your results with those for Exercise 4.4.

4.6 Determine the mean, variance, and standard deviation of weights in Table 3.1 by using the technique of Table 4.2.

4.7 (a) Calculate the coefficient of variation for height and weight in Table 3.1. (Use the results from Table 4.2 and Exercise 4.6.)
(b) Compare the two coefficients. Which one is larger? Approximately how many times larger?

4.8 (a) Calculate the mean and the standard deviation for systolic blood pressure in Table 3.1. (*Hint:* Use the technique of Table 4.2.)
(b) Calculate $\bar{x} - s$ and $\bar{x} + s$.
(c) Calculate $\bar{x} - 2s$ and $\bar{x} + 2s$.
(d) Calculate $\bar{x} - 3s$ and $\bar{x} + 3s$.
(e) What percentage of the blood pressure observations fall within each of the three intervals you calculated in (b), (c), and (d)?

4.9 (a) Find the median age of the sample represented in Table 3.1.
(b) What is the age range?

4.10 For the cholesterol values given in Table 3.1, the mean and the standard deviation are, respectively, 216.96 and 38.82. What is the variance?

4.11 If the variance of blood glucose values in Table 3.1 is 2994, what is the standard deviation?

4.12 List some practical uses for standard deviation.

4.13 Describe a situation in which it would be useful to know
(a) the mean, median, and mode
(b) primarily the median
(c) primarily the mean

4.14 (a) Refer to Table 3.1. Using Equation 4.8, calculate the mean and the standard deviation of systolic blood pressure

(i) for those who have had no education (code = 1).

(ii) for those who have had intermediate education (code = 3).

(b) Compare the standard deviations of the two groups. Which set of values has the larger standard deviation and by how much?

(c) From your computations in (b), draw a conclusion about the relative variation of the observations in the two groups.

Chapter **5**

Probability

Chapter Outline

5.1 What Is Probability?
The concept of probability as a measure of the likelihood of occurrence of a particular event is discussed.

5.2 Probability Rules
Problems involving the probability of compound events are solved by use of the addition rule or the multiplication rule.

5.3 Counting Rules
How to compute the number of possible ways an event can occur by use of permutations and combinations is explained.

5.4 Probability Distributions
The concept of a probability distribution, which lists the probabilities associated with the various outcomes of a variable, is illustrated.

5.5 Binomial Distribution
A common distribution having only two possible outcomes on each trial is described.

Learning Objectives

After studying this chapter, you should be able to

1. State the meaning of "probability" and compute it in a given situation
2. State the basic properties of probability
3. Select and apply the appropriate probability rule for a given situation
4. Distinguish between mutually exclusive events and independent events
5. Distinguish between permutations and combinations; be able to compute them for various events
6. Explain what a probability distribution is and state its major use
7. State the properties of a binomial distribution
8. Compute probabilities by using a binomial distribution
9. Interpret the symbols in the binomial term

5.1 What Is Probability?

A pregnant woman frequently wonders, "Will my baby be a boy or a girl?" An understanding of probability can throw some light on this difficult question. Any answer must be based on various assumptions. If she assumes that her bearing a boy or a girl is equally likely, she would expect one boy baby for every two births—that is, half the time. As another way of estimating her chances of having a boy, she could count the number of boys and girls born in the past year. Vital statistics indicate there are about 1056 live births of boys for every 1000 live births of girls, so she could estimate her probability of having a boy as

$$\frac{1056}{2056} = .514$$

It should be noted that the term "probability" applies exclusively to a future event, never to a past event (even if its outcome is unknown). Therefore it is really not appropriate to state that the woman's probability of bearing a boy is .514, because, upon conception, the sex of the fetus is already established. It would be more appropriate to discuss the probability *before* the baby was conceived.

Many events in life are inherently uncertain. Probability may be used to measure the uncertainty of the outcome of such events. For example, you may wish to learn the probability of survival to age 80, of developing cancer, or of becoming divorced. This chapter attempts to cover some of the basic concepts of probability and set forth some rules and models that, if followed, can provide some quantitative estimates of the occurrence of various events.

Probability statements are numeric, defined in the range of 0 to 1, never more and never less. A probability of 1.0 means that the event will happen with certainty; zero means that the event will not happen. If the probability is .5, the event should occur once in every two attempts.

There are many ways of defining probability. Here is one of the simplest definitions: **Probability** is the ratio of the number of ways the specified event can occur to the total number of **equally likely events.** This definition was implicit in our example of estimating a woman's probability of bearing a boy baby.

The probability of an event, $P(E)$, can be defined as the proportion of times a favorable event will occur in a long series of repeated trials:

$$P(E) = \frac{n}{N} = \frac{\text{number of favorable outcomes}}{\text{number of possible outcomes}} \tag{5.1}$$

EXAMPLE 1

■ *One coin:* In a toss of a fair coin, there are two possible outcomes, a head (H) or a tail (T); that is, N = 2. So the probability of having a head equals

$$P(H) = \frac{1}{2} \quad ■$$

EXAMPLE 2

■ *Two coins:* In a toss of two coins, four outcomes are possible: HT, TH, TT, HH. (HT means heads on the first coin and tails on the second.) There are two helpful ways to ensure that all possible outcomes are listed—the **tree diagram** (Figure 5.1) and the **contingency table** (Table 5.1).

Figure 5.1 A Tree Diagram

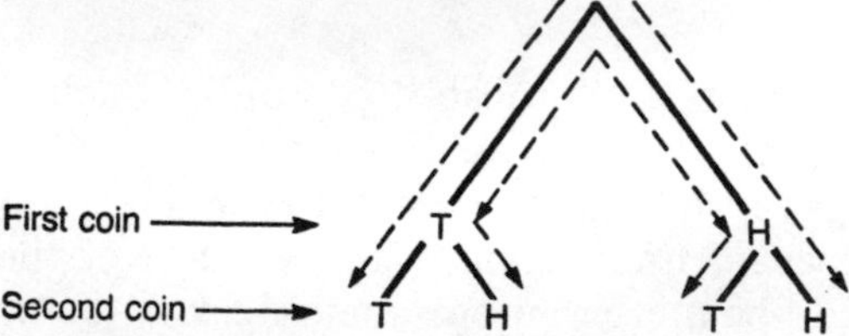

Table 5.1 A Contingency Table

		Second coin	
		H	T
First coin	H	HH	HT
	T	TH	TT

Consider the following questions: What is the probability of flipping two heads? At least one head? No heads? One head and one tail? Not more than one tail? We can tabulate the answers as follows:

Probability of an event	Favorable events
$P(2H) = \frac{1}{4}$	HH
$P(\text{at least } 1H) = \frac{3}{4}$	HT, TH, HH
$P(0H) = \frac{1}{4}$	TT
$P(1H \text{ and } 1T) = \frac{2}{4}$	HT, TH
$P(\text{not more than } 1T) = \frac{3}{4}$	HT, TH, HH ■

EXAMPLE 3

■ *Dice:* In a roll of a fair die, there are six equally possible outcomes ($N = 6$): 1, 2, 3, 4, 5, and 6. You might ask, "What is the probability of rolling a particular number?" And the answer is

$P(\text{even number}) = \frac{3}{6}$
$P(2 \text{ or } 3) = \frac{2}{6}$
$P(\text{greater than } 3) = \frac{3}{6}$ ■

Mutually exclusive events, E_i, are events that cannot happen simultaneously. That is, if one event happens, the other event cannot happen. Thus in the one-coin example, E_1 (heads) and E_2 (tails) are mutually exclusive, and their probabilities add up to 1.

Denoted symbolically, the three basic properties of probability are

$$0 \leq P(E_i) \leq 1 \tag{5.2}$$
$$P(E_1) + P(E_2) + \cdots + P(E_n) = 1 \tag{5.3}$$
$$P(\text{not } E_1) = 1 - P(E_1) \tag{5.4}$$

where $E_1, E_2, \ldots, E_n$ are mutually exclusive outcomes.

By perusing our three examples, you can see that (1) the probability of an event is always between 0 and 1 (inclusive); it is never negative and never greater than 1; and (2) the sum of the probabilities of all mutually exclusive outcomes is equal to 1.

5.2 Probability Rules

There are two indispensable rules that help answer the most common questions concerning the probability of compound events (those composed of two or more individual events). These are the **multiplication** rule and the **addition** rule.

Multiplication Rule

Two events are **independent** if the occurrence of one has no effect on the chance of occurrence of the other. The outcomes of repeated tosses of a coin illustrate independent events, for the outcome of one toss doesn't affect the outcome of any future toss. Note that "independent" and "mutually exclusive" are not the same. The occurrence of one independent event does not affect the chance of another such event occurring at the same time, whereas mutually exclusive events cannot occur simultaneously.

To determine the probability of occurrence of two independent events, we use the multiplication rule. The **multiplication rule** states that the probability of occurrence of two independent events, A and B, is equal to the product of the probabilities of the individual events.

Symbolically,

$$P(A \text{ and } B) = P(A)P(B) \tag{5.5}$$

EXAMPLE 4

■ In tossing two coins, what is the probability that a head will occur both on the first coin (H_1) *and* on the second coin (H_2)? The solution:

$$P(H_1 \text{ and } H_2) = [P(H_1)][P(H_2)] = (\tfrac{1}{2})(\tfrac{1}{2}) = \tfrac{1}{4} \quad ■$$

EXAMPLE 5

■ Suppose the probability that a typical driver will have an accident during a given year is $\frac{1}{10}$. What is the probability that two randomly selected drivers will *both* have an accident during the year? The solution:

$$P = \left(\frac{1}{10}\right)\left(\frac{1}{10}\right) = \frac{1}{100} \quad ■$$

Addition Rule

To determine the probability that one *or* another event (but not necessarily both) will occur, we use the addition rule. The **addition rule** states that the probability that event *A* or event *B* (or both) will occur equals the sum of the probabilities of each individual event less the probability of both. Symbolically,

$$P(A \text{ or } B \text{ or both}) = P(A) + P(B) - P(A \text{ and } B) \tag{5.6}$$

The reason for subtracting $P(A \text{ and } B)$ is that this portion would otherwise be included twice, as you can see from Figure 5.2a, which is an example of a

Figure 5.2 Venn Diagrams of Two Events

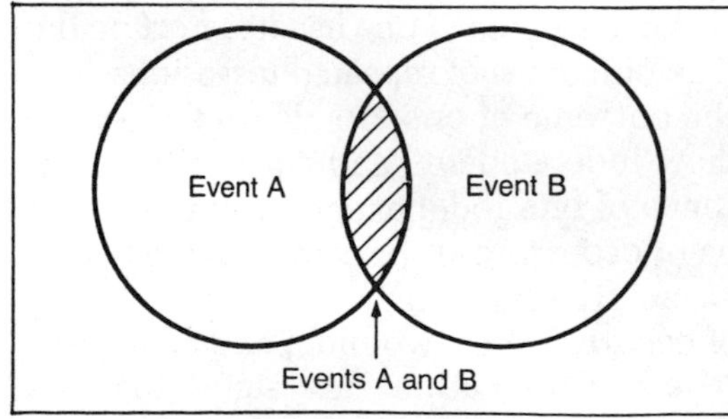

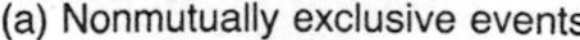

(a) Nonmutually exclusive events

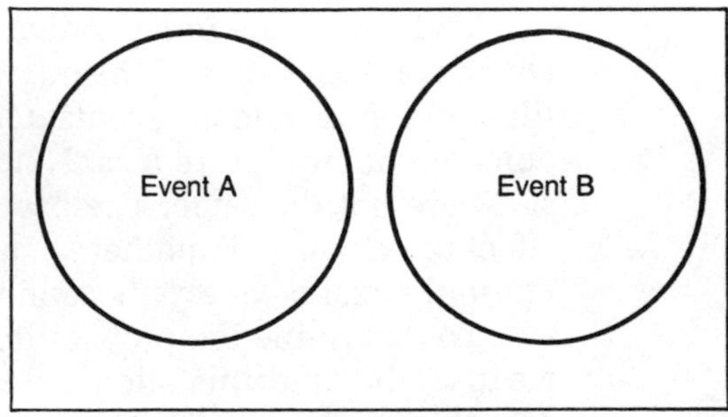

(b) Mutually exclusive events

Venn diagram. In such a diagram, circles within a rectangular space represent events; and the relationship between those events is indicated by a separation or an intersection of the circles.

EXAMPLE 6

■ In flipping two coins, you may wish to know the probability of having a head on the first coin (H_1), or on the second (H_2), or on both (H_1H_2). To get the answer, you use the addition rule:

$$P(H_1 \text{ or } H_2) = \tfrac{1}{2} + \tfrac{1}{2} - \tfrac{1}{4} = \tfrac{3}{4} \quad ■$$

EXAMPLE 7

■ What is the probability that you will obtain a 3 or 4 on one toss of a die? The addition rule gives

$$P(3 \text{ or } 4) = P(3) + P(4) - P(3 \text{ and } 4) = \tfrac{1}{6} + \tfrac{1}{6} - 0 = \tfrac{1}{3} \quad ■$$

It should be noted here that whenever two events are **mutually exclusive,** the probability of both events occurring is equal to zero. By tossing a 3, you have *excluded* the probability of tossing a 4. Likewise, you cannot simultaneously flip a head and a tail with a coin. Hence the addition rule is somewhat simplified when the two events are mutually exclusive. The rule then becomes

$$P(A \text{ or } B \text{ or both}) = P(A) + P(B) \tag{5.7}$$

The $P(A \text{ and } B)$ term of Equation 5.6 is zero; it drops out (Figure 5.2b).

EXAMPLE 8

■ At birth, the probability that a U.S. female will survive to age 65 is approximately $\frac{8}{10}$; that is, $P(F_{65}) = \frac{8}{10}$. The probability that a male will survive to age 65 is approximately $\frac{2}{3}$; that is, $P(M_{65}) = \frac{2}{3}$. What is the probability that a U.S. female will die before age 65? Using Equation 5.4, we see that the probability of dying before age 65, $P(F_d)$, is computed by subtracting from 1 the probability of surviving to age 65:

$$P(F_d) = 1 - P(F_{65}) = 1 - \tfrac{8}{10} = .2$$

Carrying the example further, the following probabilities can be computed by appropriately applying the multiplication and addition rules:

1. Probability that both will be alive at age 65:

$$P = P(M_{65})P(F_{65}) = (\tfrac{2}{3})(\tfrac{8}{10}) = .533$$

2. Probability that only the male will be alive at age 65:

$$P = P(M_{65})P(F_d) = \tfrac{2}{3}\left(1 - \tfrac{8}{10}\right)$$
$$= .133$$

3. Probability that only the female will be alive at age 65:

$$P = P(F_{65} \text{ and } M_d) = P(F_{65})\,P(M_d) = \tfrac{8}{10}\left(1 - \tfrac{2}{3}\right) = .267$$

4. Probability that at least one of the two will be alive at age 65:

$$P = P(\text{either one or both will be alive})$$

$$P = P(F_{65} \text{ and } M_{65}) + P(M_{65} \text{ and } F_d) + P(F_{65} \text{ and } M_d)$$

$$= .533 + .133 + .267 = .933$$

This answer may also be obtained by finding the probability of the complement of both the male and the female dying. That is,

$$1 - P(M_d \text{ and } F_d) = 1 - \tfrac{1}{3} \cdot \tfrac{2}{10} = .933 \quad \blacksquare$$

5.3 Counting Rules

In computing the probabilities of various events, we first need to know in how many possible ways such events can occur. For example, if one wishes to know the probability of having two girls and a boy in a three-child family, it is essential to know the order: How many different possibilities are there of having two girls and a boy? The number of different outcomes is eight:

girl girl girl	boy girl girl*
girl girl boy*	boy girl boy
girl boy girl*	boy boy girl
girl boy boy	boy boy boy

Here you can see that the three outcomes marked with asterisks qualify as successes (two girls and a boy).

You may need to know the number of different possibilities of a certain event in order to determine the denominator needed to compute a probability. Three general rules are helpful in obtaining counts.

Rule 1: Number of Ways

If an event A can occur in n_1 distinct ways and event B can occur in n_2 ways, then the events consisting of A and B can occur in $n_1 \cdot n_2$ ways.

EXAMPLE 9

■ If you had three different diet (D) choices by amount of protein (low, medium, high) and three different choices by amount of fat (low, medium, high), there would be $(n_1)(n_2) = (3)(3) = 9$ different possible diets:

D_1: protein (low), fat (low)
D_2: protein (medium), fat (low)
D_3: protein (high), fat (low)
D_4: protein (low), fat (medium)
D_5: protein (medium), fat (medium)
D_6: protein (high), fat (medium)
D_7: protein (low), fat (high)
D_8: protein (medium), fat (high)
D_9: protein (high), fat (high) ■

Rule 2: Permutations

In determining the number of ways in which you can manage a group of objects, you must first know whether the *order* of arrangement plays a role. For example, the order of arrangement of a person's missing teeth is important, but the order of selecting a group for a committee is not, because any order results in the same committee.

A **permutation** is a selection of *r* objects from a group of *n* objects, taking the order of selection into account. The number of different ways in which *n* objects may be arranged is given by *n*!. The exclamation mark stands for **factorial,** and the symbol *n*! (read "*n* factorial") means $n(n - 1)(n - 2) \cdots 3 \cdot 2 \cdot 1$. Thus 3! (i.e., three factorial) $= 3 \cdot 2 \cdot 1 = 6$, and $0! = 1$.

EXAMPLE 10

■ If one wishes to identify vials of a medication by using three different symbols, x, y, and z, how many different ways can the vials be identified? The answer is

$$3! = 3 \cdot 2 \cdot 1 = 6$$

The six different identifications are *xyz*, *xzy*, *yxz*, *yzx*, *zxy*, and *zyx*.

Suppose we want to learn the number of ways of selecting *r* objects from a set of *n* objects and *order is important*. Here we would use the equation

$$P(n,r) = \frac{n!}{(n - r)!} \quad ■ \tag{5.8}$$

EXAMPLE 11

■ If there are three effective ways of treating a cancer patient—surgery (S), radiation (R), and chemotherapy (C)—in how many different ways can a patient be treated with two different treatments if the order of treatment is important? The answer is given by

$$P(3,2) = \frac{3!}{(3-2)!} = \frac{3 \cdot 2 \cdot 1}{1} = 6$$

or SR, RS, CS, SC, RC, and CR. ■

Rule 3: Combinations

Sometimes you may wish to determine the number of arrangements of a group of objects when order is not important, as in selecting books from a shelf. A **combination** is a selection of a subgroup of distinct objects with order not being important. The equation for obtaining the number of ways of selecting r objects from n objects, disregarding order, is

$$C(n,r) = \frac{n!}{r!(n-r)!} \tag{5.9}$$

where C denotes the total number of combinations of objects.

EXAMPLE 12

■ Suppose that three patients with snakebites are brought to a physician. To his regret, he discovers that he has only two doses of antivenin. The three patients are a pregnant woman, a young child, and an elderly man. Before deciding which two to treat, he examines his choices:

$$C(3,2) = \frac{3!}{2!(3-2)!} = \frac{3 \cdot 2 \cdot 1}{2 \cdot 1} = 3$$

The three choices are wc, wm, cm. Note that cw, mw, and mc are the same as the first three because order does not matter. ■

5.4 Probability Distributions

A key application of probability to statistics is estimating the probabilities that are associated with the occurrence of different events. For example, we may wish to know the probability of having a family of two girls and one boy or the probability that two out of three patients will be cured by a certain medication. If we know the various probabilities associated with different outcomes of a given phenomenon, it is possible to determine which outcomes are common and which not. This helps us reach a decision as to whether certain events are significant. A complete list of all possible outcomes, together with the probability of each, constitutes a **probability distribution.**

Table 5.2 Examples of Probability Distribution

Toss of two coins		Roll of a die		Sex of three-child family	
E	P(E)	E	P(E)	E	P(E)
HH	$\frac{1}{4}$	1	$\frac{1}{6}$	3 boys*	.125
HT	$\frac{1}{4}$	2	$\frac{1}{6}$	2 boys, 1 girl	.375
TH	$\frac{1}{4}$	3	$\frac{1}{6}$	1 boy, 2 girls	.375
TT	$\frac{1}{4}$	4	$\frac{1}{6}$	3 girls	.125
	1.0				1.000
		5	$\frac{1}{6}$		
		6	$\frac{1}{6}$		
			1.0		

*For ease of computation, we assume that $P(\text{boy}) = .5$.

The outcome of events may be described numerically (e.g., the number of three-boy families). The symbol x usually denotes the variable of interest. This variable, which can assume any number of values, is called a **random variable** because it represents a chance (random) outcome of an experiment. Thus we can say that a probability distribution is a list of the probabilities associated with the values of the random variable obtained in an experiment. Random variables may be either discrete or continuous. Only the discrete will be discussed in this chapter.

Three examples of probability distribution are illustrated in Table 5.2. As the third example in the table shows, if a family is selected at random, the probability that it is a three-boy family is .125. In this example the number of boys is the random variable.

From the distributions in Table 5.2, you can again see that the sum of the probabilities of a set of mutually exclusive events always equals 1.

5.5 Binomial Distribution

In practice we usually work with distributions that are reasonable approximations to theoretical distributions. In constructing a frequency table, we can obtain an estimate of the probability distribution by visualizing the relative frequency associated with each possible outcome. Having this information, we can make statements about how common any given event is.

Various phenomena follow certain underlying mathematical distributions. One of the most useful, the **binomial distribution,** serves as a model for outcomes limited to two choices—sick or well, dead or alive, at risk or not at risk. For such a dichotomous population, we may wish to know the probability of having a number of r successes on n different attempts, where the probability of success on any one attempt is p.

As an example, let's again consider the probability that a couple planning three children will have two girls and one boy. Suppose we wonder whether the three children will arrive in the sequence GGB. If we assume that the probability of having a girl is .5, then the probability of the sequence GGB occurring is $(\frac{1}{2} \cdot \frac{1}{2}) \cdot \frac{1}{2} = \frac{1}{8}$. However, two girls and a boy may arrive in three different ways—GGB, GBG, BGG—as indicated by C(3,2) = 3, where C(3,2) denotes the combination of three things taken two at a time. Since the probability of each sequence is $\frac{1}{8}$, the probability of having two girls and a boy in *any* sequence is

$$3 \cdot (\tfrac{1}{8}) = 3(.125) = .375$$

as indicated in the third probability distribution in Table 5.2.

The probability distribution for this example is algebraically obtained from the expansion of the **binomial term** $(p + q)^n$, where p is the probability of a successful outcome, $q = 1 - p$ is the probability of a nonsuccessful outcome, and n is the number of trials or attempts. The binomial expansion is applicable, providing that

1. Each trial has only two possible outcomes—success or failure
2. The outcome of each trial is independent of the outcomes of any other trial
3. The probability of success, p, is constant from trial to trial

Under these conditions the probability of the sequence GGB is

$$\begin{array}{l} p \cdot p(1 - p) = p^2 q \\ \text{G} \quad \text{G} \quad \text{B} \end{array}$$

and the probability of any sequence of two girls and a boy is

$$C(3,2)p^2(q) = \frac{3!}{2!(3-2)!}\left(\frac{1}{2}\right)^2\left(\frac{1}{2}\right) = 3\left(\frac{1}{2}\right)^3 = .375$$

where C(3,2) becomes the binomial coefficient giving the number of different sequences of three children consisting of two girls and one boy.

In general, the probability of an event consisting of r successes out of n trials is

$$P = \frac{n!}{r!(n-r)!} p^r q^{n-r} \qquad (5.10)$$

where n = the number of trials in an experiment
r = the number of successes
$n - r$ = the number of failures
p = the probability of success
$q = 1 - p$, the probability of failure

The expression $(n!/(n - r)!r!)(p^r q^{n-r})$ is a term from the binomial expansion. The entire expansion lists the terms for r successes and $(n - r)$ failures from the binomial distribution:

$$
\begin{aligned}
(p + q)^3 &= q^3 + \frac{3!}{1!(3-1)!}pq^2 + \frac{3!}{2!(3-2)!}p^2q + p^3 \\
&= q^3 + 3pq^2 + 3p^2q + p^3 \qquad (5.11) \\
&= 3F \quad 1S, 2F \quad 2S, 1F \quad 3S
\end{aligned}
$$

where F = failure, and S = success. If a "success" means bearing a girl ($p = .5$), Equation 5.11 reduces to

$$
\begin{aligned}
(p + q)^3 &= (\tfrac{1}{2})^3 + 3(\tfrac{1}{2})(\tfrac{1}{2})^2 + 3(\tfrac{1}{2})^2(\tfrac{1}{2}) + (\tfrac{1}{2})^3 \\
&= .125 + .375 + .375 + .125 = 1.000 \qquad (5.12) \\
&= 3B \quad 2B, 1G \quad 1B, 2G \quad 3G
\end{aligned}
$$

Equation 5.12 shows that the binomial expansion yields the binomial distribution illustrated initially in the third example in Table 5.2 and visually portrayed in Figure 5.3.

It is essential that you gain a feeling for the meaning of a binomial term.

Figure 5.3 Example of Binomial Distribution

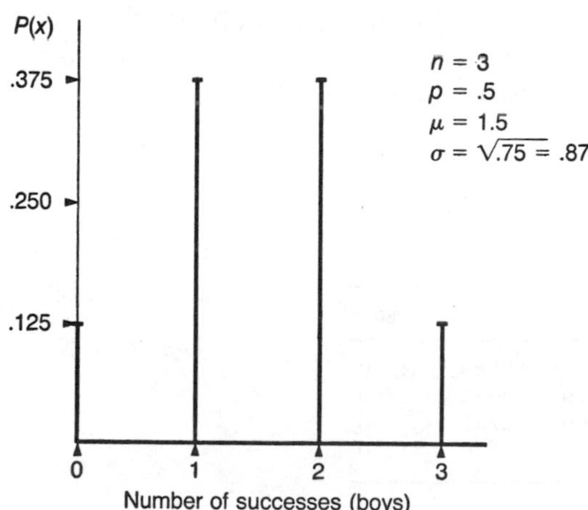

Figure 5.4 Identification of the Components of the Binomial Term

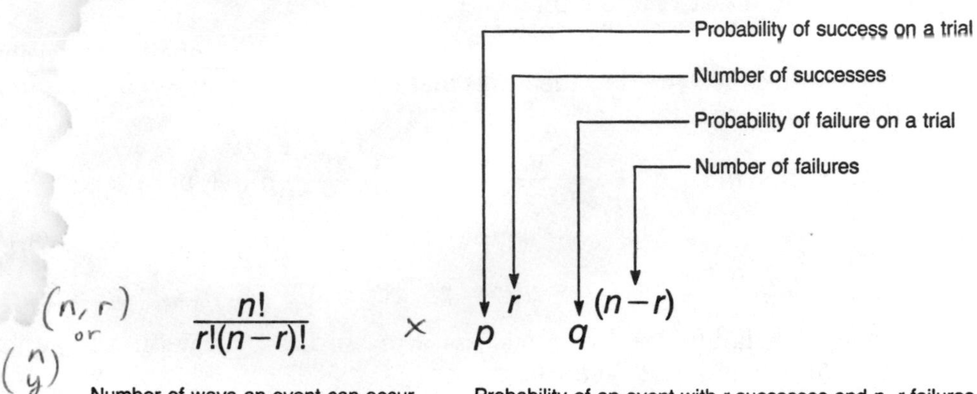

You will then be able to construct or interpret one for any occasion. Figure 5.4 should enable you to understand the anatomy of the binomial term. Note especially that in a binomial distribution, r (the number of favorable outcomes) serves as the random variable. Using the probability distribution given in Equation 5.10, you can find the following probabilities in a three-child family:

3B = .125
2G, 1B = .375
At most 2G (3B; 2B, 1G; 1B, 2G) = .125 + .375 + .375 = .875
At least 1B (3B; 2B, 1G; 1B, 2G) = .125 + .375 + .375 = .875

The probabilities of a binomial term can be obtained by reading them directly from a binomial table such as Table A (see appendix). A small portion of this table is reproduced in Table 5.3.

Table 5.3 Portion of Binomial Probability Table

		P			
n	r	.10	.25	1/3	.50
	0	.7290	.4219	.2963	.1250
	1	.2430	.4219	.4444	.3750
3	2	.0270	.1406	.2222	.3750
	3	.0010	.0156	.0370	.1250

EXAMPLE 13

■ What is the probability of having two girls and one boy in a three-child family if the probability of having a boy is .5?

From the calculations in Equation 5.12 it can be seen that

$$P(2G, 1B) = \frac{3!}{2!(3-2)!}\left(\frac{1}{2}\right)^2\left(\frac{1}{2}\right)^1 = 3(.125) = .375$$

Entering Table 5.3 with $n = 3$, $p = .5$, and $r = 2$, we again find that $P = .375$. ■

The binomial expansion is used to obtain the probability of various events when n is small, say 30 or less. When n is large, you should use the Gaussian (normal) distribution, discussed in the next chapter, as an approximation. To do this, you need to know the mean and the standard deviation of the **binomial** distribution, and we will consider these in Chapter 11.

Conclusion

Probability measures the likelihood that a particular event will or will not occur. In a long series of trials, probability is the ratio of the number of favorable outcomes to the total number of equally likely outcomes. Permutations and combinations are useful in determining the number of outcomes. If compound events are involved, we need to select and apply the addition rule or the multiplication rule to compute probabilities. The outcome of an experiment, together with its respective probabilities, constitutes a probability distribution. One very common probability distribution is the binomial. It presents the probabilities of various numbers of successes in trials where there are only two possible outcomes to each trial.

Vocabulary List

addition rule
binomial distribution
binomial term
combination
contingency table
equally likely events
factorial
independent events
multiplication rule
mutually exclusive events
permutation
probability
probability distribution
random variable
tree diagram
Venn diagram

Exercises

5.1 Two coins are tossed and the results observed. Find the probabilities of observing zero heads, one head, two heads.

5.2 Take two coins, toss them 50 times, and record the number of heads observed for each toss. Compute the proportion of zero heads, one head, and two heads, and compare the results with the expected results you computed in Exercise 5.1.

5.3 A fair coin is tossed three times and the number of heads observed. Determine the probability of observing
(a) exactly two heads
(b) at least two heads
(c) at most two heads
(d) exactly three heads

5.4 A couple is planning to have three children. Find the following probabilities by listing all the possibilities and using Equation 5.1.
(a) two boys and one girl
(b) at least one boy
(c) no girls
(d) at most two girls
(e) two boys followed by a girl
How does (e) differ from (a)?

5.5 Suppose you observe the result of a throw of a single fair die. How many times would you expect to observe a 1 in 60 throws? How many times would you expect to observe each of the other possibilities (2, 3, 4, 5, 6) in 60 throws?

5.6 Toss a die 60 times and record the frequency of occurrence of 1, 2, 3, 4, 5, 6. Compare your results with those in Exercise 5.5. In your judgment, is the die you tossed a fair one? (You will learn in Chapter 12 how to apply a statistical test to determine the fairness of a die.)

5.7 On a single toss of a pair of fair dice, what is the probability that
(a) a sum 8 is observed?
(b) a sum of 7 or 11 comes up?
(c) a sum of 8 or a double appears?
(d) a sum of 7 appears and both dice show a number less than 4?

5.8 A ball is drawn at random from a box containing 10 red, 30 white, 20 blue, and 15 orange balls. Find the probability that it is
(a) orange or red
(b) neither red nor blue
(c) not blue
(d) white
(e) red or white or blue

5.9 In an experiment involving a toxic substance, the probability that a white mouse will be alive for 10 hours is 7/10, and the probability that a black mouse will be alive for 10 hours is 9/10. Find the probability that, at the end of 10 hours,
(a) both mice will be alive
(b) only the black mouse will be alive
(c) only the white mouse will be alive
(d) at least one mouse will be alive

5.10 If an individual were chosen at random from Table 2.2, what is the probability that that person would be
(a) a vegetarian?
(b) a female?
(c) a male vegetarian?

5.11 Suppose a person is randomly selected from Table 3.1. Find the probability that he or she
(a) has completed high school or technical school
(b) is a smoker
(c) is physically inactive (code number = 1)
(d) is a physically inactive smoker
(e) has a serum cholesterol greater than 250 and a systolic blood pressure above 130
(f) has a blood glucose of 100 or less

5.12 In how many ways can five differently colored marbles be arranged in a row?

5.13 In how many ways can a roster of 4 club officers be selected from 10 nominees so that the first one selected will be president; the second, vice-president; the third, secretary; and the fourth, treasurer?

5.14 Compute
(a) $P(8,3)$
(b) $P(6,4)$

5.15 In how many ways can a committee of five people be chosen out of nine people?

5.16 Calculate
(a) $C(7,4)$
(b) $C(6,4)$
Compare (b) with 5.14b. What do you observe?

5.17 In how many ways can 10 objects be split into two groups containing 4 and 6 objects respectively?

5.18 About 50% of all persons three years of age and older wear glasses or contact lenses. For a randomly selected group of five people compute, using Equation 5.10, the probability that
(a) exactly three wear glasses or contact lenses
(b) at least one wears them
(c) at most one wears them

5.19 If 25% of 11-year-old children have no decayed, missing, or filled (DMF) teeth, find the probability that in a sample of 20 children there will be
(a) exactly 3 with no DMF teeth
(b) 3 or more with no DMF teeth
(c) fewer than 3 with no DMF teeth
(d) exactly 5 with no DMF teeth
(*Hint:* Refer to the first example in Table 5.2.)

5.20 It is known that approximately 10% of the population is hospitalized at least once during a year. If 10 people in such a community are to be interviewed, what is the probability that you will find

(a) all have been hospitalized at least once during the year?
(b) 50% have been hospitalized?
(c) at least 3 have been hospitalized?
(d) exactly 3 have been hospitalized?
(*Hint:* Refer to the first example in Table 5.2.)

5.21 Seventy-five percent of youths 12–17 years of age have a systolic blood pressure less than 136 mm of mercury. What is the probability that a sample of 12 youths of that age group will include
(a) exactly 4 who have a systolic pressure greater than 136?
(b) no more than 4 who have a blood pressure greater than 136?
(c) at least 4 who have a blood pressure greater than 136?
(*Hint:* Refer to the first example in Table 5.2.)

5.22 Assuming that, of all persons 17 years and over, half the males and one-third of the females are classified as presently smoking cigarettes, find the probability that in a randomly selected group of 10 males and 15 females
(a) exactly 10 smoke (4 males, 6 females)
(b) all smoke
(c) none smoke
(*Hint:* Refer to the first example in Table 5.2.)

Chapter **6**

The Normal Distribution

Chapter Outline

6.1 The Importance of Normal Distributions
It is explained why the normal distribution is so important in statistical analysis.

6.2 Properties of the Normal Distribution
The properties of the normal distribution, so valuable to statistical theory and methodology, are listed and explained.

6.3 Areas Under the Normal Curve
Specific examples are presented to demonstrate the interpretation and use of a table of areas that correspond to intervals of the standard score.

Learning Objectives

After studying this chapter, you should be able to

1. State why the normal distribution is so important
2. Identify the properties of the normal distribution
3. Interpret the mean and the standard deviation in the context of the normal curve
4. List the differences between the normal and the standard normal distribution
5. Explain the relative deviate $Z = (x - \mu)/\sigma$
6. Compute the percentage of areas between given points under a normal curve
7. Compute percentiles of specified variables by using a table of normal deviates

6.1 The Importance of Normal Distributions

Physicians often rely on a knowledge of **normal limits** to classify patients as healthy or otherwise. For example, a serum cholesterol level above 250 mg/dl is widely regarded as indicating a significantly increased risk of coronary heart disease. An accurate determination of such a value, whether or not based on a mathematical model, is of critical importance. The decision may be a matter of life or death, as the physician uses the findings in deciding what type of treatment to prescribe for a patient. It would be unfortunate, perhaps tragic, if the "normal limits" were faulty. In consequence, some patients might receive an unnecessary treatment, while others might fail to receive a needed treatment.

Serum albumin is the chief protein of blood plasma. For any group of persons, the concentrations of serum albumin tend to follow a **normal distribution.** The normal limits for albumin are calculated by adding and subtracting two standard deviations from the mean of a large set of observations obtained from a group of presumably healthy persons. This calculation provides the limits that contain the middle 95% (the "normal range") of observations but exclude the remaining 5%, leaving 2.5% in the lower tail and 2.5% in the upper tail. Extreme observations, those in the tails, are considered unusual and may be regarded as presumptive evidence of a health problem. However, not all variables follow a normal distribution. Two well-known counterexamples are urea and alkaline phosphatase. For these, use of the same method would give incorrect "normal limits" that would not include 2.5% of the observations in each tail. In response to this problem, medical statisticians Elveback, Guillier, and Keating (1970) have suggested that "clinical limits" rather than "normal limits" be used. **Clinical limits** are the lower and upper 2.5 percentage points for any distribution, normal or otherwise, of healthy persons. Clinical limits are obtained empirically, not by adding and subtracting two standard deviations from the mean. Use of clinical limits is greatly preferred to use of normal limits, as the 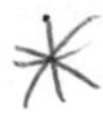 very term "normal limits" has been grossly misused and fallen into disrepute.

In the previous chapter we learned how a distribution of a variable gives an idea of the values of its population. Knowing that a variable is distributed normally can be especially helpful in drawing inferences as to how frequently certain observations are likely to occur.

The normal distribution, perhaps the most important of statistical distributions, was first discovered by the French mathematician Abraham Demoivre in 1733, and rediscovered and applied to the natural and social sciences by the French mathematician Pierre Simon de Laplace and the German mathematician and astronomer Karl Friedrich Gauss in the early nineteenth century. Sir Francis Galton, a cousin of Charles Darwin, first applied the normal curve to medicine.

Scholars like to refer to the normal curve as the **Gaussian distribution.** This preference is in reaction to a tendency of some persons to feel that anything not "normally" distributed is "abnormal." However, in popular practice, most statisticians and scientists still call it the normal distribution.

There are a legion of reasons why the normal distribution plays such a key role in statistics. For one thing, countless phenomena follow (or closely approximate) the normal distribution. Just a few of them are height, serum cholesterol, life span of light bulbs, body temperature of healthy persons, size of oranges, brightness of galaxies. But there are likewise countless phenomena that do *not* follow the normal distribution, ranging from individual annual income to clinical laboratory readings for urea, magnesium, or alkaline phosphatase. Another reason for the normal distribution's popularity is that it possesses certain mathematical properties that make it attractive and easy to manipulate. Still another reason is that much statistical theory and methodology was developed around the assumption that certain data are distributed approximately normally.

6.2 Properties of the Normal Distribution

The normal distribution has three main properties. First, it has the appearance of a symmetrical **bell-shaped curve** extending infinitely in both directions. It is symmetrical about the mean μ. Not every bell-shaped curve, however, is a normal distribution.

Second, all normal distributions have a particular internal distribution for the area under the curve. Whether the mean or standard deviation is large or small, the relative area between any two designated points is always the same. Let's look at three commonly used points along the abscissa. In Figure 6.1 we see that 68.26% of the area is contained within $\mu \pm 1\sigma$, 95.45% within $\mu \pm 2\sigma$, and 99.74% within $\mu \pm 3\sigma$ (see p. 68).

The total area under the curve in Figure 6.1 equals 1.0. This is a nice feature. Because of it, the area under the curve between any two points can
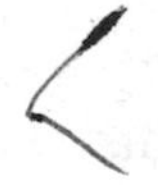
be interpreted as the relative frequency (or probability of occurrence) of the values included between those points.

Third, the normal distribution is a theoretical distribution defined by two parameters—the mean μ and the standard deviation σ. The **exponential equation** for the normal distribution is

$$y = \frac{1}{\sigma\sqrt{2\pi}} \exp\left[-\frac{1}{2}\left(\frac{x-\mu}{\sigma}\right)^2\right] \qquad (6.1)$$

Figure 6.1 Important Divisions of the Normal Distribution of IQs

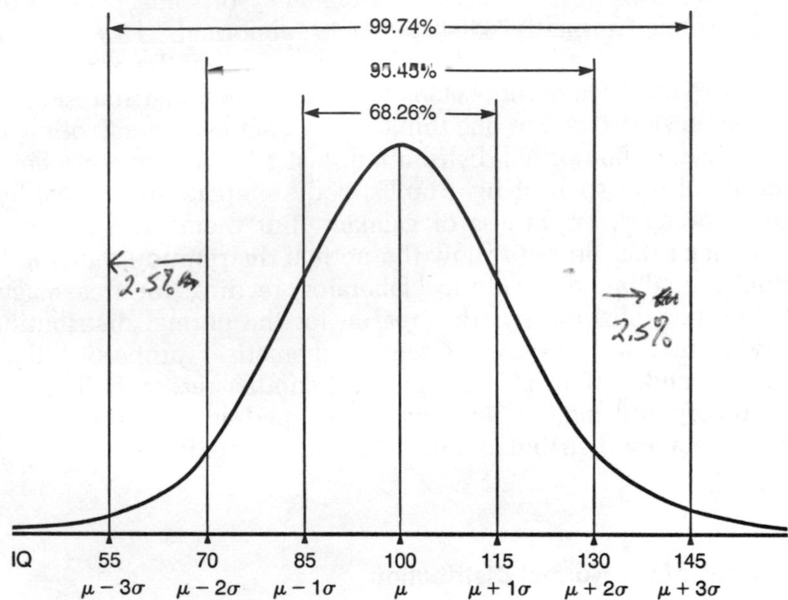

where y is the height of the curve for a given value x, exp is the base of the natural logarithms (approximately 2.71828), and π is the well-known constant (about 3.14159).

6.3 Areas Under the Normal Curve

Let us assume that the IQ of a given population is normally distributed with $\mu = 100$ and $\sigma = 15$. In that case 68.3% of the IQ scores should fall between 85 and 115 (100 ± 15) as shown in Figure 6.1. Similarly, we would expect approximately 95% of the IQs to fall between 70 and 130, 2.5% above 130 and 2.5% below 70. To find the proportion of persons with IQ scores between 130 and 135, we need a table of normal curve areas. But first, let's see how to use such a table.

Since it would be out of the question to tabulate the areas of all possible normal curves, we make use of the feature that all normal curves are symmetrical and have an area of 1.0. Thus, dealing with one normal curve is like dealing with any other, provided we use a standardized unit. Such a unit is the **relative deviate,** Z, which gives the relative position of any observation in the distribution. Sometimes Z is referred to as **Z score, Z value,** or normal deviate. Thus, for the normal curve, the relative deviate is

$$Z = \frac{x - \mu}{\sigma} \tag{6.2}$$

You can appreciate the effect of this transformation on the mean and the standard deviation of x by following a few simple steps:

		Variable	Mean	Standard deviation
Step 1:	Start with x	x	μ	σ
Step 2:	Subtract μ	$x - \mu$	$\mu - \mu = 0$	σ
Step 3:	Divide by σ	$Z = \frac{1}{\sigma}(x - \mu) = \frac{x - \mu}{\sigma}$	$\left(\frac{1}{\sigma}\right)0 = 0$	$\left(\frac{1}{\sigma}\right)\sigma = 1$

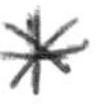

In step 1, given the variable x, the mean is μ and the standard deviation is σ. In step 2, on subtraction of μ, the mean is shifted from μ to 0, but σ is left unchanged. In step 3, the variable is divided by σ, the mean remains 0, and σ reduces to 1.

The net effect of this so-called Z transformation is to change any normal distribution to the **standard normal distribution,** where $\mu = 0$ and $\sigma = 1$. It is this distribution that takes on prominence because of its use in setting confidence limits and tests of hypotheses. Areas for the standard normal distribution are listed in Table 6.1 (p. 70). Here are a few pointers for anyone using it for the first time. Figure 6.2 (p. 71) shows areas under the standard normal curve between various points along the abscissa. The proper use of Table 6.1 may be demonstrated by finding the areas between different points along the abscissa. The area under the curve, A, is tabulated in the body of the table; it is that area between zero and some point Z to the right of zero. Z values are given in the left margin. Whole numbers and tenths are read at the left; hundredths at the upper horizontal margin. Further, since the normal curve is symmetrical, the area between zero and any negative point is equal to the area between zero and the corresponding positive point. Remember that since the area under the curve is equal to 1 and the curve is symmetrical about zero, the area to the right of Z can be computed by subtracting from .5.

Now let's extend our IQ score example to illustrate various uses of Table 6.1.

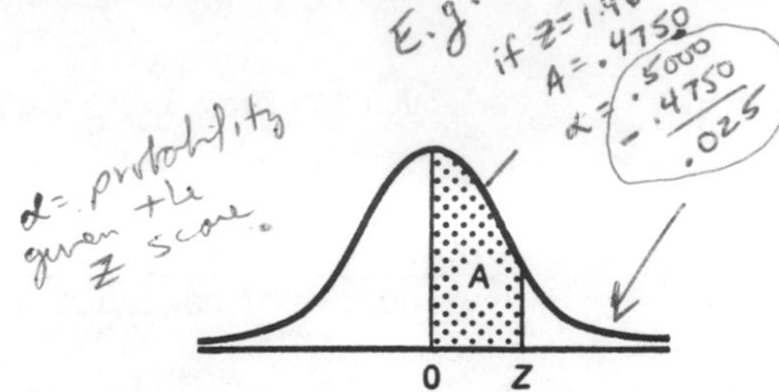

Table 6.1 Areas Under the Normal Curve

Z	.00	.01	.02	.03	.04	.05	.06	.07	.00	.09
0.0	.0000	.0040	.0080	.0120	.0160	.0199	.0239	.0279	.0319	.0359
0.1	.0398	.0438	.0478	.0517	.0557	.0596	.0636	.0675	.0714	.0753
0.2	.0793	.0832	.0871	.0910	.0948	.0987	.1026	.1064	.1103	.1141
0.3	.1179	.1217	.1255	.1293	.1331	.1368	.1406	.1443	.1480	.1517
0.4	.1554	.1591	.1628	.1664	.1700	.1736	.1772	.1808	.1844	.1879
0.5	.1915	.1950	.1985	.2019	.2054	.2088	.2123	.2157	.2190	.2224
0.6	.2257	.2291	.2324	.2357	.2389	.2422	.2454	.2486	.2517	.2549
0.7	.2580	.2611	.2642	.2673	.2704	.2734	.2764	.2794	.2823	.2852
0.8	.2881	.2910	.2939	.2967	.2995	.3023	.3051	.3078	.3106	.3133
0.9	.3159	.3186	.3212	.3238	.3264	.3289	.3315	.3340	.3365	.3389
1.0	.3413	.3438	.3461	.3485	.3508	.3531	.3554	.3577	.3599	.3621
1.1	.3643	.3665	.3686	.3708	.3729	.3749	.3770	.3790	.3810	.3830
1.2	.3849	.3869	.3888	.3907	.3925	.3944	.3962	.3980	.3997	.4015
1.3	.4032	.4049	.4066	.4082	.4099	.4115	.4131	.4147	.4162	.4177
1.4	.4192	.4207	.4222	.4236	.4251	.4265	.4279	.4292	.4306	.4319
1.5	.4332	.4345	.4350	.4370	.4382	.4394	.4406	.4418	.4429	.4441
1.6	.4452	.4463	.4474	.4484	.4495	.4505	.4515	.4525	.4535	.4545
1.7	.4554	.4564	.4573	.4582	.4591	.4599	.4608	.4616	.4625	.4633
1.8	.4641	.4649	.4656	.4664	.4671	.4678	.4686	.4693	.4699	.4706
1.9	.4713	.4719	.4726	.4732	.4738	.4744	.4750	.4756	.4761	.4767
2.0	.4772	.4778	.4783	.4788	.4793	.4798	.4803	.4808	.4812	.4817
2.1	.4821	.4826	.4830	.4834	.4838	.4842	.4846	.4850	.4854	.4857
2.2	.4861	.4864	.4868	.4871	.4875	.4878	.4881	.4884	.4887	.4890
2.3	.4893	.4896	.4898	.4901	.4904	.4906	.4909	.4911	.4913	.4916
2.4	.4918	.4920	.4922	.4925	.4927	.4929	.4931	.4932	.4934	.4936
2.5	.4938	.4940	.4941	.4943	.4945	.4946	.4948	.4949	.4951	.4952
2.6	.4953	.4955	.4956	.4957	.4959	.4960	.4961	.4962	.4963	.4964
2.7	.4965	.4966	.4967	.4968	.4969	.4970	.4971	.4972	.4973	.4974
2.8	.4974	.4975	.4976	.4977	.4977	.4978	.4979	.4979	.4980	.4981
2.9	.4981	.4982	.4982	.4983	.4984	.4984	.4985	.4985	.4986	.4986
3.0	.4987	.4987	.4987	.4988	.4988	.4989	.4989	.4989	.4990	.4990

EXAMPLE 1

■ What is the proportion of persons having IQs between 100 and 120?

Sketch a curve like the one in Figure 6.3. Shade in the area desired. Transform the IQ variable to a normal deviate. The Z corresponding to $x = 100$ is

$$Z = \frac{x - \mu}{\sigma} = \frac{100 - 100}{15} = 0$$

Figure 6.2 Areas Under the Standard Normal Curve

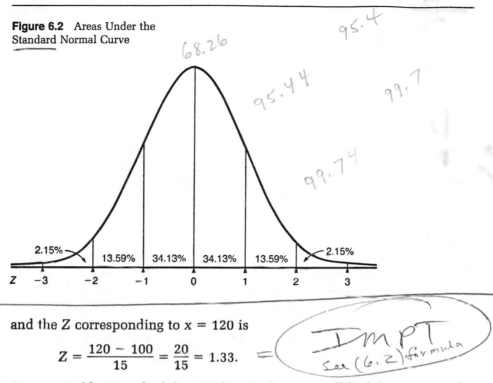

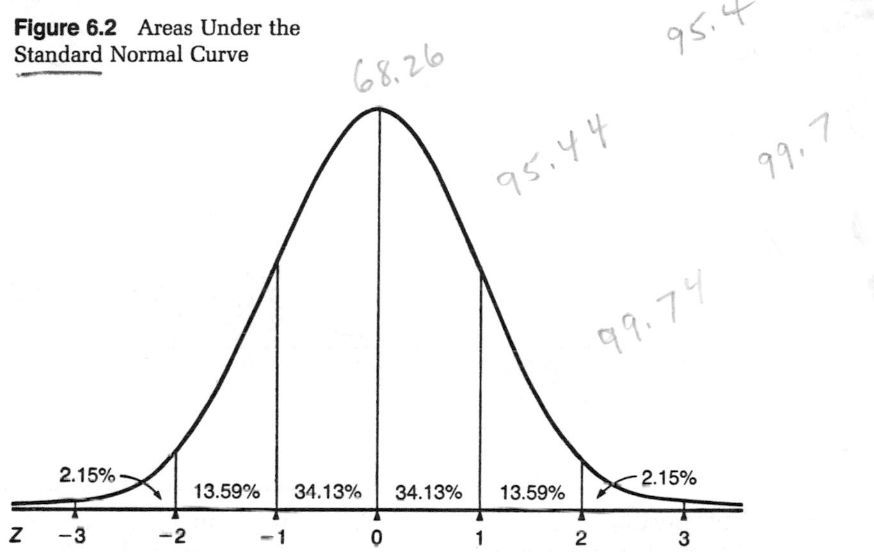

and the Z corresponding to x = 120 is

$$Z = \frac{120 - 100}{15} = \frac{20}{15} = 1.33.$$

By using Table 6.1 to find the area for a Z of 1.33, you'll find the answer to be .4082. Therefore the proportion of persons having IQs between 100 and 120 is .4082, about 41%. ■

Figure 6.3 Area Corresponding to IQs Between 100 and 120

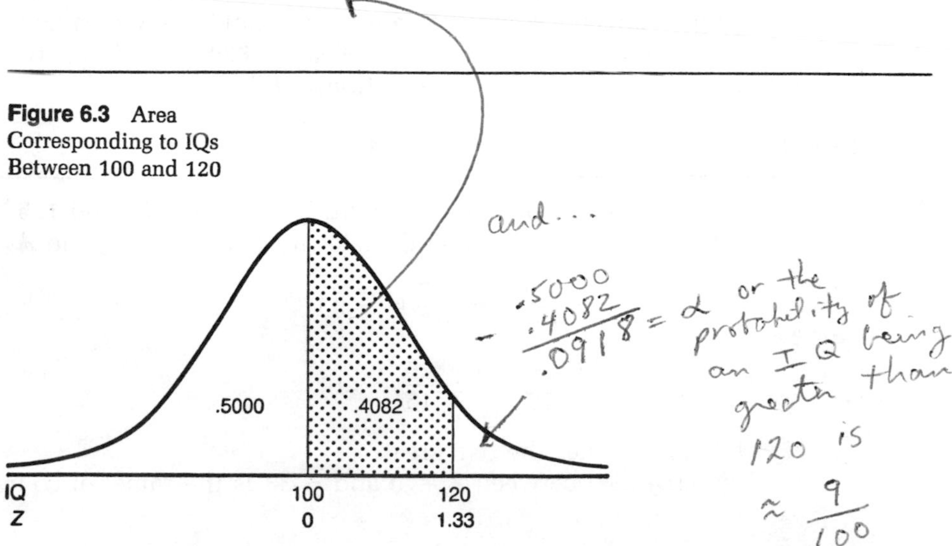

Figure 6.4 Area Corresponding to IQs Above 120

Figure 6.5 Area Corresponding to IQs Between 80 and 120

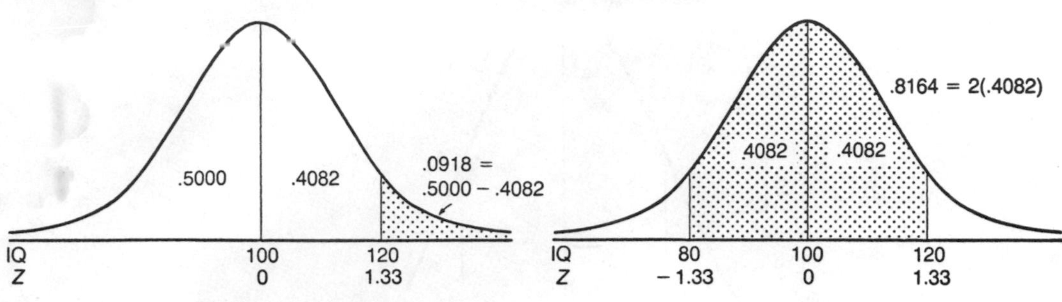

EXAMPLE 2

■ What proportion of persons have IQs greater than 120?

Again, sketch a curve, this time following the model of Figure 6.4. Since the area to the right of $Z = 0$ is .50, and the area between $Z = 0$ and 1.33 is 0.4082, by subtraction you will obtain the area beyond a Z of 1.33, namely, $.5000 - .4082 = .0918$. So the answer is that about 9% have IQs over 120. ■

EXAMPLE 3

■ What is the proportion of persons with IQs between 80 and 120?

This is the same as asking what proportion is found under the normal curve between the standardized values of Z between -1.33 and $+1.33$. Using the symmetry argument, you simply double the area between $Z = 0$ and 1.33, namely, $2(.4082) = .8164$. That is, 82% have IQs between 80 and 120. Figure 6.5 illustrates this solution. ■

EXAMPLE 4

■ What is the proportion of persons with IQs between 95 and 125?

The corresponding normal deviates for two areas, A_1 and A_2, are

$$A_1\text{: } Z = \frac{95 - 100}{15} = \frac{-5}{15} = -.33$$

$$A_2\text{: } Z = \frac{125 - 100}{15} = \frac{25}{15} = 1.67$$

Figure 6.6 illustrates the two areas.

The area (A_1) between $Z = 0$ and $-.33$ is the same, of course, as that

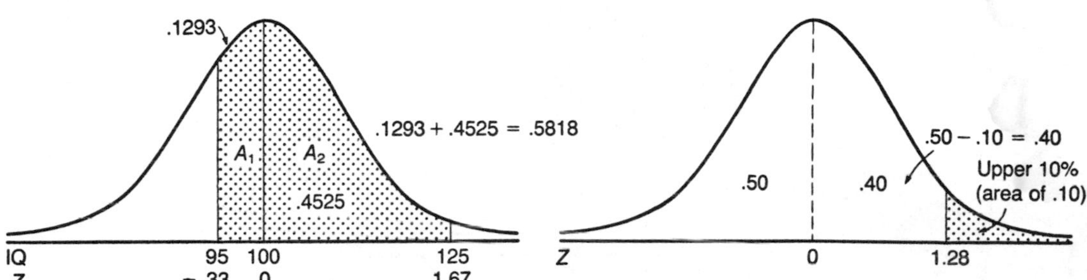

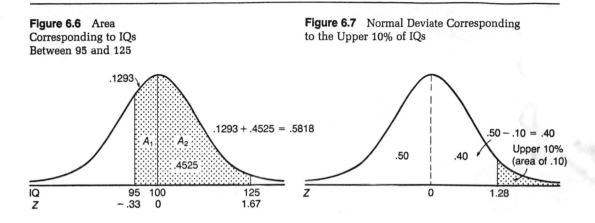

Figure 6.6 Area Corresponding to IQs Between 95 and 125

Figure 6.7 Normal Deviate Corresponding to the Upper 10% of IQs

between 0 and +.33. In Table 6.1, we see that A_1 is .1293 and that A_2, between $Z = 0$ and 1.67, is .4525. Thus $A_1 + A_2 = .1293 + .4525 = .5818$. The answer, then, is that about 58% of this population have IQs between 95 and 125. ■

Table 6.1 may also be used to determine the Z value that corresponds to any given area, as, for instance, the upper 10% of the curve. Consequently, we can obtain the value on the abscissa that corresponds to the 90th **percentile,** P_{90}.

EXAMPLE 5

■ What is the Z value of the normal curve that marks the upper 10% of the area?

The desired normal deviate is that value corresponding to .40 of the area, as Figure 6.7 illustrates. In Table 6.1 the value is found to be approximately $Z = 1.28$. ■

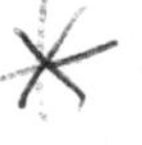

EXAMPLE 6

■ What is the 90th percentile of IQ scores?

This is the logical extension of Example 5. We just found the Z of the 90th percentile to be 1.28. But what does this mean in terms of IQs? The answer is found by a simple application of Equation 6.2.

$$Z = \frac{X - \mu}{\sigma}$$

$$1.28 = \frac{X - 100}{15}$$

Figure 6.8 90th Percentile of the Distribution of IQs

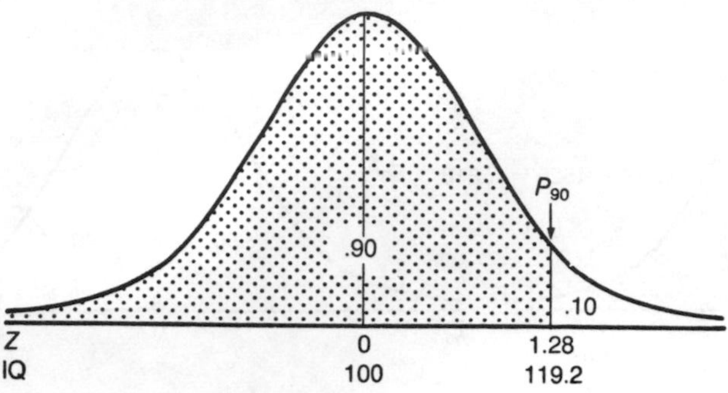

Therefore

$$x = 1.28\,(15) + 100 = 119.2$$

Thus 119.2 is the 90th percentile of IQ scores, as illustrated in Figure 6.8. ■

Knowing how to compute areas under a normal curve makes it easy to find the proportion (**probability**) of persons possessing certain cholesterol values, heights, or any other variable that is normally distributed. Knowing the probability of a given event allows us to draw appropriate inferences as to the expected occurrence of that event.

Conclusion

The normal distribution is an important concept for a number of reasons. It has been used to define "normal limits" for clinical variables. Many variables follow a normal distribution. The assumption of normality proves extremely useful because of the exceptional properties of the distribution. We can quickly reduce any normal distribution to the standard normal distribution by transforming the variable to a normal deviation Z score. Because these Z scores and the normal curve areas corresponding to them are conveniently tabulated, we are able to compute the probability of occurrence of various events and thus to decide about the degree of uniqueness of those events.

Vocabulary List

bell-shaped curve
clinical limits
exponential equation
normal distribution (Gaussian distribution)
normal limits
percentile
relative deviate
standard normal distribution
standard score
Z score (Z value; normal deviate)

Exercises

6.1 Find the areas under the normal curve that lie between the given values of Z:
(a) $Z = 0$ and $Z = 2.37$
(b) $Z = 0$ and $Z = -1.94$
(c) $Z = -1.85$ and $Z = 1.85$
(d) $Z = -0.76$ and $Z = 1.13$
(e) $Z = 0$ and $Z = 3.09$
(f) $Z = -2.77$ and $Z = -0.96$

6.2 Determine the areas under the normal curve falling to the right of Z (or to the left of $-Z$).
(a) $Z = 1.73$
(b) $Z = -2.41$ and $Z = 2.41$
(c) $Z = 2.55$
(d) $Z = -3$ and $Z = 3$
(e) $Z = 5$

6.3 What Z scores correspond to the following areas under the normal curve?
(a) Area of .05 to the right of $+Z$
(b) Area of .01 to the left of $-Z$
(c) Area of .05 beyond $\pm Z$
(d) Area of .01 beyond $\pm Z$
(e) Area of .90 between $\pm Z$
(f) Area of .95 between $\pm Z$

6.4 Find the standard normal score for
(a) the 95th percentile
(b) the 80th percentile
(c) the 50th percentile

6.5 The figure at the top of the next page shows the assumed distribution for systolic blood pressure readings of a large male population.
(a) Determine the relative deviates Z for the various cutoff points.
(b) Find the equivalent cutoff points in terms of systolic blood pressures if the mean reading is 130 and the standard deviation is 17.

6.6 If the heights of male youngsters are normally distributed with a mean of 60 in. and a standard deviation of 10, what percentage of the boys' heights (in inches) would we expect to fall

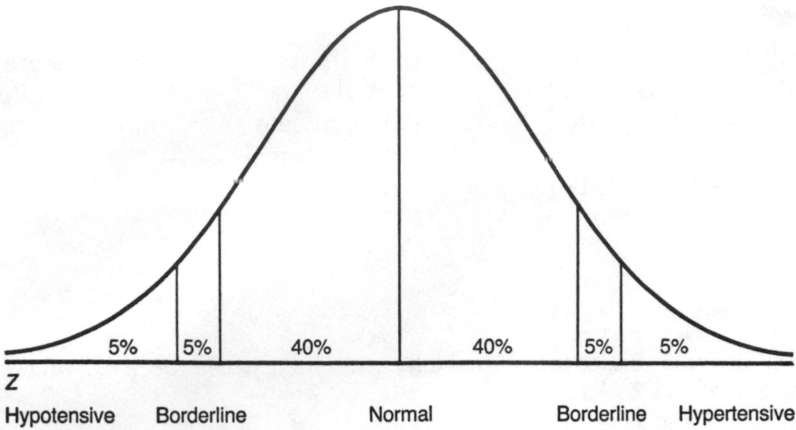

(a) between 45 and 75?
(b) between 30 and 90?
(c) less than 50?
(d) 45 or more?
(e) 75 or more?
(f) between 50 and 75?

6.7 For Exercise 6.5, find the 95th percentile.

6.8 An instructor is administering a final examination. She tells her class that she will give an A to the 10% of the students who earn the highest grades. Past experience with the same examination has shown that the mean grade is 75 and the standard deviation is 8. If the present class runs true to form, what grade would a student need in order to earn an A?

6.9 Assume that the age at onset of disease X is distributed normally with a mean of 50 years and a standard deviation of 12 years. What is the probability that an individual afflicted with X had developed it before age 35?

6.10 For Table 2.2, $\overline{X} = 73$ and $s^2 = 121$. If a person were chosen at random, what is the probability that she or he would have a diastolic blood pressure
(a) between 80 and 100?
(b) less than 70?
(c) greater than 90?

6.11 The mean blood glucose in Table 3.1 is 152 and $s = 55$. Find the probability that a randomly selected individual would have a glucose value
(a) between 80 and 120
(b) less than 80
(c) greater than 200

6.12 If the mean serum cholesterol in Table 3.1 is 217 and the variance is 1507, determine the probability that a randomly selected person would have a cholesterol value
(a) between 150 and 250
(b) greater than 250
(c) less than 150

Chapter **7**

Sampling Distribution of Means

Chapter Outline

7.1 The Distribution of a Population and the Distribution of Its Sample Means
A population distribution of observations is compared and contrasted with the distribution of sample means selected from it.

7.2 Central Limit Theorem
It is explained why an astonishing idea, the central limit theorem, plays a pivotal role in inferential statistics.

7.3 Standard Error of the Mean
The standard error is discussed as a key to computations of areas of the sampling curve.

7.4 Student's *t* Test
It is explained when and how to use the *t* distribution instead of the normal distribution to determine the relative position of $\bar{x}$ in its sampling distribution.

7.5 Application
The principles of the central limit theorem are applied to a specific example.

Learning Objectives

After studying this chapter, you should be able to

1. Distinguish between the distribution of a population and the distribution of its sample means
2. Explain the importance of the central limit theorem
3. Identify the main parts of the central limit theorem
4. Apply the principles of sampling distributions to predict the behavior of sample means
5. Compute and interpret the standard error of the mean
6. Determine when to use a *t* distribution

7.1 The Distribution of a Population and the Distribution of Its Sample Means

Statisticians are always interested in drawing inferences about a population. For example, it would be prohibitively expensive to conduct a health status survey by giving everyone in the United States a standardized comprehensive physical examination. Instead, a statistician would recommend that a sample be examined to estimate the important health parameters of the population. Such estimates would be expected to vary from sample to sample. In fact, if we were to select a large number of samples from a population and tabulate the sample means, the result would be a dis-

Table 7.1 Distribution of the Population and Distribution of Means from Samples for Blood Glucose Measurements of Men in the Honolulu Heart Study

Blood glucose (mg/100 ml)	Number of observations (frequency)	Sample means (n = 25) (frequency)
30.1–45.0	2	
45.1–60.0	15	
60.1–75.0	40	
75.1–90.0	210	
90.1–105.0	497	
105.1–120.0	977	
120.1–135.0	1073	5
135.1–150.0	1083	62
150.1–165.0	849	201
165.1–180.0	691	109
180.1–195.0	569	23
195.1–210.0	440	
210.1–225.0	343	
225.1–240.0	291	
240.1–255.0	153	
255.1–270.0	115	
270.1–285.0	82	
285.1–300.0	60	
300.1–315.0	38	
315.1–330.0	18	
330.1–345.0	26	
345.1–360.0	19	
360.1–375.0	20	
375.1–390.0	9	
390.1–405.0	13	
405.1–420.0	11	
420.1–435.0	6	
435.1–450.0	5	
450.1–465.0	4	
465.1–480.0	24	
Total	7683	400

tribution of sample means. And we might be surprised at the shape of that distribution.

It is of fundamental importance to make a clear distinction between a distribution of **sample means** and the **population distribution** of observations. A **distribution of sample means** is the set of values of sample means obtained from all possible samples of the same size (n) from a given population.

A distribution of sample means can be readily illustrated by again using the data of blood glucose measurements from the Honolulu Heart Study (Table 7.1 and Figures 7.1 and 7.2). Figure 7.1 illustrates the distribution of blood glucose values for the entire population of 7683 men. The population mean μ is 161.52, and its standard deviation σ is 58.15. These parameters are based on all 7683 cases. Suppose you select a sample of size 25 from this population and compute its sample mean $\bar{x}$, and standard deviation s. If, with $n = 25$, you repeat this random sampling scheme a number of times, you will generate a new distribution, that of the means of the samples. This particular random sampling was done 400 times to generate the distribution of sample means, as shown in the right-hand column of Table 7.1. Were it possible to select all possible samples of size 25 from the population of 7683,

Figure 7.1 Distribution of Blood Glucose Values from the Honolulu Heart Study Population ($N = 7683$)

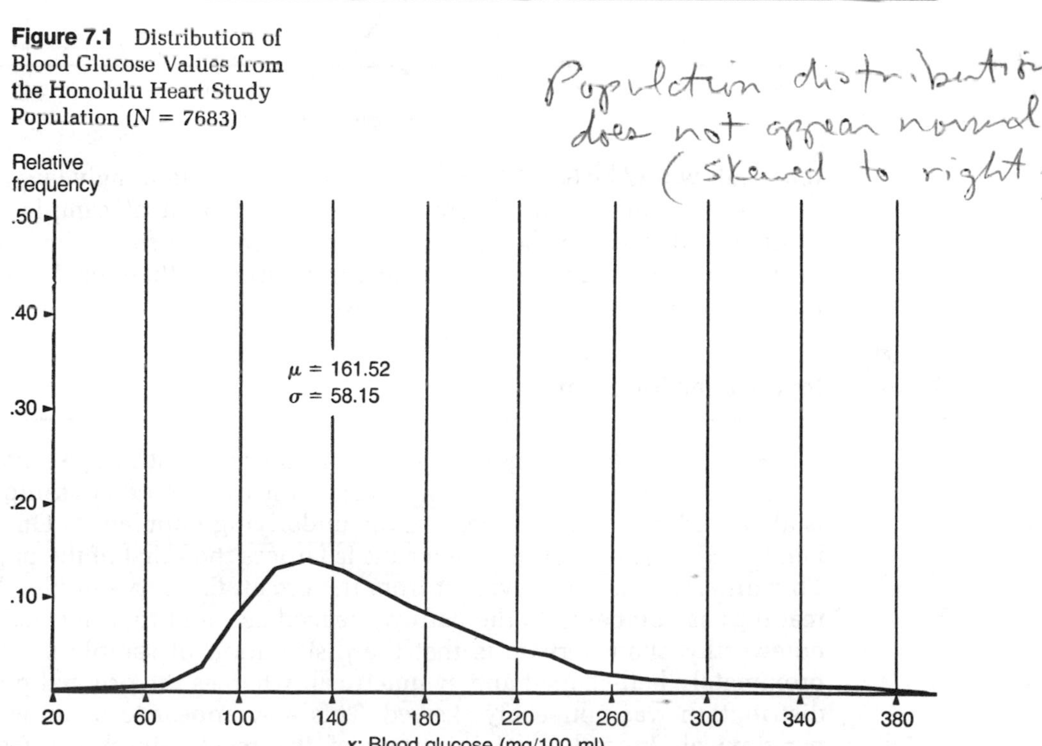

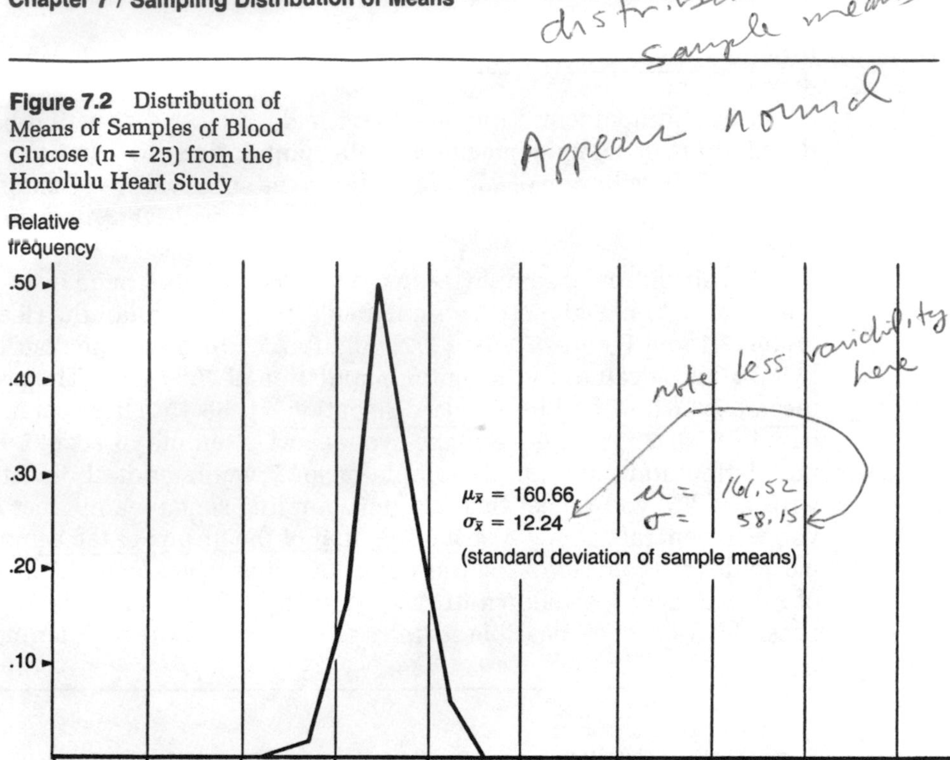

Figure 7.2 Distribution of Means of Samples of Blood Glucose (n = 25) from the Honolulu Heart Study

the result would be 8.524×10^{71} samples, an overwhelmingly large number!

As you can see in Figure 7.2, the distribution of sample means is symmetrical, roughly bell-shaped, and centered close to the population mean of 161.52, but with considerably less variation than the distribution of individual glucose values.

7.2 Central Limit Theorem

A quick glance at Figures 7.1 and 7.2 shows one striking similarity and an equally striking difference. The mean of the distribution of sample means is almost identical to the mean of the underlying population. On the other hand, the variability of sample means is far less than that of the population. This difference is quite evident from the broad, flat curve of blood glucose readings as compared to the narrow, peaked curve of their means. Another noteworthy characteristic is that the distribution of sample means is approximately bell-shaped and symmetrical, whereas the original population distribution was noticeably skewed. This may appear to be unusual, even paradoxical. Indeed it is! It is one of the most remarkable features of mathematical statistics, and it is called the **central limit theorem.**

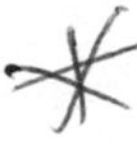

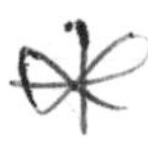

The **central limit theorem** states the following principles for a randomly selected sample of size n (n should be at least 25, but the larger n is, the better the approximation) with a mean μ and a standard deviation σ:

1. The distribution of sample means $\bar{x}$ is approximately normal regardless of whether the population distribution was normal or not.
2. The mean of the distribution of sample means is equal to the mean of the population distribution—that is, $\mu_{\bar{x}} = \mu$.
3. The standard deviation of the distribution of sample means is equal to the standard deviation of the population divided by the square root of the sample size. That is,

$$\sigma_{\bar{x}} = \frac{\sigma}{\sqrt{n}} \tag{7.1}$$

The principles of the central limit theorem are illustrated in Figure 7.3. Four very different population distributions are shown (p. 82). For each, as the sample size n increases, the sampling distribution of the mean approaches normality, regardless of whether the original population distribution was normal. A close scrutiny also reveals that, for any population distribution, the mean of each sampling distribution is the same as the mean (μ) of the population itself. Note also that as the sample size increases, the variability of the sampling distribution becomes progressively smaller.

7.3 Standard Error of the Mean

The measure of variation of the distribution of sample means, $\sigma/\sqrt{n}$, referred to as the **standard error of the mean,** is denoted as SE($\bar{x}$). That is,

$$\text{SE}(\bar{x}) = \sigma_{\bar{x}} = \frac{\sigma}{\sqrt{n}} \tag{7.2}$$

SE($\bar{x}$) is a counterpart of the standard deviation in that it is a measure of variation, but variation of sample means rather than of individual observations. It is an important statistical tool because it is a measure of the amount of sampling error. Sampling error differs from other errors in that it can be reduced at will, provided one is willing to increase the sample size. A nearly universal application of the standard error of the mean in medical literature is to specify an interval of $\bar{x} \pm 2\text{SE}(\bar{x})$, which covers approximately 95% of the sample means.

To prove the central limit theorem requires a considerable mathematical background beyond the level of this book. However, the sampling experiment of Figures 7.1 and 7.2 is in itself convincing evidence regarding the theorem's truthfulness. In these figures we can see the following:

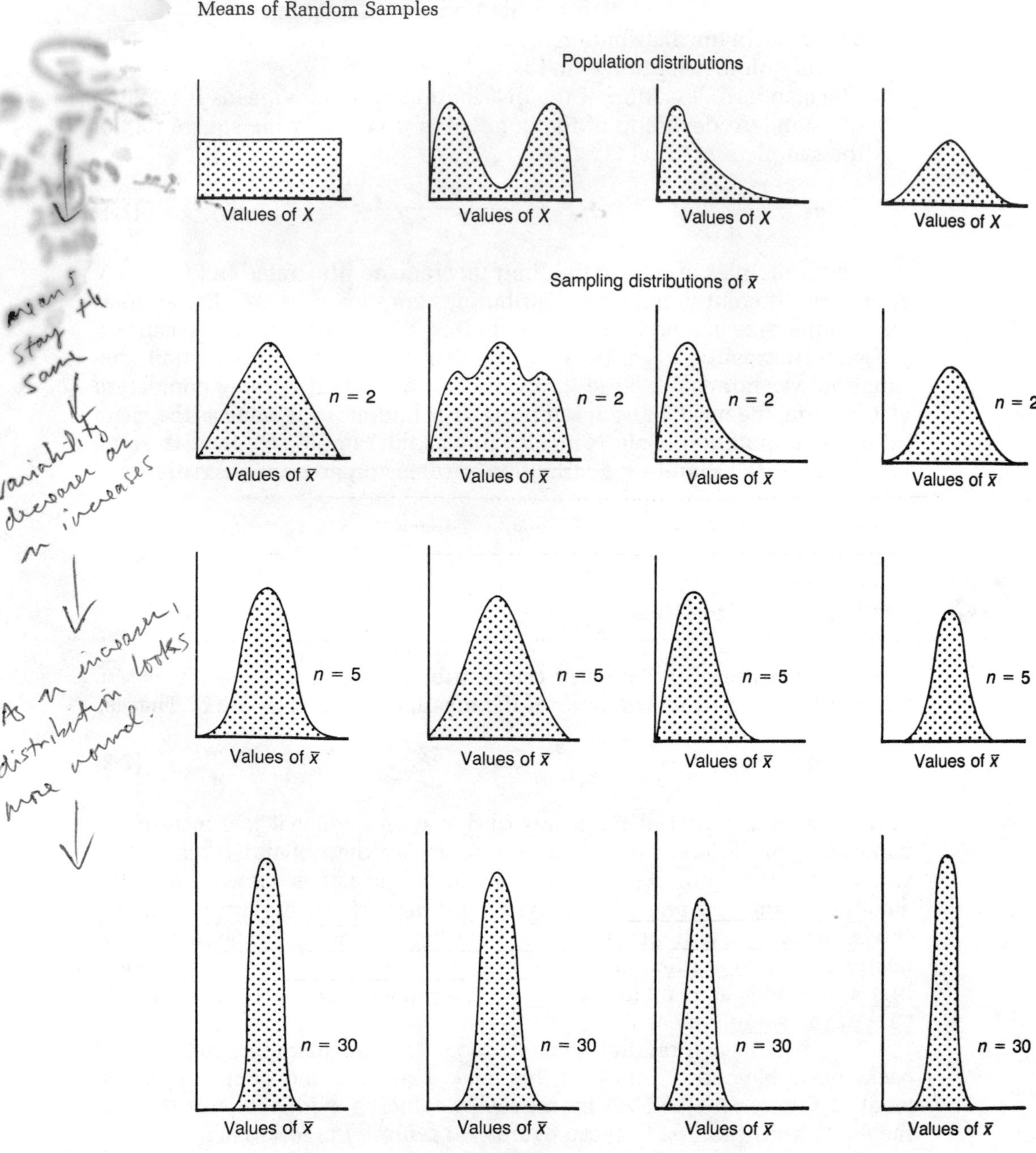

Figure 7.3 The Effect of Shape of Population Distribution and Sample Size on the Distribution of Means of Random Samples

1. The mean of the distribution of sample means $\mu_{\bar{x}}$ is almost identical to the population mean μ.
2. The standard deviation of the sample means computed by use of the traditional formula $\sqrt{\Sigma(\bar{x} - \mu_{\bar{x}})^2/(n-1)}$ is 12.24, very close to the standard error of the mean computed by using $\sigma_{\bar{x}} = \sigma/\sqrt{n} = 11.63$. This is an impressive result; it is now possible to compute the standard error of the mean knowing only the sample size and the population σ or its estimate s.
3. The distribution of sample means is approximately normally distributed.

In practice σ is seldom known. We estimate it from the sample standard deviation s; consequently, the equation most commonly used for computing the standard error of the mean is

$$s_{\bar{x}} = \frac{s}{\sqrt{n}} \tag{7.3}$$

Often we encounter data that are not normally distributed. This may present a problem in the statistical analysis; but by working with sample means, we can meet the assumption of normality, providing the sample size is sufficient (about 25 or more).

Since the central limit theorem states that sample means are approximately normally distributed, it is possible to find the area under the curve for the normal distribution of sample means. To find it, we must again use the Z transformation, that is, computation of a relative deviate. For sample means, the equation for Z is

$$Z = \frac{\bar{x} - \mu}{\sigma/\sqrt{n}} \tag{7.4}$$

This computed Z also establishes the relative position of $\bar{x}$ in a distribution of sample means.

7.4 Student's *t* Distribution

All too often the population standard deviation σ is unknown. Without σ we are unable to calculate the normal deviate. As we already know, when σ is unknown it may be estimated by s, the sample standard deviation. In Chapter 3, we calculated s like this:

$$s = \sqrt{\frac{\Sigma(x - \bar{x})^2}{n - 1}}$$

Can this s be used instead of the σ in Equation 7.4? Fortunately, yes. But we no longer have the standard normal distribution. Instead we have a distribution that was discovered in 1906 and published in 1908 by William S. Gossett, an English chemist and statistician employed by the Guinness Brewery in Dublin. Because the brewery, fearing release of trade secrets, rarely permitted publications by its employees, Gossett published under the pseudonym "Student." So his distribution is commonly referred to as **Student's *t* distribution.** The equation for its relative deviate is

$$t = \frac{\bar{x} - \mu}{s/\sqrt{n}} \tag{7.5}$$

This t distribution is similar to the standard normal distribution in that it is unimodal, bell-shaped, and symmetrical, and extends infinitely in either direction. Although the curve has more variance than the normal distribution, its area is still equal to 1.0. Areas under the curve, designated as α in Table 7.2, are a function of a quantity called **degrees of freedom** (df), where

$$\text{df} = n - 1 \tag{7.6}$$

Degrees of freedom measure the quantity of information available in one's data that can be used in estimating the population variance σ^2. Therefore, they are an indication of the reliability of s, in that the larger the sample size, the more reliable s will be as an estimate of σ. It follows that the variance of the t distribution of a large sample is less than that of a small sample. Note that when the sample size exceeds about 25, the t distribution so closely approximates the normal distribution that for practical purposes the normal distribution may be used. In other words, for large samples, s becomes a quite reliable estimate of σ, as graphically illustrated in Figure 7.4.

Figure 7.4 Comparison of *t* Distributions and Normal Distributions

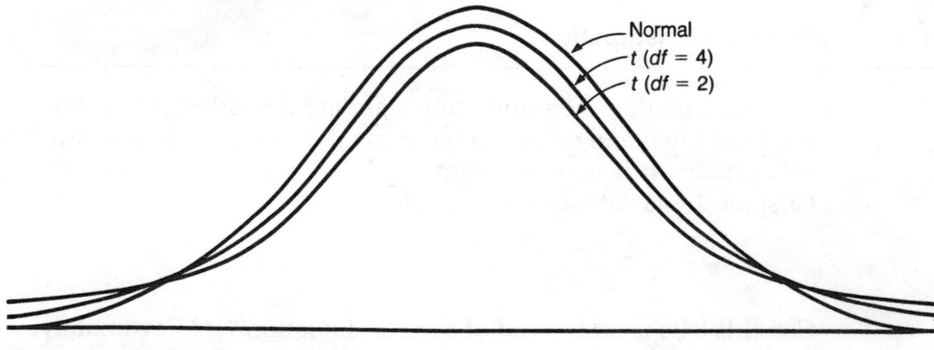

The *t* distribution introduces the concept of infinite degrees of freedom for large sample sizes. In fact, the *t* distribution for infinite degrees of freedom is precisely equal to the normal distribution. This equality is readily seen by comparing the critical values for df = ∞ (infinity) of Table 7.2 for various values of α with those of Table 6.1 (p. 70). The approximation is good beginning with 25 df and nearly identical at 30 df. The percentage points of the *t* distribution in Table 7.2 are given for a limited number of areas. For example, the *t* value for α = .05 with 15 df equals 1.753. It is found

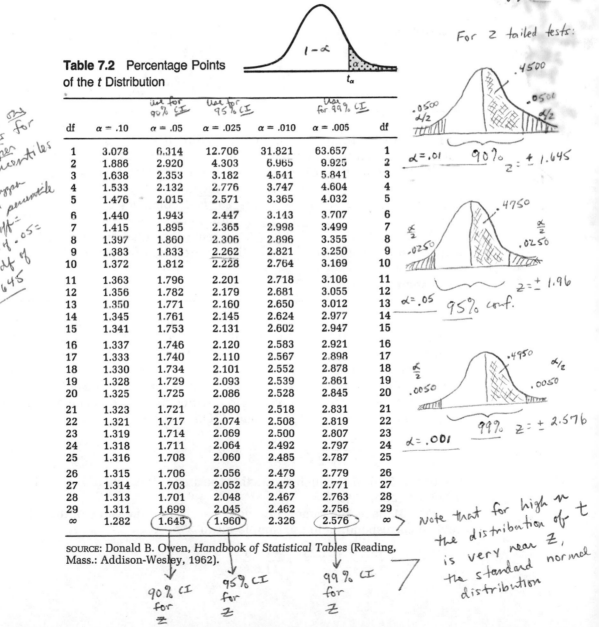

Table 7.2 Percentage Points of the *t* Distribution

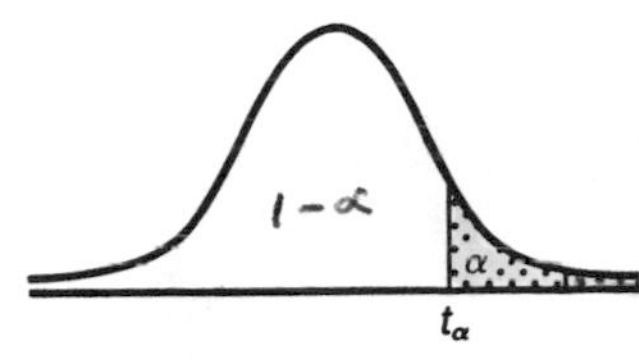

df	α = .10	α = .05	α = .025	α = .010	α = .005	df
1	3.078	6.314	12.706	31.821	63.657	1
2	1.886	2.920	4.303	6.965	9.925	2
3	1.638	2.353	3.182	4.541	5.841	3
4	1.533	2.132	2.776	3.747	4.604	4
5	1.476	2.015	2.571	3.365	4.032	5
6	1.440	1.943	2.447	3.143	3.707	6
7	1.415	1.895	2.365	2.998	3.499	7
8	1.397	1.860	2.306	2.896	3.355	8
9	1.383	1.833	2.262	2.821	3.250	9
10	1.372	1.812	2.228	2.764	3.169	10
11	1.363	1.796	2.201	2.718	3.106	11
12	1.356	1.782	2.179	2.681	3.055	12
13	1.350	1.771	2.160	2.650	3.012	13
14	1.345	1.761	2.145	2.624	2.977	14
15	1.341	1.753	2.131	2.602	2.947	15
16	1.337	1.746	2.120	2.583	2.921	16
17	1.333	1.740	2.110	2.567	2.898	17
18	1.330	1.734	2.101	2.552	2.878	18
19	1.328	1.729	2.093	2.539	2.861	19
20	1.325	1.725	2.086	2.528	2.845	20
21	1.323	1.721	2.080	2.518	2.831	21
22	1.321	1.717	2.074	2.508	2.819	22
23	1.319	1.714	2.069	2.500	2.807	23
24	1.318	1.711	2.064	2.492	2.797	24
25	1.316	1.708	2.060	2.485	2.787	25
26	1.315	1.706	2.056	2.479	2.779	26
27	1.314	1.703	2.052	2.473	2.771	27
28	1.313	1.701	2.048	2.467	2.763	28
29	1.311	1.699	2.045	2.462	2.756	29
∞	1.282	1.645	1.960	2.326	2.576	∞

SOURCE: Donald B. Owen, *Handbook of Statistical Tables* (Reading, Mass.: Addison-Wesley, 1962).

Table 7.3 Characteristics of a Population Distribution and Its Distribution of Sample Means

Characteristic	Population distribution	Distribution of sample means
Mean	μ	$\mu_{\bar{x}} = \mu$
Measure of variation	σ	$\sigma_{\bar{x}} = \dfrac{\sigma}{\sqrt{n}}$
Relative deviate	$Z = \dfrac{x - \mu}{\sigma}$	$Z = \dfrac{\bar{x} - \mu}{\sigma/\sqrt{n}}$
t statistic		$t = \dfrac{\bar{x} - \mu}{s/\sqrt{n}}$

by locating df = 15 in the margin and reading the value of t = 1.753 in the column labeled $\alpha = .05$. Here α denotes the area in the tail under the curve.

When should the *t* distribution be used? Use it for small samples when the population standard deviation is not known. If you know the population's σ, or your sample exceeds 25, feel confident to use the normal distribution. Otherwise, the *t* test is indicated.

As a recapitulation, Table 7.3 presents the equations for Student's *t* distribution, along with other equations introduced in this chapter.

7.5 Application

Using the blood glucose observations from the entire Honolulu Heart Study population (Figure 7.1), we find that $\mu = 161.52$ and $\sigma = 58.15$. Suppose that we select samples of size 25 from this population. (a) What proportion of sample means would have values of 170 or greater? (b) What proportion of sample means would have values of 155 or lower?

For (a), we reduced the problem to Z scores so that we can determine the proportion of the area that is beyond Z. On obtaining

$$Z = \frac{170 - 161.52}{58.15/\sqrt{25}} = \frac{8.48}{11.63} = .73$$

we turn to Table 6.1, which shows that the area to the right of Z = .73 is .5 − .2673, or about 23%.

For (b), using the same technique, we can find the value of the relative deviate corresponding to the sample mean 155:

$$Z = \frac{155 - 161.25}{58.15/\sqrt{25}} = \frac{-6.25}{11.63} = -.54$$

Table 6.1 reveals that the area below $Z = -.54$ is $.5 - .2054 = .2946$, or about 29%.

Conclusion

A distinction exists between the distribution of a population's observations and the distribution of its sample means. A powerful tool called the central limit theorem gives reassuring results: no matter how unlike normal a population distribution may be, the distribution of its sample means will be approximately normal, provided only that the sample size is reasonably large ($n \geq 25$). The mean of the sampling distribution is equal to the mean of the population distribution. The standard error of sample means equals the standard deviation of the observations divided by the square root of the sample size. In sampling experiments these results are often applied to determine how unusual a sample mean is.

Vocabulary List

central limit theorem
degrees of freedom
distribution of sample means
population distribution
standard error of the mean
Student's *t* distribution

Exercises

7.1 Suppose samples of size 36 were drawn from the population of Exercise 6.5. Describe the distribution of the means of these samples.

7.2 If samples of size 25 were selected from the population of Exercise 6.6, what percentage of the sample means would you expect to be
(a) between 57 and 63?
(b) less than 55?
(c) 64 or larger?
(d) 75 or larger?

7.3 (a) Compare the results of Exercise 7.2a with those of Exercise 6.6a and explain.
(b) Compare the results of Exercise 7.2d with those of Exercise 6.6e and explain.

7.4 Compute the 95th percentile for Exercise 7.2.

7.5 Refer to the population of Exercise 6.9.
(a) What is the standard error of the mean for $n = 16$?
(b) What is the standard error of the mean for $n = 64$?
(c) What is true about the relationship between n and $SE(\bar{x})$?

7.6 Suppose heights of 20-year-old men are approximately normally distributed with a mean of 71 in. and a standard deviation of 8 in. A random sample of fifteen 20-year-old men is selected and measured. Find the probability that the sample mean $\bar{x}$

(a) is at least 77 in.
(b) lies between 65 and 75 in.
(c) is not more than 63 in.

7.7 If the length of normal infants is 52.5 cm and the standard deviation is 4.5 cm, what is the probability that the mean of a sample of (a) size 10, and (b) size 15 is greater than 56 cm?

7.8 Suppose that the mean weight of infants born in a community is $\mu = 3360$ g and $\sigma = 490$ g.

(a) Find $P(2300 < x < 4300)$.
(b) Find $P(x \leq 2500)$.
(c) Find $P(x \geq 5000)$.
(d) What must you assume about the distribution of birthweights to make the answers to (a), (b), and (c) valid?

7.9 Suppose you select a sample of 49 infants from the population described in Exercise 7.8.

(a) What is the mean and standard error of this sampling distribution?
(b) Find $P(3100 < \bar{x} < 3600)$.
(c) Find $P(\bar{x} < 2500)$.
(d) Find $P(\bar{x} > 3540)$.
(e) What must you assume about the distribution of birthweights to make the answers to (b), (c), and (d) valid?

7.10 If the mean number of cigarettes smoked by pregnant women is 16 and the standard deviation 8, find the probability that in a random sample of 100 pregnant women the mean number of cigarettes smoked will be greater than 24.

Chapter **8**

Estimation of Population Means

Chapter Outline

8.1 Estimation
It is explained why estimation is a primary statistical tool.

8.2 Point Estimates and Confidence Intervals
Point estimates and confidence intervals are discussed as two ways of estimating population parameters where only sample statistics are known.

8.3 Two Independent Samples
The difference between sample means is described as a modification of the estimate of a single-sample mean.

8.4 Confidence Intervals for the Difference Between Two Means
It is shown how confidence intervals help estimate the difference between two population parameters.

8.5 The Before-and-After Experiment
Pros and cons are presented for using a treatment group as its own control.

8.6 Determination of Sample Size
Methods are offered for determining in advance the sample size needed to design an efficient study.

Learning Objectives

After studying this chapter, you should be able to

1. Compute a confidence interval from a set of data for
   (a) a single population mean
   (b) the difference between two population means
2. State three ways of narrowing the confidence interval
3. Determine the sample size required to estimate a variable at a given level of accuracy
4. Distinguish between a probability interval and a confidence interval
5. List the pros and cons of performing a before-and-after experiment

8.1 Estimation

One of the principal objectives of research is comparison: How does one group differ from another? Specifically, we may encounter such questions as: What is the mean serum cholesterol level of a group of middle-aged men? How does it differ from that of women? From that of men of other ages? How does today's level differ from that of a decade ago? What is the mean number of children per family in the United States? What is the difference in the mean number of cavities between children who drink fluoridated and those who drink nonfluoridated water? What is the difference in oxygen uptake between joggers and nonjoggers?

These are typical questions that can be handled by the primary tools of classical statistical inference—**estimation** and **hypothesis testing.** The unknown characteristic (parameter) of a population is usually estimated from a statistic computed from data of a sample. Ordinarily, we are interested in estimating the mean and the standard deviation of some characteristic of the population. Estimation is the main focus of this chapter. In the next chapter, we move on to hypothesis testing.

In both estimation and hypothesis testing we may deal either with the characteristic of a population or with the differences in two population characteristics. The latter is more typical; the former is nevertheless in quite common use. Either approach can be followed in one of two ways: (1) by estimating the difference in means between an experimental group and a control group or (2) by estimating the difference in means between one group before treatment and the same group after treatment.

In the first case, we deal with two random samples from two different populations; in the second, with two samples obtained from the same group before and after treatment. Whereas in the first case the observations are independent, in the second the observations are not independent because they were obtained from the same source although at two different times. Since the estimation procedures are different for the two cases, they are treated separately.

8.2 Point Estimates and Confidence Intervals

There are two ways of estimating a population parameter: a **point estimate** and a **confidence interval** estimate.

A **point estimate** of the population mean μ is the sample mean $\bar{x}$ computed from a random sample of the population. A frequently used point estimate for the population standard deviation σ is s, the sample standard deviation. For example, in attempting to assess the physical condition of joggers, an investigator used the maximal volume oxygen (VO_2) uptake method. He found that the point estimate of VO_2 for joggers was $\bar{x} = 47.5$ ml/kg. As $\bar{x}$ is a statistic, the point estimate varies from sample to sample. In fact, if the investigator had repeated the experiment a number of times, he would have found a range of $\bar{x}$'s, any one of which would be a point estimate of the same population parameter. So a weakness of the point estimate idea is that it fails to make a probability statement as to how close the estimate is to the population parameter. This flaw is remedied by use of a **confidence interval** (CI), the interval of numbers in which we have a specified degree of assurance that the value of the parameter can be found. Using nothing more complicated than the normal deviate, it is possible to derive the equation for an interval that has a known probability of including the population mean μ. By using this method, you can be confident, say, that 95% of all sample means based on a given sample size will fall within ± 1.96 standard errors of the population mean. This outcome can be stated algebraically in terms of normal deviates:

$$P(-1.96 \leq \frac{\bar{x} - \mu}{\sigma/\sqrt{n}} \leq 1.96) = .95 \tag{8.1}$$

A few simple manipulations lead from Equation 8.1 to Equation 8.2, an important expression. First, multiply by $\sigma/\sqrt{n}$:

$$P(-1.96 \frac{\sigma}{\sqrt{n}} \leq \bar{x} - \mu \leq 1.96 \frac{\sigma}{\sqrt{n}}) = .95$$

Next, change signs:

$$P(1.96 \frac{\sigma}{\sqrt{n}} \geq -\bar{x} + \mu \geq -1.96 \frac{\sigma}{\sqrt{n}}) = .95$$

Finally, add $\bar{x}$:

$$P(\bar{x} + 1.96 \frac{\sigma}{\sqrt{n}} \geq \mu \geq \bar{x} - 1.96 \frac{\sigma}{\sqrt{n}}) = .95$$

For convenience, reverse the inequality signs. The result is

$$P(\bar{x} - 1.96 \frac{\sigma}{\sqrt{n}} \leq \mu \leq \bar{x} + 1.96 \frac{\sigma}{\sqrt{n}}) = .95 \tag{8.2}$$

Using Equation 8.2 on repeated sampling, you can expect (with a probability of .95) the true population mean μ to fall in the interval $\bar{x} - 1.96(\sigma/\sqrt{n})$ to $\bar{x} + 1.96(\sigma/\sqrt{n})$. The interval is referred to as the **95% confidence interval** of the population mean and is usually denoted as

$$95\% \text{ CI of } \mu = \bar{x} \pm 1.96 \frac{\sigma}{\sqrt{n}} \tag{8.3}$$

This procedure can be used for other probabilities. For example, the 99% confidence interval for μ is given by

$$99\% \text{ CI of } \mu = \bar{x} \pm 2.58 \frac{\sigma}{\sqrt{n}} \tag{8.4}$$

These confidence interval equations are not used very frequently because they suffer from a drawback: σ is usually unknown. But we have already established that when σ is unknown, we can estimate it by s, the sample standard deviation. Let's say we use the **(1 − α) 100% confidence interval** for a population mean μ, which is an interval constructed from sample data such that, upon repeated sampling, it will have a probability $1 - \alpha$ of containing the population mean. As before, to construct the interval, we use a t value (with $n - 1$ df) instead of the Z value. By using a procedure parallel to the one employed for Equations 8.3 and 8.4, we can obtain the confidence interval when only s (not σ) is known:

$$(1 - \alpha)100\% \text{ CI for } \mu = \bar{x} \pm t \frac{s}{\sqrt{n}} \tag{8.5}$$

EXAMPLE 1

■ If we wished to estimate the mean VO_2 uptake for a population of joggers from a sample of 25, we could use the 95% confidence interval for μ. We already know that $\bar{x} = 47.5$ ml/kg and $s = 4.8$ for a sample of 25. In Table 7.2 we find that the t value for 24 df for the central 95% of the t distribution is 2.064. The 95% confidence interval is thus

$$\begin{aligned} 95\% \text{ CI of } \mu &= \bar{x} \pm 2.064 \frac{s}{\sqrt{n}} \\ &= 47.5 \pm 2.064 \frac{4.8}{\sqrt{25}} \\ &= 47.5 \pm 1.98 \\ &= (45.5, 49.5) \end{aligned}$$

The result: Upon many repetitions of this experiment, we would expect the population mean μ to fall between $\bar{x} - 2.064s/\sqrt{n}$ and $\bar{x} + 2.064s/\sqrt{n}$ about 95% of the time. The values 45.5 and 49.5 are the lower and upper 95% **confidence limits.** The interval, 45.5 to 49.5 ml/kg, is the 95% confidence interval. ■

The confidence interval provides a range in which $\bar{x}$ may be above or below the true value of the population mean. Even though there is a 5% chance that the interval does not capture μ, there is a 2.5% chance that μ actually lies above $Z = 1.96$ (or below $Z = -1.96$). Therefore we use $Z_{.975} = 1.96$ and $Z_{.025} = -1.96$ in calculating the upper and lower confidence limits.

It is important to note an interesting distinction: these intervals are referred to as **confidence intervals,** not **probability intervals.** Before we actually obtain specific confidence limits based on a sample, the equation is properly referred to as a probability statement. But once the specific confidence limits are calculated, the **a posteriori probability** (i.e., the probability derived from observed facts) that the interval contains the mean μ is either 100% or 0%. Therefore, with typical caution, statisticians refer to it as a 95% confidence interval because there is 95% confidence that in the long run the intervals constructed in such a way will indeed contain the population mean. The 95% confidence interval is used quite commonly, as is the 99% confidence interval. Other percentages may be used but are less frequently encountered in practice.

8.3 Two Independent Samples

Suppose we wish to extend our example of comparing the physical condition of joggers and nonjoggers, again using the VO_2 uptake criterion. To obtain two independent samples, we first compute VO_2 uptake means for the two groups: joggers ($\bar{x}_1$) and nonjoggers ($\bar{x}_2$). The next logical step is to compute $\bar{x}_1 - \bar{x}_2$, the difference in mean VO_2 uptake for the two samples. As you might expect, $\bar{x}_1 - \bar{x}_2$ is an estimate of $\mu_1 - \mu_2$, the difference between means of the two underlying populations. Just as we computed confidence intervals for the mean, so do we compute them for the difference between two means.

From the central limit theorem, mathematical statisticians are able to demonstrate that $\bar{x}_1 - \bar{x}_2$ is normally distributed with a mean of $\mu_1 - \mu_2$ and a variance equal to $\sigma_1^2/n_1 + \sigma_2^2/n_2$. Its square root is the **standard error of the difference** between two means and is often denoted as

$$\text{SE}(\bar{x}_1 - \bar{x}_2) = \sqrt{\frac{\sigma_1^2}{n_1} + \frac{\sigma_2^2}{n_2}} \tag{8.6}$$

This equation should not be too surprising since $\bar{x}_1$ and $\bar{x}_2$ are each normally distributed with respective variances of σ_1^2/n_1 and σ_2^2/n_2. But the variance of the difference is the **sum** of the two individual variances. This is certainly reasonable if we realize that the variation of $\bar{x}_1 - \bar{x}_2$ can't help but be more than that which would be expected for either $\bar{x}_1$ or $\bar{x}_2$ separately.

Finally, the equation for the calculation of the normal deviate is

$$Z = \frac{(\bar{x}_1 - \bar{x}_2) - (\mu_1 - \mu_2)}{\sqrt{\sigma_1^2/n_1 + \sigma_2^2/n_2}} \tag{8.7}$$

In many cases, we compare a given phenomenon in a treated and an untreated population. The cases and controls being drawn from the same population, it is reasonable to assume that $\sigma_1^2 = \sigma_2^2$, thereby simplifying Equation 8.7 to

$$Z = \frac{(\bar{x}_1 - \bar{x}_2) - (\mu_1 - \mu_2)}{\sigma\sqrt{1/n_1 + 1/n_2}} \tag{8.8}$$

As before, σ^2 is seldom known. So again we estimate it by a sample variance obtained from the data. This procedure again moves us from the normal to the t distribution. In such a case, we actually obtain two different estimates of σ^2, namely, s_1^2 and s_2^2. If it is safe to assume that these two are an estimate of a common variance, σ^2, we can pool the two sample variances and obtain the **pooled standard deviations,** s_p, a single improved estimate of σ^2 (improved because it is based on a larger sample). We get the **pooled sample variance** by taking a weighted average of s_1^2 and s_2^2:

$$s_p^2 = \frac{s_1^2(n_1 - 1) + s_2^2(n_2 - 1)}{n_1 + n_2 - 2} \tag{8.9}$$

What Equation 8.9 does is to take the sum of weighted squares of the two separate samples and divide them by the sum of the degrees of freedom. This procedure for computing s_p^2 is nice in that it provides an unbiased estimate of σ^2.

After computing s_p^2, we can obtain s_p simply by extracting the square root. We will need s_p to compute the t score:

$$t = \frac{(\bar{x}_1 - \bar{x}_2) - (\mu_1 - \mu_2)}{s_p\sqrt{1/n_1 + 1/n_2}} \tag{8.10}$$

with $n_1 + n_2 - 2$ df.

8.4 Confidence Intervals for the Difference Between Two Means

After estimating the difference between two population means, we take the next logical step and establish a confidence interval around the difference. The point estimate of the difference was given by $\bar{x}_1 - \bar{x}_2$; the confidence interval equation may be derived from the probability statement:

$$P\left(-1.96 \le \frac{(\bar{x}_1 - \bar{x}_2) - (\mu_1 - \mu_2)}{\sigma\sqrt{1/n_1 + 1/n_2}} \le 1.96\right) = .95 \tag{8.11}$$

This derivation, parallel to that of Equation 8.2, yields the following equation for the 95% confidence interval:

$$95\%\ \text{CI for } \mu_1 - \mu_2 = \bar{x}_1 - \bar{x}_2 \pm 1.96\left(\sigma\sqrt{\frac{1}{n_1} + \frac{1}{n_2}}\right) \tag{8.12}$$

The general equation for the confidence interval with an unknown σ is

$$(1 - \alpha)100\% \text{ CI for } \mu_1 - \mu_2 = \bar{x}_1 - \bar{x}_2 \pm t\left(s_p \sqrt{\frac{1}{n_1} + \frac{1}{n_2}}\right) \quad (8.13)$$

which uses a t score, where t is the value corresponding to the $1 - \alpha$ proportion of the central area with $n_1 + n_2 - 2$ df.

EXAMPLE 2

■ In estimating physical condition by means of maximal VO_2 uptake, it was found that for a random sample of 25 joggers, $\bar{x}_1 = 47.5$ ml/kg with $s_1 = 4.8$ and that for 26 nonjoggers, $\bar{x}_2 = 37.5$ ml/kg with $s_2 = 5.1$. From these results, it is possible to compute a confidence interval. This computation will help us estimate the magnitude of the true difference, $\mu_1 - \mu_2$. The 99% confidence interval is calculated as follows by using Table 7.2 for an $\alpha/2$ of .005 with df = 49. The t value = 2.576 or 2.58.

To proceed with the computation of the confidence interval, we will need the value of s_p, which we obtain using Equation 8.9.

$$\begin{aligned} s_p &= \sqrt{\frac{s_1^2(n_1 - 1) + s_2^2(n_2 - 1)}{n_1 + n_2 - 2}} \\ &= \sqrt{\frac{4.8^2(24) + 5.1^2(25)}{25 + 26 - 2}} \\ &= \sqrt{\frac{1203.21}{49}} = \sqrt{24.56} = 4.96 \end{aligned}$$

It follows that

$$\begin{aligned} 99\% \text{ CI for } (\mu_1 - \mu_2) &= \bar{x}_1 - \bar{x}_2 \pm t_{.005}\left(s_p \sqrt{\frac{1}{n_1} + \frac{1}{n_2}}\right) \\ &= 47.5 - 37.5 \pm 2.58(4.96)\sqrt{\frac{1}{25} + \frac{1}{26}} \\ &= 10.0 \pm 3.58 \\ &= (6.42, 13.58) \end{aligned}$$

Hence we have 99% confidence that the difference of the population mean for VO_2 uptake for joggers versus nonjoggers falls between 6.42 ml/kg and 13.58 ml/kg. So $\mu_1 - \mu_2$, which is estimated to be 10.0 ml/kg, is quite likely to be within this confidence interval. Since both of the confidence limits are positive, the interval does not include the value zero. This means that whatever the true difference really is, joggers almost surely have a higher VO_2 uptake than nonjoggers. ■

Figure 8.1 Ninety-Nine Percent Confidence Intervals for Differences in Systolic Blood Pressure $\mu_1 - \mu_2$ for 50 Samples of Size 25 from Each Group of Nonsmokers and Smokers

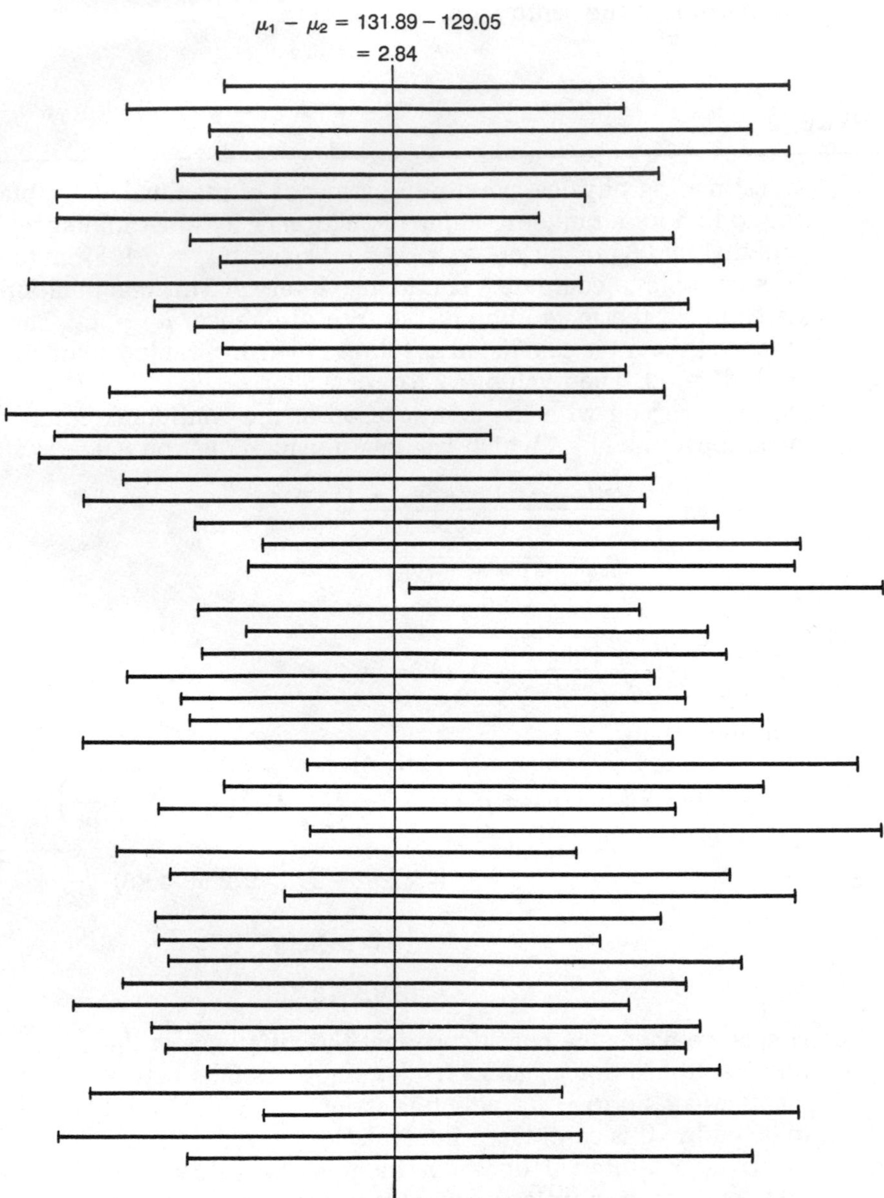

If more samples were obtained from the same populations as those in our example, we would find different means, different standard deviations, and consequently different confidence intervals. On average we would expect that 99% of them would contain the true difference ($\mu_1 - \mu_2$) and 1% would not.

Figure 8.1 shows 50 confidence intervals for the differences in mean systolic blood pressure between smokers and nonsmokers, as given in Table 3.1. Here we know the true value of $\mu_1 - \mu_2$: 131.89 − 129.05 = 2.84. So in this case we can determine how many of these confidence intervals actually include the known value of $\mu_1 - \mu_2 = 2.84$. And we find that only the 24th one does not. One out of 50 is 2%—a bit higher than expected. However, in a longer series we would expect the result to be closer to 1%.

Narrow confidence intervals are of the greatest value in making estimates, because they allow us to estimate an unknown parameter with little room for error. This attribute moves us to consider all possible ways of narrowing confidence intervals. As seen from the confidence interval for the single population mean, $\bar{x} \pm Z\,(\sigma/\sqrt{n})$, the quantities that affect the width of the interval are the sample size, the Z value, and the standard deviation.

A confidence interval can be narrowed by

1. Increasing the sample size
2. Reducing the significance (for example, instead of using $Z = 2.58$ for 99% confidence, use $Z = 1.96$ for 95% confidence)
3. Increasing precision and thereby reducing error in the observations, thus producing less variance

8.5 The Before-and-After Experiment

In many investigations the treatment group is used as its own control. This technique often generates quite appropriate comparisons because variability due to extraneous factors is reduced. It is not unusual for extraneous factors to account for many of the differences between means obtained from two independent samples. Given extraneous factors that add to variability, use of the treatment group as its own control will reduce the variability and give a smaller standard error, hence a narrower confidence interval. But one pays a price. First, independence is sacrificed. Second, one is left with about half the degrees of freedom as would obtain using two independent samples. With fewer degrees of freedom the *t* value is larger, and consequently the confidence interval is wider. So you must take these pros and cons into consideration when planning an experiment. Only then can you tell which procedure—two independent samples or a **before-and-after experiment**—would be more advantageous.

Data from before-and-after experiments must never be thought of as coming from two independent samples. We can, however, handle the data statistically as a one-sample problem, then proceed with the confidence interval determination as for a single population mean. The procedure is to reduce the data to a one-sample problem by computing before-and-after differences for each subject. By doing this with paired observations, we get a list of differences that can be handled as a single-sample problem.

EXAMPLE 3

■ To determine whether a person's physical condition improves after taking up jogging, an investigator obtains maximal VO_2 uptake values before subjects start jogging and six months later. Table 8.1 lists the values for VO_2 uptake for 25 randomly selected joggers. The difference between the before (x) and after (x′) value is given as $d = x' - x$. The mean of the difference, $\bar{d}$, is 12.42, and the standard deviation is $s_d = 1.57$. These values represent sample estimates of population parameters δ and σ_δ, respectively, where δ (delta) signifies the mean difference of population observations. We now can test whether jogging has been effective in improving physical condition as measured by the change in VO_2 uptake over time. Using the procedure for obtaining a single-sample confidence interval, we find that (with df = $n - 1 = 24$),

$$\begin{aligned} 99\% \text{ CI for } \delta &= \bar{d} \pm t_{.005} \frac{s_d}{\sqrt{n}} \\ &= 12.42 \pm 2.797 \frac{1.57}{\sqrt{25}} \\ &= 12.42 \pm .88 \\ &= (11.54, 13.30) \end{aligned}$$

The sample estimate of δ, $\bar{d} = 12.42$, indicates a gain in VO_2 uptake after jogging. The 99% confidence interval suggests that this gain is not likely to be less than 11.54 ml/kg or greater than 13.30 mg/kg. Note again that zero (i.e., the possibility that the before mean equals the after mean) is not included in the interval. The conclusion: six months of jogging improves one's physical fitness as measured by VO_2 uptake. ■

Before-and-after experiments are one of several classes of experiments used with nonindependent samples. Other types include twin studies, studies of siblings of the same sex, litter mates in animal studies, and pairs of individuals who are matched on several characteristics such as age, race, sex, and condition of health. Because of the pairing, the test is known as a *paired t-test*.

Table 8.1 Maximal Volume Oxygen Uptake Values of 25 Persons Age 30–40 Before and After They Became Joggers

Case	Before x	After x'	$d = x' - x$	d^2
1	34.1	47.9	13.8	190.44
2	32.3	44.6	12.3	151.29
3	36.5	47.3	10.8	116.64
4	38.6	50.6	12.0	144.00
5	39.6	51.9	12.3	151.29
6	31.8	43.3	11.5	132.25
7	31.0	43.3	12.3	151.29
8	38.8	51.9	13.1	171.61
9	29.3	41.2	11.9	141.61
10	35.3	47.6	12.3	151.29
11	41.3	54.0	12.7	161.29
12	43.3	55.6	12.3	151.29
13	33.8	45.6	11.8	139.24
14	28.3	39.4	11.1	123.21
15	36.8	48.9	12.1	146.41
16	30.6	42.4	11.8	139.24
17	28.8	46.3	17.5	306.25
18	40.0	52.8	12.8	163.84
19	39.8	48.9	9.1	82.81
20	44.8	56.7	11.9	141.61
21	30.8	46.5	15.7	246.49
22	25.8	38.7	12.9	166.41
23	32.7	44.2	11.5	132.25
24	35.3	47.2	11.9	141.61
25	37.9	51.0	13.1	171.61
	$\Sigma x = 877.3$	$\Sigma x' = 1187.8$	$\Sigma d = 310.5$	$\Sigma d^2 = 3915.27$
	$\bar{x} = 35.1$	$\bar{x}' = 47.5$	$\bar{d} = 12.42$	

$$s_d = \sqrt{\frac{\Sigma d^2 - (\Sigma d)^2/n}{n-1}} = \sqrt{\frac{3915.27 - (310.5)^2/25}{24}} = 1.57$$

8.6 Determination of Sample Size

The daily life of a modern statistician involves a lot more than manipulating data and running computer programs. The statistician serves as a resource, sometimes to scientists, sometimes to administrators, almost always to persons less sophisticated in statistics. The statistician has to be prepared to answer many questions, and one of the foremost goes something like this: "How large a sample size do I need to obtain a statistically meaningful result?"

Now that's a tough question. It's analogous, in a sense, to "How many runs must we score to win the ball game?" In the ball park, you couldn't field that one without more information, so you would have to ask a few questions yourself: "What's the score? What inning? Who's at bat? How many outs?" Similarly, in approaching the sample-size question you first need to ask: "How much error can I live with in estimating the population mean? What level of confidence is needed in the estimate? How much variability exists in the observations?" Once you have the answers to these questions, you can attack the sample-size question.

Arithmetically, the sample size can be obtained by solving for n in the now-familiar equation

$$Z = \frac{\bar{x} - \mu}{\sigma/\sqrt{n}} \tag{8.14}$$

which could be rewritten as

$$Z = \frac{d}{\sigma/\sqrt{n}}$$

where $d = \bar{x} - \mu$ and is a measure of how close we need to come to the population mean μ. Put another way, the estimate should be within d units of the population mean. Solving for n, we obtain

$$n = \left(\frac{Z\sigma}{d}\right)^2 \tag{8.15}$$

EXAMPLE 4

■ You need to estimate the mean serum cholesterol level of a population within 10 mg/dl of the true mean. You learn that $\sigma = 20$, and you want to state with 95% confidence that $\bar{x}$ is within 10 units of μ. So you obtain n as follows:

$$n = \frac{[(1.96)(20)]^2}{10^2} = 15.36$$

As fractional sample sizes are not available, you conservatively round up to the next integer and get busy obtaining a sample of 16. If σ is unknown, you estimate it by s and use the t distribution. ■

Knowing how to determine sample size in advance of an experiment is wise planning, because your financial resources might limit you to, say, only 10 guinea pigs. If 16 are needed to gain significant results, it would be unwise to proceed. Alternatively, you could conserve resources by advance knowledge of the number of animals needed. If 16 guinea pigs would suffice, it wouldn't be cost-effective to do the experiment with 25 or 30 animals.

Equation 8.15 is the simplest way of estimating sample size. In the next chapter, we look at other, somewhat more complicated approaches. Taken together, all these approaches underscore an important counsel to researchers: consult a statistician to determine your sample size.

Conclusion

A point estimate is something of a "best guess" at a population parameter. A confidence interval gives us a range of values to which we can append a probability statement as to whether the population parameter is included. Differences between population means may be estimated in two ways: by use of two independent samples or by a single sample measured before and after the experiment. But first consider the pros and cons.

You'd better be prepared to answer the statistician's toughest and most common question: "How large a sample . . . ?" The answer is both easy and difficult: easy, in employing a simple equation; difficult, in getting the right input to that equation.

Vocabulary List

a posteriori probability
before-and-after experiment
confidence interval
confidence limits
point estimate
pooled sample variance
pooled standard deviation
standard error of the difference
two independent samples

Exercises

8.1 Mice of a given strain were assigned randomly to two experimental groups. Each mouse was injected with a measured amount of tumor pulp. The pulp came from a large, suitable tumor excised from another mouse. After the tumor injections, the two groups received different chemotherapy treatments. Forty days after injection, the tumor volumes (in cubic centimeters) were measured as a comparison of the treatments. The data were as follows:

	Chemotherapy "A" treatment	Chemotherapy "B" treatment
n	27	30
$\bar{x}$	.51 cc	.64 cc
s^2	.010	.045
	$s_p = .17$	

Estimate $\mu_1 - \mu_2$; calculate its 95% confidence interval.

8.2 The standard hemoglobin reading for healthy adult men is 15 g/100 ml with a standard deviation of 2 g. For a group of 25 men in a certain occupation, we find an average hemoglobin of 16.0 g. Obtain a 95% confidence interval for μ and give its interpretation.

8.3 The standard serum cholesterol for adult males is 200 mg/100 ml with a standard deviation of 16.67. For a sample of 49 overweight men the mean reading was 225.
(a) Construct a 95% confidence interval for μ.
(b) What size sample would you need to have 95% confidence that the estimate of μ is within 10 mg/100 ml?

8.4 The standard urine creatinine for healthy adult males is .25 to .40 g/6 hr.
(a) If we assume the range encompasses six standard deviations, what is the estimate of the mean and the standard deviation of the standard?
(b) Construct the 99% confidence interval for μ. Pg. 17

✓ **8.5** The mean diastolic blood pressure in Table 2.2 is 73 mmHg with a standard deviation of 11.6 mmHg. Construct a 99% confidence interval for μ.

✓ **8.6** The mean weight of the sample of 100 men from the Honolulu Heart Study was 64 kg with the standard deviation s = 8.61. Obtain a point estimate and a 95% confidence interval for μ.

8.7 Compute 99% confidence intervals for $\mu_1 - \mu_2$ as between males and females if for 38 males $\bar{x}_1 = 74.9$ and $s_1^2 = 144$; and for 45 females $\bar{x}_2 = 71.8$ and $s_2^2 = 121$.

8.8 Cholesterol measurements from 54 vegetarians and 51 nonvegetarians yielded the following data:

Vegetarians: 115, 125, 125, 130, 130, 130, 130, 135, 135, 140,
140, 140, 140, 145, 145, 150, 150, 150, 155, 160,
160, 160, 160, 160, 165, 165, 165, 165, 165, 165,
165, 170, 170, 170, 170, 170, 170, 170, 175, 175,
175, 180, 180, 180, 180, 180, 185, 185, 185, 200,
215, 215, 225, 230

Nonvegetarians: 105, 110, 115, 125, 125, 130, 135, 145, 145, 150,
150, 160, 165, 165, 165, 170, 170, 170, 170, 170,
175, 175, 175, 180, 180, 180, 180, 185, 185, 190,
190, 190, 190, 195, 200, 200, 200, 200, 200, 205,
210, 210, 210, 210, 215, 220, 230, 230, 240, 240,
245

Find an estimate of $\mu_1 - \mu_2$ and calculate the 99% confidence interval for the difference between the population parameters.

Chapter **9**

Tests of Significance

Chapter Outline

9.1 Definitions
Important concepts involved in a test of significance are explained and an analogy is presented before launching into a formal discussion of the technique.

9.2 Basis for a Test of Significance
By use of a specific example, the rationale for a test of significance is illustrated.

9.3 Procedure for a Test of Significance
A formal description is given of the steps that constitute a test of significance, and an example from the Honolulu Heart Study is used to illustrate the procedure.

9.4 One-Tailed Versus Two-Tailed Tests
It is explained how to decide whether a test of significance is to be unidirectional or bidirectional.

9.5 Meaning of "Statistically Significant"
It is emphasized that "significance" in a statistical sense differs from the ordinary meaning of the word and is related to the testing procedures.

9.6 Type I and Type II Errors
The two types of errors one is liable to make in the performance of a test of significance are discussed.

9.7 Test of Significance of Two Independent Sample Means
An example of the difference in oxygen uptake of joggers and nonjoggers is used to illustrate the most common method of comparing sample means—the t test.

9.8 Relationship of Tests of Significance to Confidence Intervals
This section demonstrates how confidence intervals can be used to perform tests of significance.

Learning Objectives

After studying this chapter, you should be able to

1. Outline and explain the procedure for a test of significance
2. Explain the meaning of a null hypothesis and its alternative
3. Define statistical significance

4. Find the value of Z or t corresponding to a specified significance level, α
5. Distinguish between a one-tailed and a two-tailed test
6. Distinguish between the critical value and the test statistic
7. Determine when to use a Z test and when to use a t test
8. Distinguish between the meaning of practical and technical significance
9. Determine whether the difference between two means is statistically significant for both independent and dependent sample means
10. Explain the meaning and relationship of the two types of errors made in testing a hypothesis
11. Be able to list the reasons it is inappropriate to perform the

$$t = (\bar{x}_1 - \bar{x}_2 - 0)/\text{SE}(\bar{x}_1 - \bar{x}_2)$$

test on dependent sample means
12. Explain the meaning of a p value
13. Explain the relationship between a confidence interval and a test of significance and how the confidence interval can be used in testing a given hypothesis

9.1 Definitions

Before getting into the step-by-step procedure of a test of significance, you should find it helpful to peruse the following definitions.

Hypothesis. A statement of belief used in the evaluation of population values.

Null hypothesis, H_0. A claim that there is no difference between the population mean μ and the hypothesized value μ_0.

Alternative hypothesis, H_1. A claim that disagrees with the null hypothesis. If the null hypothesis is rejected, we are left with no choice but to accept the alternative that μ is not equal to μ_0.

Test statistic. A statistic used to determine the relative position of the mean in the hypothesized frequency distribution of sample means.

Critical region. The region on the far end of the distribution. If only one end of the distribution is involved, the region is referred to as a **one-tailed test;** if both ends are involved, the region is known as a **two-tailed test.** When the computed Z falls in the critical region designated by α, we reject the null hypothesis. The critical region is sometimes called the **rejection region.**

Significance level. The level that corresponds to the area in the critical region. By choice this area is usually small; the implication is that results falling in it do so infrequently. Consequently, such events are deemed unusual or statistically significant. When a test statistic falls in this area, the result is referred to as **significant** at the α level.

***p* value.** The area that falls in the tail or tails of a distribution beyond the value of the test statistic. The probability that the value of the calculated test statistic, or a larger one, occurred by chance alone is denoted by p.

Acceptance region. The region of the sampling distribution not included in α. That is, it is located under the middle portion of the curve. Whenever a test statistic falls in this region, the evidence does not permit us to reject the null hypothesis. The implication is that results falling in this region are not unexpected. The acceptance region is denoted by $(1 - \alpha)$.

Test of significance. A procedure used to establish the validity of a claim by determining whether or not the test statistic falls in the critical region. If it does, the results are referred to as significant. This test is sometimes called the **hypothesis test.**

To reinforce some of these definitions, let's consider an analogy. In a criminal court, the jury's duty is to evaluate the evidence of the prosecution and the defense to determine whether a defendent is guilty or innocent. By use of the judge's instructions, which provide guidelines for their reaching a decision, the members of the jury can arrive at one of two verdicts, guilty or not guilty. Their decision may be correct or they could make one of two possible errors: convict an innocent person or exonerate a guilty one.

Statisticians have found a lot in common between a court trial and a **test of significance.** By a statistical test of significance, one attempts to determine whether a certain claim is valid. The claim is usually stated as a **null hypothesis,** H_0, which holds that the mean of a certain population is some value, μ_0 (the defendent is innocent). Using the data obtained in the sample (the evidence), one computes a **test statistic** (the jury) and uses it to determine whether it supports the null hypothesis claim (innocence) that the sample comes from a population with a mean of μ_0. The basis for finding out whether the test statistic supports the null hypothesis is the **critical region** (judge's instructions). The critical region sets guidelines for rejecting or failing to reject the null hypothesis. If the computed statistic falls in the critical region of the distribution curve, where it is unlikely to occur by chance, the claim is not supported (conviction). If the test statistic falls in the **acceptance region,** where it is quite likely to occur by chance, the claim is not rejected (exoneration).

9.2 Basis for a Test of Significance

To illustrate the basic concepts of a test of significance, let's again consider the Honolulu Heart Study. Suppose someone claims that the mean age of the population of 7683 individuals is 53 years. How can you verify (or reject) this claim? Start by drawing a sample of, say, 100 persons. Suppose

Figure 9.1 Distribution of Sample Means

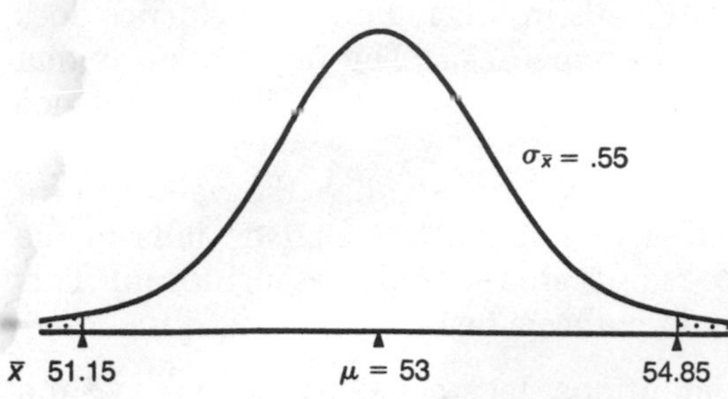

Figure 9.2 Critical Region of a Test Statistic

Critical region α/2

Acceptance region (or fail-to-reject region) 1 − α

α/2 Critical region

−Z 0 Z

the sample mean equals 54.85. Now the question is, What is the likelihood of finding a sample mean of 54.85 in a sample of 100 from a distribution whose true mean, μ, is 53? You can determine the answer by examining the relative position of $\bar{x}$ (54.85) on the scale of possible sample means. In Figure 9.1 you can see that 54.85 falls considerably above the hypothesized population mean of 53.

If the probability of such an occurrence is small as judged by the areas (in either direction) in the tails beyond this point, the occurrence is considered unusual or statistically significant. Why consider the areas in *both* directions? Remember that $\bar{x}$ could have fallen either above or below the mean μ. If $\bar{x}$ fell close to the center of the distribution, the probability of its occurring by chance would be fairly high. Events that have a high probability of occurrence are common and consequently *not significant*. The likelihood (probability) of the chance occurrence of a certain event can be obtained by performing a test of significance.

9.3 Procedure for a Test of Significance

To perform a test of significance, we take the following steps:

1. State H_0: $\mu = \mu_0$ versus H_1: $\mu \neq \mu_0$.
2. Choose a significance level $\alpha = \alpha_0$ (usually $\alpha_0 = .05$ or $.01$).
3. Compute the test statistic (the Z score):

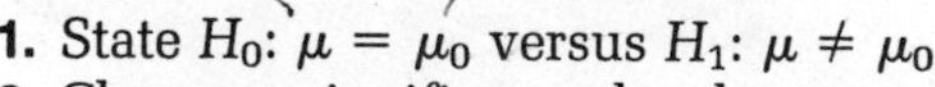

$$Z = \frac{\bar{x} - \mu}{\sigma/\sqrt{n}}$$

4. Determine the critical region, which is the region of the Z distribution with $\alpha/2$ in each tail, as shown in Figure 9.2.

5. Reject the null hypothesis if the test statistic Z falls in the critical region. Do not reject the null hypothesis if it falls in the acceptance region.
6. State appropriate conclusions.

EXAMPLE 1

■ Using the Honolulu Heart Study sample of $n = 100$, which has a mean age $\bar{x} = 54.85$, we can perform a test of significance to determine the likelihood that such a sample mean comes from a population whose mean is 53, given that $\sigma = 5.50$. Using the procedure just outlined, we obtain the following:

1. H_0: $\mu = 53$ versus H_1: $\mu \neq 53$.
2. Significance level $\alpha = .05$.
3. Test statistic:

$$Z = \frac{\bar{x} - \mu}{\sigma/\sqrt{n}} = \frac{54.85 - 53}{5.5/\sqrt{100}} = \frac{1.85}{.55} = 3.36$$

4. Critical region: From the Z distribution (Table 6.1), we find, for a two-tailed test where $\alpha/2 = .025$, the corresponding $Z = \pm 1.96$ (Figure 9.3).
5. Since the computed test statistic $Z = 3.36$ (step 3) falls within the critical region (beyond the critical values ±196), we are compelled to reject the null hypothesis that the sample comes from a population with a mean of 53 and to accept the alternative hypothesis that the sample comes from a population with a mean not equal to 53.

This result is considered to be significant at the $\alpha = .05$ level because the probability of its occurring by chance is less than .05. The actual probability of obtaining a Z of 3.36 or larger is much smaller.

Figure 9.3 Critical Region for Example 1

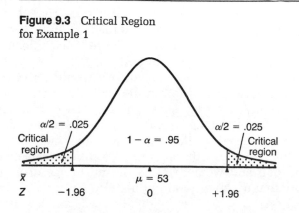

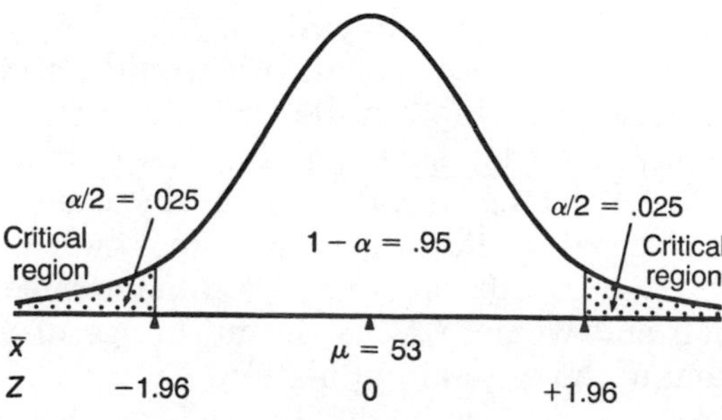

Since the computed test statistic falls 3.36 standard errors from the mean, we could say that the probability of having a sample mean of 54.85 or larger in either direction (that is, above or below $\mu = 53$) is less than .002. This figure is usually denoted by p and is obtained by summing the area beyond $Z = \pm 3.36$, which is at most $2(.5 - .4990) = 2(.001) = .002$. (Observe that since 3.36 does not appear in Table 6.1, we use the area .4990 corresponding to 3.09, the largest value in the table.)

The p value of .002 indicates that the probability of selecting by chance a mean that falls 3.36 standard errors above or below the population mean of 53, is quite small, that is, less than .002. You could ask yourself, "How could I be so lucky as to have obtained such a result?" Your logical conclusion: the sample probably came from another population with a mean other than 53. ■

9.4 One-Tailed Versus Two-Tailed Tests

In testing statistical hypotheses, you must always ask a vital question: "Am I interested in the deviation of $\bar{x}$ from μ in one or both directions?" The answer is usually implicit in the way H_0 and H_1 are stated. If you are interested in determining whether the mean age is significantly *different* from a given μ, you would perform a **two-tailed** test, since the deviation, $\bar{x} - \mu$, could be either negative or positive.

If you are interested in whether the mean age is significantly *larger* than the given μ, you would perform a **one-tailed** test. Likewise, you would go to the one-tailed test for mean ages *smaller* than μ.

Figure 9.4 illustrates the use of each kind of test. Figure 9.4a indicates that a two-tailed test is called for in testing the null hypothesis that $\mu = \mu_0$ against the alternative hypothesis that $\mu \neq \mu_0$. One half of the rejection region α is placed in each tail of the distribution. That is, we would reject H_0 if the value of the calculated test statistic fell in either of the outlying regions. Figure 9.4b indicates a one-tailed test for testing the null hypothesis that $\mu \leq \mu_0$ against the alternative hypothesis that $\mu > \mu_0$. Here, the critical region falls entirely in the positive tail; we would reject H_0 if the test statistic were so large as to fall in the critical region. Figure 9.4c indicates a left-handed one-tailed test for testing the null hypothesis that $\mu \geq \mu_0$. Here, the critical region falls entirely in the negative tail; we would reject H_0 if the calculated statistic were negative and fell in the critical region.

A one-tailed test is indicated for questions like these: Is a new drug superior to a standard drug? Does the air pollution level exceed safe limits? Has the death rate been reduced for those who quit smoking? A two-tailed test is indicated for questions like these: Is there a difference between the cholesterol levels of men and women? Does the mean age of a group of volunteers differ from that of the general population?

Figure 9.4 Two-Tailed Versus One-Tailed Test ($\alpha = .05$)

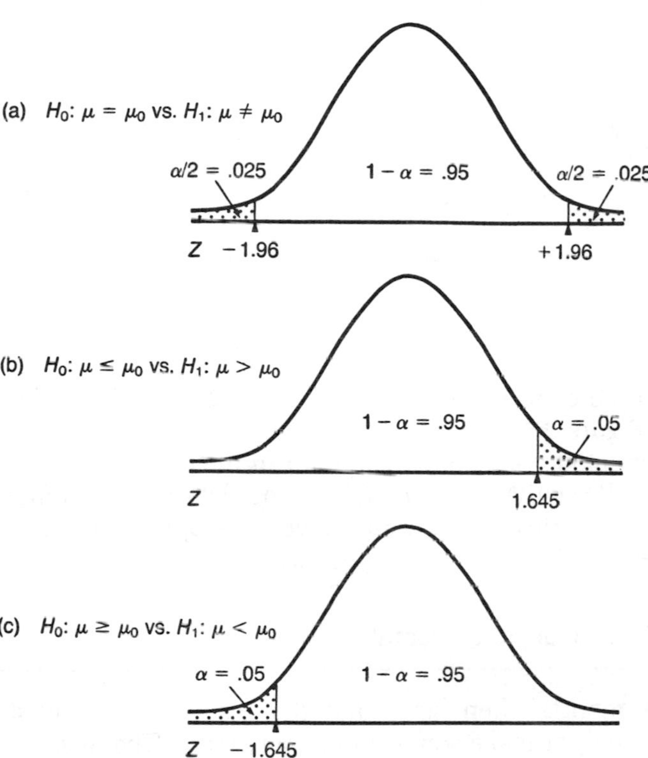

EXAMPLE 2

The criterion for issuing a smog alert is established at greater than 7 ppm of a particular pollutant. Samples collected from 16 stations give an $\bar{x}$ of 7.84 with an s of 2.01. Do these findings indicate that the smog alert criterion has been exceeded, or can the results be explained by chance? Since σ is estimated by s, we rely on the t test.

1. H_0: $\mu \leq 7.0$ and H_1: $\mu > 7.0$.
2. $\alpha = .05$.
3. Test statistic:

$$t = \frac{\bar{x} - \mu}{s/\sqrt{n}} = \frac{7.84 - 7.0}{2.01/\sqrt{16}} = \frac{.84}{.50} = 1.68$$

4. Critical region: Since the H_1: $\mu > 7.0$ indicates a one-tailed test, we place

Figure 9.5 Critical Region for Example 2

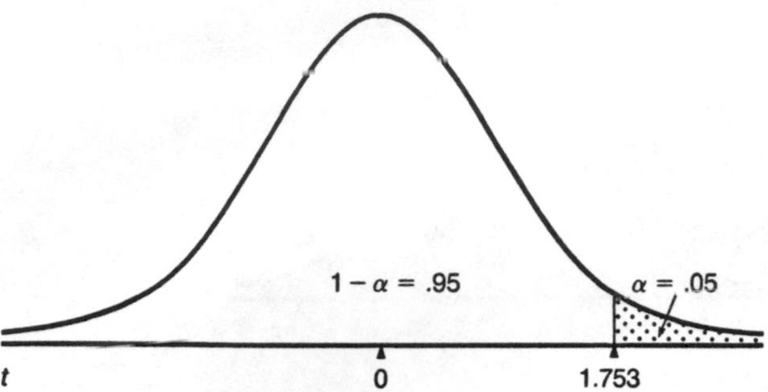

all of $\alpha = .05$ on the positive side. From Table 7.2 we find that, for 15 df, $t_{.05} = 1.753$ (Figure 9.5).

5. Since the calculated $t = 1.68$ does not fall in the critical region, we do not reject H_0; alternatively, we conclude the data were insufficient to indicate that the critical air pollution level of 7 ppm was significantly exceeded. ■

9.5 Meaning of "Statistically Significant"

Research reports often state that the results were **statistically significant,** ($p < .05$), or make some similar statement. The meaning of such a comment is that the observed difference is likely to be real rather than easily explainable by chance. The level of significance, somewhat arbitrarily selected at such values of α as .05, .025, .01, or .001, is a measure of how good H_0 is. The significance level α is also the magnitude of error that one is willing to take in making the decision to reject the null hypothesis. Some investigators prefer to report their results in terms of the p value alone and let the reader conclude whether the results are significant.

In Section 9.3, a p value was calculated for the test of $\mu = 53$. Since it was a two-tailed test, we doubled the area in the tails beyond $Z = \pm 3.36$, namely, $p < .002$. For a one-tailed test the p value would be the area beyond $Z = 3.36$, that is, $p < .001$. Researchers and statisticians generally agree on the following conventions for interpreting p values:

p value	Interpretation
$p > .05$	Result is not significant
$p < .05$	Result is significant
$p < .01$	Result is highly significant

Some investigators would consider $p < .10$ to be marginally significant. "Statistically significant" means that the evidence obtained from the sample is not compatible with the null hypothesis; consequently, we reject H_0. However, just because a result is "not statistically significant" does not prove that H_0 is true. We may not be able to reject H_0 simply because the sample was too small to provide enough evidence to do so. In that sense, the decision to reject a null hypothesis is stronger than the decision not to reject it. Nor does "statistically significant" imply clinically significant. That is, the difference, although technically "significant," may be so small that it has little biological or practical consequence.

9.6 Type I and Type II Errors

In our analogy between hypothesis testing and a criminal trial, we noted that the jury could make one of two errors: (1) reject the claim of innocence when the defendent is indeed innocent or (2) fail to reject the claim of innocence when the defendent is indeed guilty. Likewise, in testing a null hypothesis (H_0), you have two possible decisions:

1. H_0 is false and consequently rejected. That is, the evidence is that the sample comes from another population than one having $\mu = \mu_0$.
2. H_0 is true and consequently accepted. The observed difference between μ and μ_0 is relatively small and may be reasonably ascribed to chance variation.

If your decision is that H_0 is false when indeed it is, you have reached a correct decision. If you decide that H_0 is false when it is actually true, an event likely to occur α proportion of the time, you have committed a **type I error** (i.e., **α error**)—rejecting a true hypothesis that in the court analogy corresponds to convicting an innocent person. If your decision is that H_0 is true when indeed it is, you have also reached a correct decision. If you decide that H_0 is true when it is actually false, an event likely to occur β proportion of the time, you have committed a **type II error** (i.e., **β error**)—accepting a false hypothesis that in the court analogy corresponds to freeing a guilty person. These two errors are summarized in Figure 9.6.

In the test of a null hypothesis, some specific value for the parameter, say μ_0, is proposed. If this value happens to be correct but we reject it based on the observed sample, we have committed a Type I error. If the proposed value happens to be incorrect but we accept it based on the observed sample, we have committed a Type II error. Therefore, we can say that the type I error is the probability of rejecting a true null hypothesis and that the type II error is the probability of accepting a false null hypothesis.

Let's apply this test to the Honolulu Heart Study. The mean age for the population was $\mu = 54.36$. If we didn't know this, but guessed that μ was 53,

Figure 9.6 Possible Errors in Hypothesis Testing

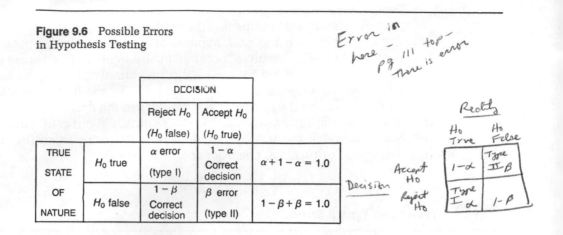

		DECISION		
		Reject H_0 (H_0 false)	Accept H_0 (H_0 true)	
TRUE STATE OF NATURE	H_0 true	α error (type I)	$1 - \alpha$ Correct decision	$\alpha + 1 - \alpha = 1.0$
	H_0 false	$1 - \beta$ Correct decision	β error (type II)	$1 - \beta + \beta = 1.0$

the upper critical point for the distribution under the null hypothesis of 53 would be 54.08, since

$$1.96 = \frac{\bar{x} - 53}{5.5/\sqrt{100}}$$

reduces to $\bar{x} = 54.08$. Figure 9.7 illustrates that if we had randomly arrived at an $\bar{x}$ below 54.08, we would have accepted the false H_0 (that $\mu = 53$) β proportion of the time. This β error is represented by the area to the left of $\bar{x} = 54.08$. This area for an $\bar{x}$ of 54.08 and an s of 5.5, based on a sample of 100, is equal to the area corresponding to

$$Z = \frac{54.08 - 54.36}{5.5/\sqrt{100}} = \frac{-.28}{.55} = -.51$$

Using Table 6.1, we find that $\beta = .30$.

In Figure 9.7 it is seen that we would have rejected the false H_0 about 70% of the time $(1 - \beta = .70)$. The quantity $1 - \beta$ is referred to as the **power of a test**, which is the probability of rejecting H_0 when H_0 is indeed false. Generally, statisticians try to design statistical tests that have high power; that is, β is small. We can infer from Figure 9.7 that this goal could be accomplished either by decreasing the significance level (α) from .01 to .05 or by increasing the sample size.

From the foregoing discussion, it should be clear that the α level represents the probability of a type I error, and β the probability of a type II error. There is a sort of reciprocal relationship between the two types of error. Figure 9.7 suggests that the smaller you choose α to be, the larger β will be. The reason for this is that as the critical region moves farther to the right, more β area is generated to the left of the critical point. The only way to

Figure 9.7 Distribution of Sample Means for $\mu_0 = 53$ and $\mu = 54.36$

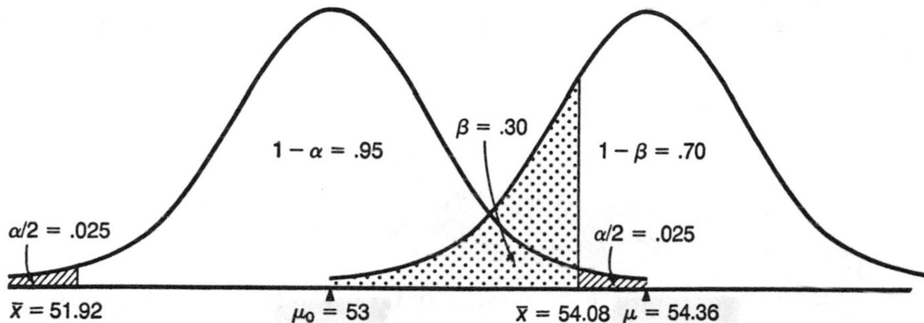

reduce both α and β errors is to reduce the overlap, that is, the area common to the two distributions. This can be done by increasing the sample size, which will reduce $s_{\bar{x}} = s/\sqrt{n}$ and thus narrow the sampling distributions.

9.7 Test of Significance of Two Independent Sample Means

We learned in Chapter 8 of the frequent need to compare sample means. As we seldom know the value of σ, we estimate it by s_p (see Equation 8.9) and compute the test statistic, which we defined as

$$t = \frac{\bar{x}_1 - \bar{x}_2 - (\mu_1 - \mu_2)}{s_p\sqrt{1/n_1 + 1/n_2}} \tag{9.1}$$

with $n_1 + n_2 - 2$ df. Using this test statistic, we compare $\bar{x}_1 - \bar{x}_2$, the difference between the sample means (an estimate of the difference between population means), with $\mu_1 - \mu_2$, the unknown difference between the population means. Since under the null hypothesis the difference between the two means $\mu_1 - \mu_2$ equals zero, in Equation 9.1 the expression $\mu_1 - \mu_2$ vanishes.

This situation was illustrated in Example 2 of Chapter 8. Recall that a random sample (n_1) of 25 from a population of joggers provided an estimate of mean maximal VO_2 uptake ($\bar{x}_1$) of 47.5 ml/kg with $s_1 = 4.8$, and for a sample of $n_2 = 26$ from a population of nonjoggers a mean maximal VO_2 uptake of $\bar{x}_2 = 37.5$ ml/kg with an s_2 of 5.1. Is this difference statistically significant or can it be explained by chance? Using the test statistic, we can proceed as follows:

1. H_0: $\mu_1 = \mu_2$; H_1: $\mu_1 \neq \mu_2$.

   Another way of writing $\mu_1 = \mu_2$ is $\mu_1 - \mu_2 = 0$, giving H_0: $\mu_1 - \mu_2 = 0$ and H_1: $\mu_1 - \mu_2 \neq 0$

2. $\alpha = .01$.
3. To proceed with the test statistic, we compute s_p by using Equation 8.9.

$$s_p = \sqrt{\frac{s_1^2(n_1 - 1) + s_2^2(n_2 - 1)}{n_1 + n_2 - 2}}$$

$$= \sqrt{\frac{(4.8)^2\,(24) + (5.1)^2(25)}{25 + 26 - 2}} = \sqrt{\frac{1203.21}{49}}$$

$$= \sqrt{24.56} = 4.96$$

4. The test statistic is computed by using Equation 9.1, which is modified only to the extent of dropping $\mu_1 - \mu_2$:

$$t = \frac{\bar{x}_1 - \bar{x}_2 - 0}{s_p\sqrt{1/n_1 + 1/n_2}} \qquad (9.2)$$

$$= \frac{47.5 - 37.5 - 0}{4.96\sqrt{1/25 + 1/26}}$$

$$= \frac{10.00}{1.39} = 7.2$$

5. The critical region for a t with $n_1 + n_2 - 2 = 49$ df is shown in Figure 9.8. Since this is a two-tailed test, the t value is found in the column labeled $\alpha = .01/2 = .005$, that is, 2.58.
6. As the computed t of 7.2 falls well into the critical region, we reject the null hypothesis and conclude that joggers have significantly better physical condition than nonjoggers as judged by their VO_2 uptake.

Figure 9.8 Critical Region for a Test Statistic

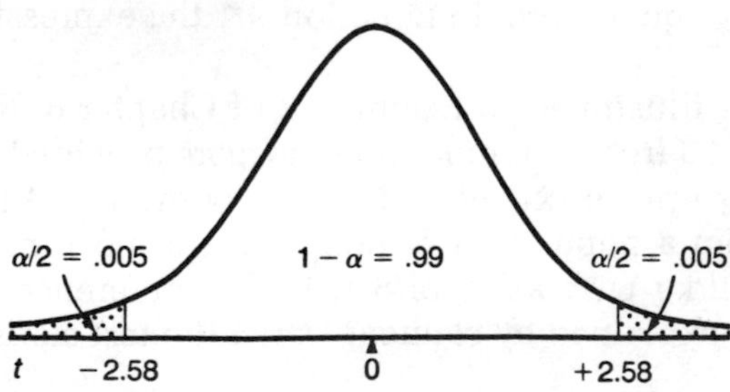

There is a temptation for persons with little experience in statistics to use Equation 9.2 to test the difference between the two means obtained in a before-and-after experiment, as alluded to in Section 8.5. This is a faulty approach because the assumption behind Equation 9.2 presupposes two independent samples, whereas the before-and-after case yields two sample means that are dependent. A desirable way to handle such a case is to reduce it to a single population statistic (as illustrated by Table 8.1) and apply the following test statistic:

$$t = \frac{\bar{d} - 0}{s_d/\sqrt{n}} \tag{9.3}$$

with $n - 1$ df. The value $\bar{d}$ is the mean difference between x (before) and x′ (after) for each of the cases; s_d is the estimate of the standard deviation of the differences; and zero is used for the difference between the mean before the experiment and the mean after the experiment.

9.8 Relationship of Tests of Significance to Confidence Intervals

Since confidence intervals are determined from Z or t statistics, you might suspect that the decision reached by use of a significance test would be the same as that reached by use of a confidence interval. And it is indeed the same whenever the hypothesis test is two-tailed. When the significance test was performed on the difference of mean VO_2 uptake between joggers and nonjoggers, it was found that the difference was highly significant. The 99% confidence interval for the difference $\mu_1 - \mu_2$ was 6.42 to 13.58, which did not include the hypothesized mean of zero. Consequently, since zero was not likely to have occurred in this interval, we reached the conclusion that it was not likely to have occurred by chance alone at the 1% significance level. Both confidence limits being positive, we concluded that the difference was significant.

Generally, there are two rules to follow in using confidence intervals to determine whether a difference is significant:

1. If a hypothesized difference in means such as $\mu_1 - \mu_2 = 0$ is included in the confidence interval, H_0 is *not* rejected.
2. If the hypothesized difference is *not* included, H_0 is rejected.

So far we have considered tests of significance in which we compare either sample means with population means or the differences between sample means for two groups. It is also possible to compare simultaneously the differences among three or more sample means. The technique for doing this is described in the next chapter.

Conclusion

Tests of significance are performed to determine the validity of claims regarding the parameters (e.g., μ_1 or $\mu_1 - \mu_2$) of a population. From the nature of each claim we can decide whether the test should be one-tailed or two-tailed. The decision determines how the null and alternative hypotheses are stated and the manner in which the test is performed. Together with the choice of significance level, the decision defines the critical region. The critical region is the decision-making feature of the test, and the computed test statistic is compared to it. If the value of the test statistic falls in the critical region, we reject the null hypothesis and accept the alternative; if it falls outside the critical region, we fail to reject the null hypothesis and cannot accept the alternative. In the former case the evidence supports the claim; in the latter it is insufficient to support the claim. It is possible to commit one of two errors in executing these tests. In rejecting a true null hypothesis we make a type I error (α error), whereas in accepting a false hypothesis we make a type II error (β error). If we do not wish to define a critical region, it is possible to compute a p value, which indicates the probability of the chance occurrence of this or a larger value of the test statistic.

Vocabulary List

acceptance region
alternative hypothesis
critical region
(rejection region)
null hypothesis
one-tailed test
power of a test
p value
significance level
statistical significance
test of significance
(hypothesis test)
test statistic
two-tailed test
type I error (α error)
type II error (β error)

Exercises

9.1 What would be the critical value for a test of significance in each of the following situations?

(a) One-tailed test, $\alpha = .05$, σ known, $n = 20$
(b) One-tailed test, $\alpha = .05$, σ unknown, $n = 10$
(c) Two-tailed test, $\alpha = .01$, σ unknown, $n = 14$
(d) Two-tailed test, $\alpha = .01$, σ known, $n = 25$
(e) Two-tailed test, $\alpha = .05$, σ unknown, $n = 35$

9.2 In which of the situations in Exercise 9.1 would you use a (a) Z test? (b) t test? Why?

9.3 For each part, state the null (H_0) and alternative (H_1) hypotheses:

(a) Has the average community level of suspended particulates for the month of August exceeded 30 mcg per cubic meter?

(b) Does mean age of onset of a certain acute disease for school children differ from 11.5?

(c) A psychologist claims that the average IQ of a sample of 60 children is significantly above the normal IQ of 100.

(d) Is the average cross-sectional area of the lumen of coronary arteries for men, ages 40 to 59, less than 31.5% of the total arterial cross section?

(e) Is the mean hemoglobin level of a group of high-altitude workers different from 16 g/cc?

(f) Does the average speed of 50 cars as checked by radar on a particular highway differ from 55 mph?

9.4 Determine the critical value that would be used to test a hypothesis under the conditions given in each of the following.

(a) $H_0{:}\mu = 220$, $H_1{:}\mu \neq 220$, $\alpha = .05$, $n = 20$, σ known

(b) $H_0{:}\mu \leq 15$, $H_1{:}\mu > 15$, $\alpha = .01$, $n = 35$, σ known

(c) $H_0{:}\mu = 70$, $H_1{:}\mu \neq 70$, $\alpha = .01$, $n = 18$, σ known

(d) $H_0{:}\mu = 120$, $H_1{:}\mu \neq 120$, $\alpha = .05$, $n = 25$, σ unknown

(e) $H_0{:}\mu \geq 100$, $H_1{:}\mu < 100$, $\alpha = .01$, $n = 16$, σ unknown

(f) $H_0{:}\mu \geq 55$, $H_1{:}\mu < 55$, $\alpha = .05$, $n = 49$, σ unknown

9.5 In each of the following situations choose an α appropriate to the seriousness of the potential error involved should the null hypothesis be rejected when it is actually true.

(a) You wish to decide if a new treatment for pancreatic cancer, known to be a usually fatal disease, is superior to the standard treatment.

(b) It is claimed that the mean income for families of size four is greater than $20,000.

9.6 For each of the parts of Exercise 9.4 decide if you should reject H_0 or fail to reject H_0 according to the corresponding test statistic:

(a) $Z = -1.79$

(b) $Z = 2.01$

(c) $Z = 3.63$

(d) $t = 2.77$

(e) $t = -2.14$

(f) $t = -1.82$

9.7 Boys of a certain age have a mean weight of 85 lb. A complaint was made that in a municipal children's home the boys were underfed. As one bit of evidence, all 25 boys of the given age were weighed and found to have a mean weight of 80.94 lb.

(a) If it is known in advance that the population standard deviation for weights of boys this age is 11.6 lb, what would you conclude regarding the complaint? Use $\alpha = .05$.

(b) Suppose that the population standard deviation is unknown. If the sample standard deviation is found to be 12.3 lb, what conclusion regarding the complaint might you draw? Use $\alpha = .05$.

9.8 In Table 3.1 the mean systolic blood pressure is 130 mmHg and the variance is 448. Is this an indication that the group is significantly different from the standard if the population standard is known to be 120 mmHg? Test at $\alpha = .05$.

9.9 (a) Calculate the p value for each case in Exercises 8.2, 8.3, 9.7, 9.8, and 9.17.
(b) For each test, what do the p values tell you about statistical significance?
(c) Do your answers to (b) agree with the decisions and conclusions you made in each exercise? Why? Why not?

9.10 (a) State the value of the type I error for each case in Exercises 8.2, 8.3, 9.7, 9.8, and 9.17.
(b) What does the type I error tell you?
(c) What does the type II error tell you?
(d) From the information stated in the problems, are you able to state the type II errors?
(e) If in any given problem you should decide to decrease the type I error (say from .05 to .01), what would happen to the type II error?
(f) What is usually done to avoid type II errors?
(g) What could you do to reduce simultaneously both types of error?

9.11 In Table 2.2 the means and standard deviations of some subgroups of the sample are as follows:

	Mean	Standard deviation	n
Vegetarians	72.9	11.7	40
Nonvegetarians	73.5	11.4	43
Males	74.9	12.0	38
Females	71.8	11.0	45

Is there a significant difference in the mean diastolic blood pressures, at $\alpha = .05$, between
(a) vegetarians and nonvegetarians?
(b) males and females?

9.12 Birth lengths of male and female infants in a small clinic gave the following results:

Group	Sample size	$\bar{x}$ (cm)	s (cm)
Males	12	52.2	8.6
Females	9	50.7	9.5

Assuming normally distributed populations with equal variances, do these data justify the conclusion, at $\alpha = .05$, that the mean birth length is greater for males than for females? Also calculate the p value for the computed *t*.

9.13 For Exercise 8.2, determine whether the mean hemoglobin level of the group of 25 men is significantly different from $\mu = 15$ at the $\alpha = .05$ level.

9.14 Ten experimental animals were subjected to conditions simulating disease. The number of heartbeats per minute, before and after the experiment, were recorded as follows:

Heartbeats per minute				Heartbeats per minute			
Animal	Before	After	d	Animal	Before	After	d
1	70	115	45	6	100	178	78
2	84	148	64	7	110	179	69
3	88	176	88	8	67	140	73
4	110	191	81	9	79	161	82
5	105	158	53	10	86	157	71

Do these data provide sufficient evidence to indicate that the experimental condition increases the number of heartbeats per minute? Let $\alpha = .05$. Also calculate the p value for the computed *t*.

9.15 Blood samples from 10 persons were sent to each of two labs for cholesterol determinations.

	Serum cholesterol (mg/ml)	
Subject	Lab 1	Lab 2
1	296	318
2	268	287
3	244	260
4	272	279
5	240	245
6	244	249
7	282	294
8	254	271
9	244	262
10	262	285
Σx	2,606	2,750
Σx^2	682,316	760,706
s_x	18.83	22.25

Is there a statistically significant difference (at the $\alpha = .01$ level) in the cholesterol levels as reported by lab 1 and lab 2?

(a) Should one use the pooled *t* test or the paired *t* test to answer this question?
(b) Perform the test you chose for (a) and answer the question.
(c) Perform the test you did *not* choose for (a) and compare the result with (b). What do you observe?
(d) Determine the p values for both (b) and (c) and compare them. Discuss the relationship of the p values to what you have already concluded about the two *t* tests.

9.16 If in Exercise 8.4 you found for the group of 25 men a mean of .35 g/6 hr, would you conclude that this group is significantly different from the standard group at the $\alpha = .01$ level?

9.17 The mean diastolic blood pressure in Table 2.2 is 73 mmHg with a standard deviation of 11.6 mmHg. For an α of .01, test whether the mean blood pressure of this group is significantly greater than 70.

9.18 The mean weight of the sample of 100 persons from the Honolulu Heart Study was 64 kg. If the ideal weight was known to be 60 kg, is the group significantly overweight? Assume $\sigma = 10$ kg and $\alpha = .05$.

9.19 (a) For the data in Exercise 8.8, indicate at an α of .05 whether the mean cholesterol level of the vegetarian group is significantly lower than that of the nonvegetarians.

(b) Compute a p value for the test statistic.

Chapter **10**

Analysis of Variance

Chapter Outline

10.1 Function of ANOVA
The general usefulness of ANOVA (analysis of variation) for comparing means of several groups is discussed.

10.2 Rationale for ANOVA
It is explained how ANOVA utilizes a comparison of variations between and within groups by means of an F ratio.

10.3 ANOVA Calculations
The equations for the various sources of variation are shown.

10.4 Assumptions
The assumptions necessary for performing the tests of hypotheses—independence, normality, and homogeneity of variance—are described.

10.5 Application
The testing of the hypothesis of equality of mean birthweights among the infants of three groups of mothers classified by smoking status is used to test the one-way ANOVA classification.

Learning Objectives

After studying this chapter, you should be able to

1. Indicate the circumstances that call for an ANOVA rather than a t test
2. Set up an ANOVA table that partitions the total sum of squares into between-group and within-group sums of squares
3. Compute the F ratio and its appropriate degrees of freedom
4. List the two assumptions that need to be made to perform an ANOVA
5. Indicate the type of hypothesis that can be tested with an ANOVA
6. Find the critical region for an F-ratio test
7. Indicate the reason for performing multiple-range tests

10.1 Function of ANOVA

Analysis of variance (**ANOVA**) is one of the most powerful methods of analyzing differences among a number of groups. It deals with the comparison of means from several groups. In Chapter 9 we discussed the technique for testing the significance of the difference between means for two groups. But how do you determine, for instance, whether there is a significant difference in birthweight among three groups of infants—the first group born to nonsmoking mothers, the second to light-smoking mothers, and the third to heavy-smoking mothers?

It is possible to perform *t* tests between the means of each pair of groups and determine which pairs differ significantly. But this approach presents a number of difficulties—the choice of a proper significance level for "overtesting," the numerous tests needed if many groups are involved, and the lack of one overall measure of significance for the differences among the means.

ANOVA, which is in fact a generalization of the *t* test to more than two independent groups, is able to handle these problems elegantly. The results obtained with ANOVA for two groups is identical to the results obtained with a *t* test. So it is fair to say that ANOVA is an extension of the *t* test to handle more than two groups.

For the birthweight example, the null hypothesis being tested is

$$H_0: \mu_1 = \mu_2 = \mu_3$$

the alternative hypothesis, H_1, being that H_0 is not true; that is, either one of the means is not equal to the others or none of them are equal to one another. The three smoking-status groups would be commonly referred to as the treatment groups, with smoking exposure considered as the "treatment." The theoretical basis for performing this test is the partitioning of the available variance of all observations into two sources of variation—variation *between** the group means and variation *within* each of the groups. The sampling distribution used for testing these means is not the *t* distribution but rather the ***F* distribution** (named in honor of the celebrated R.A. Fisher, who developed the *F* statistic).

10.2 Rationale for ANOVA

Analysis of variance is unique in that it simultaneously compares two different estimates of the population variance to test a hypothesis con-

*When comparing more than two groups that are not reciprocally related, the term "among" is grammatically preferable to "between." In the present context, we owe the somewhat ungrammatical but traditional use of "between" to the work of some pioneer statisticians.

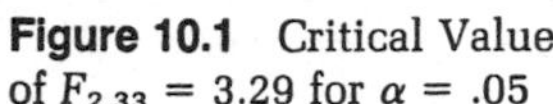

Figure 10.1 Critical Value of $F_{2,33} = 3.29$ for $\alpha = .05$

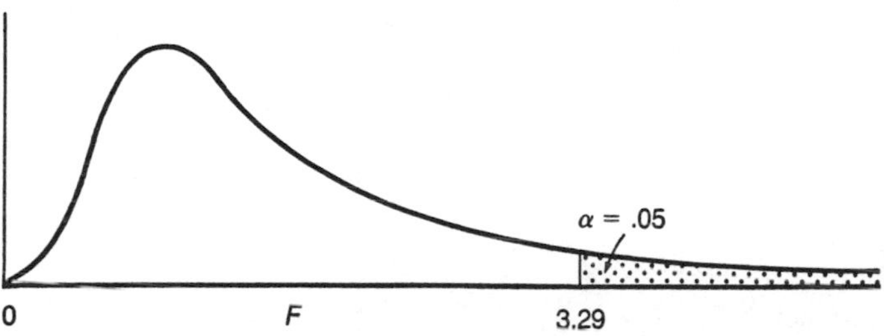

cerning the population mean. One of these estimates is **within-group variance**, which is simply the sum of the variances of each of the groups. It is analogous to the s_p^2 used in t tests, extended to the sum of the sample variances of more than two groups. It is called *within* variance because it is the collective variance of all observations within each group. By convention, within variance is denoted by s_w^2. The other estimate of variance is the **between-group variance** that measures the variation between the means of the various groups and is denoted by s_b^2. Using mathematical statistics, we can demonstrate that the between variance is equal to the within variance if the observations in each group are normally distributed and the means of each are equal: that is, there is *no* treatment effect.

With this knowledge we can move toward performing a test of the hypothesis of equality of means by comparing the ratio of the two variance estimates, s_b^2/s_w^2. If the two variances are indeed equal, the ratio s_b^2/s_w^2 should be approximately 1. Since we are dealing with s^2, an estimate of σ^2, the ratio will sometimes be greater and sometimes smaller than 1 even if the hypothesis of equal means is true. The ratio s_b^2/s_w^2 follows the F distribution and is illustrated in Figure 10.1.

In fact, there is a family of F distributions, one for each pair of degrees of freedom. The F statistic follows a skewed distribution, with two sets of degrees of freedom. The variance estimate s_b^2 has $k - 1$ df (where k is the number of groups); s_w^2 has $k(n - 1)$, where n is the number of observations in each group. Table B in the appendix gives critical values for the F distribution. Note that separate tabulations are provided for $\alpha = .05$ and $\alpha = .01$. For example, the critical F values for 2 and 33 df are 3.29 for an α of .05 and 5.32 for an α of .01.

10.3 ANOVA Calculations

We need a systematic procedure for computing ANOVA. To illustrate the procedure, we will use data from the general case shown in Table 10.1. It

Table 10.1 Symbolic Representation of Data in a One-Way Analysis of k Groups, with Equal Numbers of Observations per Group

	Group						
	1	2		i		k	
	x_{11}	x_{21}	⋯	x_{i1}	⋯	x_{k1}	
	x_{12}	x_{22}	⋯	x_{i2}	⋯	x_{k2}	
	x_{13}	x_{23}	⋯	x_{i3}	⋯	x_{k3}	
	⋮	⋮		⋮		⋮	
	x_{1j}	x_{2j}	⋯	x_{ij}	⋯	x_{kj}	
	⋮	⋮		⋮		⋮	
	x_{1n}	x_{2n}	⋯	x_{in}	⋯	x_{kn}	
Total	$x_{1\cdot}$	$x_{2\cdot}$	⋯	$x_{i\cdot}$	⋯	$x_{k\cdot}$	$x_{\cdot\cdot}$ (grand total)
Mean	$\bar{x}_{1\cdot}$	$\bar{x}_{2\cdot}$	⋯	$\bar{x}_{i\cdot}$	⋯	$\bar{x}_{k\cdot}$	$\bar{x}_{\cdot\cdot}$ (grand mean)

can be seen that there are an equal number of observations for each k group. The observations within each group are indicated with **double notation,** where the first subscript indicates the group number and the second subscript indicates the observation in that group: for example, x_{12} is the second observation in group 1. By extension, the jth observation in the ith group is indicated by x_{ij}. Furthermore, by convention, the dot notation is used to indicate the total. The mean for group 1 is denoted by $\bar{x}_{1\cdot}$ and is shown by

$$\bar{x}_{1\cdot} = \sum_{j=1}^{n} \frac{x_{1j}}{n} = \frac{x_{1\cdot}}{n} \tag{10.1}$$

The sum of all observations is given by

$$\sum_{i=1}^{k} \sum_{j=1}^{n} x_{ij} = \sum_{i=1}^{k} (x_{i\cdot}) = x_{\cdot\cdot} \tag{10.2}$$

The overall mean is obtained by dividing the total of all observations by the total number of observations, k times n. Therefore, the overall mean is

$$\bar{x}_{\cdot\cdot} = \frac{x_{\cdot\cdot}}{kn}$$

Now the **between-group sum of squares** (SS_b)—that is, the sum of the squared deviations between groups—is needed for computing the between-group variance. This SS_b can be obtained from Table 10.1 by use of

$$\begin{aligned} SS_b &= n \sum_{i=1}^{k} [(\bar{x}_{i\cdot} - \bar{x}_{\cdot\cdot})^2] \\ &= n[(\bar{x}_{1\cdot} - \bar{x}_{\cdot\cdot})^2 + (\bar{x}_{2\cdot} - \bar{x}_{\cdot\cdot})^2 + \cdots + (\bar{x}_{k\cdot} - \bar{x}_{\cdot\cdot})^2] \end{aligned} \tag{10.3}$$

The **within-group sum of squares,** SS_w, needed for computing the within-group variance, can be obtained by use of

$$SS_w = n \sum_{i=1}^{k} \left[\sum_{j=1}^{n} (x_{ij} - \bar{x}_{i\cdot})^2 \right] \tag{10.4}$$

The total sum of squares, SS_t, which measures the amount of variation about the overall mean, is the sum of the squared deviations of each x_{ij} from the overall mean. To obtain it, we use

$$SS_t = \sum_{i=1}^{k} \left[\sum_{j=1}^{n} (x_{ij} - \bar{x}_{\cdot\cdot})^2 \right]$$

A little algebraic manipulation shows that $SS_t = SS_b + SS_w$. That is,

$$\sum_{i=1}^{k} \left[\sum_{j=1}^{n} (x_{ij} - \bar{x}_{\cdot\cdot})^2 \right] =$$

$$n \sum_{i=1}^{k} \left[(\bar{x}_{i\cdot} - \bar{x}_{\cdot\cdot})^2 \right] + \sum_{i=1}^{k} \left[\sum_{j=1}^{n} (x_{ij} - \bar{x}_{i\cdot})^2 \right] \tag{10.5}$$

which suggests that the total variation of observations from the overall mean can be partitioned into two parts—the variation of the sum of squares between groups and that of the sum of squares within groups. The total number of degrees of freedom ($kn - 1$) is equal to the sum of the between group ($k - 1$) plus the within group $k(n - 1)$.

From Equations 10.3 and 10.4 it follows that the F statistic used to test the hypothesis of equality of means is

$$F_{k-1,k(n-1)} = \frac{s_b^2}{s_w^2} = \frac{SS_b/k - 1}{SS_w/k(n - 1)}$$

To complete an ANOVA table we usually calculate only SS_t and SS_b. The SS_w is obtained by $SS_w = SS_t - SS_b$. To calculate we use

$$SS_t = \sum_{i=1}^{k} \sum_{j=1}^{n} x_{ij}^2 - \frac{\left[\sum_{i=1}^{k} \sum_{j=1}^{n} x_{ij} \right]^2}{kn} \tag{10.6}$$

and

$$SS_b = n \sum_{i=1}^{k} \bar{x}_{i\cdot}^2 - \frac{\left[\sum_{i=1}^{k} \sum_{j=1}^{n} x_{ij} \right]^2}{kn} \tag{10.7}$$

10.4 Assumptions

To perform tests of hypotheses we need to make two assumptions:

1. The observations are independent. That is, the value of one observation is not correlated with that of another.
2. The observations in each group are normally distributed and the variance of each group is equal to that of any other group. That is, the variances of the various groups are **homogeneous.**

It should be pointed out that ANOVA is a **robust** technique, insensitive to departures from normality and homogeneity, and is particularly so if the sample sizes are nearly equal for each group.

10.5 Application

Let's return now to the question posed at the beginning of this chapter: Is there a significant difference in birthweight among three groups of infants classified by the smoking status of the mothers? The analysis procedure would be as follows:

1. H_0: $\mu_1 = \mu_2 = \mu_3$.
   H_1: that one or more mean is different from the others.

Table 10.2 Infant Birthweights (grams) and Means Classified by Smoking Status of Three Groups of Mothers

	Smoking status			
	None	1 Pack/day	1+ Pack/day	
Subject	1	2	3	
1	3,515	3,444	2,608	
2	3,420	3,827	2,509	
3	3,175	3,884	3,600	
4	3,586	3,515	1,730	
5	3,232	3,416	3,175	
6	3,884	3,742	3,459	
7	3,856	3,062	3,288	
8	3,941	3,076	2,920	
9	3,232	2,835	3,020	
10	4,054	2,750	2,778	
11	3,459	3,460	2,466	
12	3,998	3,340	3,260	
$x_{i\cdot}$	43,352	40,351	34,813	$x_{\cdot\cdot}$ = 118,516 (grand total)
$\bar{x}_{i\cdot}$	3,613	3,363	2,901	$\bar{x}_{\cdot\cdot}$ = 3,292 (grand mean)

Table 10.3 ANOVA Table for a One-Way Classification with an Equal Number of Observations per Group

Source of variation	Sum of squares	df	Mean squares	F ratio
Between	$SS_b = n\Sigma(\bar{x}_{i.} - \bar{x}_{..})^2$	$k - 1$	$MS_b = \frac{SS_b}{k-1}$	$F_{k-1,k(n-1)} = \frac{MS_b}{MS_w}$
Within	$SS_w = SS_t - SS_b$	$k(n-1)$	$s_p^2 = \frac{SS_w}{k(n-1)}$	
Total	$SS_t = \sum_{i=1}^{k} \sum_{j=1}^{n}[(x_{ij} - \bar{x}_{..})^2]$	$kn - 1$		

2. Test statistic: $F = s_b^2/s_w^2$ for $k - 1, k(n - 1)$ df.
3. Rejection region: We reject H_0 if the computed F statistic is greater than the tabulated value for α with the given degrees of freedom.

Using the observations of Table 10.2 and the equations of Table 10.3, we can set things up in a conventional ANOVA table. Note that in Table 10.3 the **mean squares** are the sums of squares divided by their respective degrees of freedom.

Using equation 10.6, we have

$$SS_t = \Sigma\Sigma\, x_{ij}^2 - \frac{(\Sigma\Sigma x_{ij})^2}{kn}$$

$$= 398{,}915{,}214 - \frac{(118{,}516)^2}{(3)(12)}$$

$$= 8{,}747{,}373.4$$

and using Equation 10.7, we obtain

$$SS_b = n\Sigma\bar{x}_{i.}^2 - \frac{(\Sigma\Sigma x_{ij})^2}{kn}$$

$$= 12\left[(3613)^2 + (3363)^2 + (2901)^2\right] - \frac{(118{,}516)^2}{(3)(12)}$$

$$= 3{,}184{,}227.4$$

and the within sum of squares is

$$SS_w = SS_t - SS_b$$

$$= 8{,}747{,}373.4 - 3{,}184{,}227.4$$

$$= 5{,}563{,}146.0$$

Table 10.4 ANOVA for Infant Birthweight Classified by Mother's Smoking Status

Source	SS	df	MS	F
Between	3,184,227.4	2	1,592,113.7	9.44
Within	5,563,146.0	33	168,580.2	
Total	8,747,373.4	35		

Now we're able to set up the ANOVA table for our illustration of the effect of maternal smoking (Table 10.4). From this table we can see that the computed F ratio is greater than the tabulated value of $F_{2,33} = 3.29$. This indicates that at least one of the means is significantly different from the others—that is, that maternal smoking appears to have an effect on infant birthweight. To find out which means are significantly different, we may be tempted to perform a number of multiple t tests between the various pairs of means. But it would be inappropriate to do so unless we wanted to know whether there was a significant difference between the nonsmokers and the heavy smokers before seeing the results. Multiple t tests are inappropriate because the probability of incorrectly rejecting the hypothesis increases with the number of t tests performed. So even though we may be performing a test of significance at $\alpha = .05$, the actual α level is, in effect, made considerably higher. Special **multiple tests** for comparison have been developed to deal with this problem. You can find a discussion of these in more advanced textbooks. (See, for example, Snedecor, 1979, or Steel and Torrie, 1980.)

In this chapter we have discussed ANOVA on the basis of an equal number of observations per group. The equations can, however, be modified to accommodate unequal numbers. We have also considered only the one-way ANOVA classification. It is possible to work with two-way, three-way, or multiple-way classifications as well. For example, a two-way ANOVA might consider four treatment groups for each sex group, with the second classification being by sex. With this kind of approach it is possible to partition the total variance three ways: compare between treatment groups, compare between sex groups, and compare either or both of those to the within variance. For a more detailed discussion and a more advanced treatment of ANOVA, see Snedecor (1973) or Armitage (1971).

Conclusion

The analysis of variance is so named because its test procedure is based on a comparison of the estimate of the between-group variance to the estimate of the within-group variance. These two estimates of σ^2 are obtained by partitioning the overall variance. An F statistic is used to determine the critical region for the test. If the computed F ratio falls in the critical region, we conclude that at least one of the means is significantly different from the others. To determine which specific pairs of means are significant, we utilize a multiple-range test, not multiple t tests. To test the hypothesis, we must assume independence of observations, normality of each group, and homogeneous variances. An important interpretation of ANOVA is that it tests whether there is a treatment effect, where the treatment is drug dosage, smoking exposure, or some other factor.

In this chapter we have discussed the one-way classification of variance. To be able to account for the many possible sources of variation in a particular experiment, you may wish to perform a two-way or a three-way ANOVA.

Vocabulary List

ANOVA	F distribution	robust technique
between-group sum of squares	homogeneous variances	within group sum of squares
between-group variance	mean squares	within-group variance
double notation	multiple tests	

Exercises

10.1 A survey was done in a community to assess who had a felt need for family planning. Residents were asked if they felt that family planning counseling was needed in the community. The following tabulation gives the opinions and the number of children of the respondents.

	Great need	Some need	No need	
No. of children	0	10	17	
	1	5	10	
	3	7	9	
	4	3	3	
	2	9	15	
	1	8	10	
	3	7	11	
	0	9	10	
	1	10	9	
	2	9	8	
Σx	17	77	102	196 (grand total)
$\bar{x}$	1.7	7.7	10.2	6.53 (grand mean)

Determine whether there is a difference in mean number of children of respondents:

(a) What is the null hypothesis?

(b) Construct an ANOVA table.

(c) What are your results and conclusions?

10.2 Five samples were taken randomly from each blood type, and the white cell counts were noted to be as follows:

	Blood type				
	A	B	AB	O	
White cell counts	5,000	7,000	7,000	5,325	
	5,500	8,000	7,125	7,985	
	8,000	5,000	9,000	6,689	
	10,000	9,900	9,235	9,321	
	7,735	6,342	7,699	6,666	
Σx	36,235	36,242	40,059	35,986	148,522 (grand total)
$\bar{x}$	7247.0	7248.4	8011.8	7197.2	7426.1 (grand mean)

Are the four blood types the same with respect to white cell counts?

10.3 Seven samples of individuals were selected randomly from three communities. The ages of the persons were as tabulated below.

	Community A	Community B	Community C	
Age	16	65	45	
	15	43	30	
	25	77	22	
	30	90	66	
	39	82	47	
	20	69	33	
	16	73	50	
Σx	161	499	293	953.00 (grand total)
$\bar{x}$	23	71.29	41.86	45.38 (grand mean)

Is there a significant difference in the ages?

10.4 Measurements on cumulative radiation dosage were made on workers at an atomic weapons plant over a six-month period. The table below presents data for workers whose dosage was assessed at three different locations. Determine whether there was a significant difference in the mean dosage level among the three locations.

	Location A	Location B	Location C	
Cumulative radiation dosage	11	29	37	
	27	41	51	
	19	19	42	
	21	39	28	
	31	24	35	
	14	35	48	
	28	46	75	
	22	64	49	
	18	52	61	
	10	23	52	
Σx	201	372	478	1051 (grand total)
$\bar{x}$	20.1	37.2	47.8	35.03 (grand mean)

Chapter **11**

Inferences Regarding Proportions

Chapter Outline

11.1 Introduction
The problem of inference in qualitative data is discussed.

11.2 Mean and Standard Deviation of the Binomial Distribution
How to compute a mean and a standard deviation for the binomial distribution is explained.

11.3 Approximation of the Normal to the Binomial Distribution
It is shown that, using the normal approximation, it is possible to compute a Z score for a number of successes.

11.4 Test of Significance of a Binomial Proportion
Instructions are given on how to test hypotheses regarding proportions if the distribution of the proportion of successes is known.

11.5 Test of Significance of the Difference Between Two Proportions
This section illustrates that, since the difference between two proportions is approximately normally distributed, a hypothesis test for the difference may be easily set up.

11.6 Confidence Intervals
Confidence intervals for p and $p_1 - p_2$ are discussed and illustrated.

Learning Objectives

After studying this chapter, you should be able to

1. Compute the mean and the standard deviation of a binomial distribution
2. Compute Z scores for specific points on a binomial distribution
3. Perform significance tests of a binomial proportion and of the difference between two binomial proportions
4. Calculate confidence intervals for a binomial proportion and for the difference between two proportions

11.1 Introduction

Is there a significant difference in the risk of death from leukemia between males and females? Is the proportion of persons who smoke now less than it was at the time of publication of the Surgeon General's Report on the hazards of smoking? These are typical of questions that cannot be easily answered by the methods discussed in the previous chapters. Why not? The methods previously discussed are applicable to **quantitative** data such as height, weight, and blood pressure for which a mean and standard error can be computed. The new questions deal with **qualitative** data, data for which individual quantitative measurements are not available, but which relate to the presence or absence of some characteristic such as smoking. For these data we have a new statistic, $\hat{p}$ (read "p-hat"), the estimate of the proportion of individuals who possess a certain characteristic. Previously we dealt with $\bar{x}$, the mean value of some characteristic for a group of individuals.

This chapter focuses on (1) the mean and the standard deviation of x, the number of successful events in a binomial experiment, and (2) the mean and the standard error of $\hat{p}$, the proportion of successful events. To best understand the difference between the distribution of binomial events (x) and the distribution of the **binomial proportion** ($\hat{p}$), try comparing these distributions to those in the analogous quantitative situation. The x's of a binomial distribution correspond to the quantitative x's in a distribution with a mean μ and a standard deviation σ. The $\hat{p}$'s of the binomial correspond to the $\bar{x}$'s in a distribution with a mean $\mu_{\bar{x}}$ and a standard error $\sigma/\sqrt{n}$.

This chapter considers the tests of significance for proportions, differences between two proportions, and the confidence intervals for both.

11.2 Mean and Standard Deviation of the Binomial Distribution

In Chapter 5 we learned that the probability of x successful outcomes in n independent trials is given by

$$\binom{n}{x}p^x(1-p)^{n-x}$$

where p is the probability of a success in one individual trial.

Using mathematical statistics, we can show that in a binomial distribution the mean for the number of successes, x, is

$$\mu = np \tag{11.1}$$

? standard error (Ross)

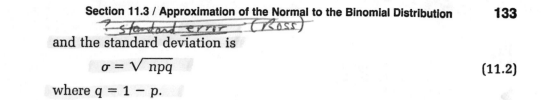

and the standard deviation is

$$\sigma = \sqrt{npq} \tag{11.2}$$

where $q = 1 - p$.

11.3 Approximation of the Normal to the Binomial Distribution

The normal distribution is a reasonable approximation to the binomial when n is large. Therefore we can find the point on the Z distribution that corresponds to a point x on the binomial distribution by using

$$Z = \frac{x - np}{\sqrt{npq}} \tag{11.3}$$

In Chapter 5 we showed that when the number of trials or cases is greater than 30, it would be quite cumbersome to evaluate the binomial expansion to find the exact probability of the occurrence of a certain event. Mathematical statisticians have demonstrated that the continuous normal distribution is a good approximation to the discrete binomial. Hence, with the use of the well-known equations for the mean and the standard deviation 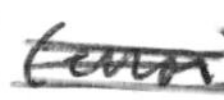 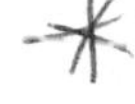 of the binomial distribution, it is a simple task to approximate the probability of a binomial event.

EXAMPLE 1

■ A group of physicians treated 25 cases of chronic leukemia, a disease for which the five-year survival rate was known to be .20. They observed that 9 of their patients had survived for five years or more. They wanted to know whether such an event was unusual. What is the probability, out of 25 cases, of observing 9 or more "successes" (i.e., survival for five or more years)?

First, we compute the mean and the standard deviation:

$$\mu = np = (25)(.2) = 5$$

$$\sigma = \sqrt{npq} = \sqrt{25(.2)(.8)} = 2$$

Then we compute the Z score:

$$Z = \frac{x - np}{\sqrt{npq}} = \frac{9 - 5}{\sqrt{25(.2)(.8)}} = \frac{4}{2} = 2.0$$

The result: 9 five-year survivals on the binomial corresponds to a Z of 2.0 on the normal distribution, as shown in Figure 11.1 (p. 134). The area beyond $Z = 2.0$ is .023. Therefore, the probability of five-year survival for at least 9 of 25 patients is .023, whereas the probability of five-year survival for 1 is .20. ■

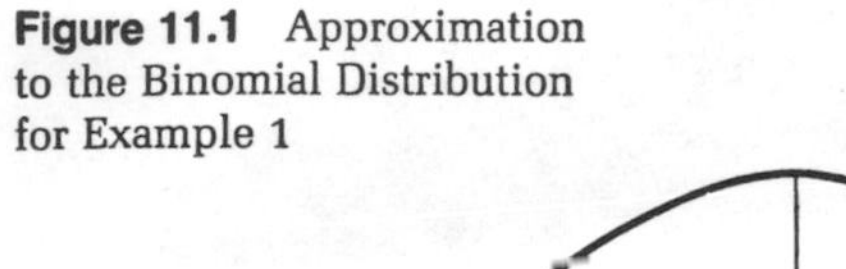

Figure 11.1 Approximation to the Binomial Distribution for Example 1

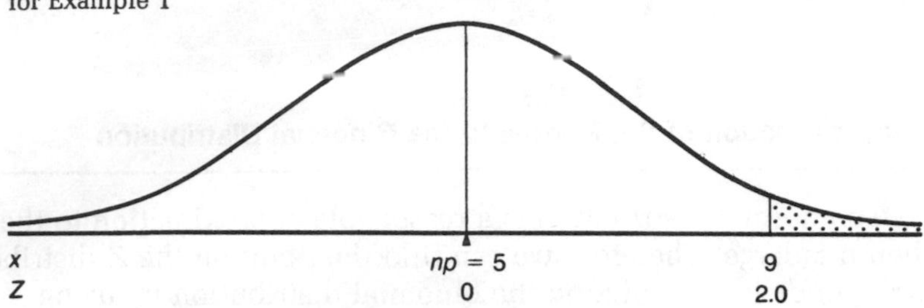

When n is very large and p is very small, another important distribution, the **Poisson distribution,** is a good approximation to the binomial. It deals with discrete events that occur infrequently. For a treatment of this subject, see more advanced textbooks, such as Armitage (1971).

11.4 Test of Significance of a Binomial Proportion

The previous section considered the distribution of the binomial event x. This section considers the distribution of the binomial proportion $\hat{p}$, which is similar to considering the distribution of $\bar{x}$ for quantitative data.

The mean of the distribution of a binomial proportion $\hat{p}$ is given by the population parameter

$$p = \frac{x}{n} = \frac{\text{number of successes in the population}}{\text{number of cases in the population}} \tag{11.4}$$

and the standard error of $\hat{p}$ is given by

$$\sigma_{\hat{p}} = \sqrt{\frac{pq}{n}} \tag{11.5}$$

Since $\hat{p}$ appears to be normally distributed, providing n is reasonably large (i.e., np and nq are both greater than 5), we can find the Z score corresponding to a particular $\hat{p}$ and perform a test of significance.

EXAMPLE 2

■ There were 245 deaths from leukemia in California in 1977. Of these 145 were males,

$$\hat{p} = \frac{145}{245} = .59$$

and 100 were females,

$$\hat{q} = \frac{100}{245} = .41$$

Is .59, the observed proportion of male deaths, significantly different from the expected .49, the proportion of males in the California population?

$$p = .49 \qquad q = .51 \qquad n = 245$$

$$\text{SE}(\hat{p}) = \sqrt{\frac{pq}{n}} = \sqrt{\frac{(.49)(.51)}{245}} = .032$$

Using the steps of a test of a hypothesis, we get the following results:

1. H_0: $p = .49$; there is no sex difference in the proportion of deaths.
2. $\alpha = .05$.
3. Test statistic:

$$Z = \frac{\hat{p} - p}{\text{SE}(\hat{p})} = \frac{.59 - .49}{.032} = \frac{.10}{.032} = 3.12 \qquad (11.6)$$

4. Critical region: From the Z distribution (Table 7.2), we find Z is ± 1.96 (Figure 11.2).
5. The computed Z of 3.12 is greater than the critical value of 1.96, so we reject the null hypothesis that the proportion of deaths from leukemia is the same for both sexes and conclude that the risk of dying from this disease is greater for males than for females. ■

11.5 Test of Significance of the Difference Between Two Proportions

In practice you seldom have a convenient population proportion for comparison. More commonly, you will be called upon to compare pro-

Figure 11.2 Critical Region for Example 2

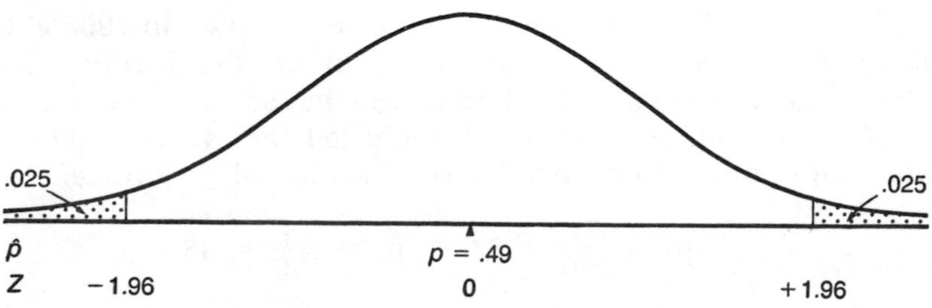

portions from two different samples, possibly one from a control group and the other from a treatment group. In such a case, you want to learn if $\hat{p}_1$, the proportion with the given characteristic in one sample, differs significantly from $\hat{p}_2$, the proportion with the same characteristic in the other sample. To do this, you need to know the distribution of the differences $(\hat{p}_1 - \hat{p}_2)$ and the mean and the standard error of this distribution. Mathematical statisticians have shown that $\hat{p}_1 - \hat{p}_2$ follows a nearly normal distribution. The mean is

$$\mu = \hat{p}_1 - \hat{p}_2 \tag{11.7}$$

The standard error is

$$SE(\hat{p}_1 - \hat{p}_2) = \sqrt{\frac{p'q'}{n_1} + \frac{p'q'}{n_2}} \tag{11.8}$$

where

$$p' = \frac{x_1 + x_2}{n_1 + n_2} \quad \text{and} \quad q' = 1 - p' \tag{11.9}$$

and

$$\hat{p}_1 = \frac{x_1}{n_1} \tag{11.10}$$

and

$$\hat{p}_2 = \frac{x_2}{n_2} \tag{11.11}$$

Knowing the mean and the standard error of the distribution of differences, we can calculate a Z score:

$$Z = \frac{\hat{p}_1 - \hat{p}_2 - (p_1 - p_2)}{SE(\hat{p}_1 - \hat{p}_2)} \tag{11.12}$$

EXAMPLE 3

■ A public health official wishes to know how effective health education efforts are regarding smoking. Of 100 males sampled in 1965 at the time of release of the Surgeon General's Report on the Health Consequences of Smoking, 51 were found to be smokers. In 1980 a second random sample of 100 males, similarly gathered, indicated that 43 were smokers. Is the reduction in proportion from .51 to .43 statistically significant?

$$\hat{p}_1 = \frac{51}{100} = .51 \qquad \hat{p}_2 = \frac{43}{100} = .43$$

$$p' = \frac{51 + 43}{100 + 100} = \frac{94}{200} = .47$$

$$\text{SE}(\hat{p}_1 - \hat{p}_2) = \sqrt{\frac{(.47)(.53)}{100} + \frac{(.47)(.53)}{100}}$$

$$= \sqrt{.004982} = .071$$

Again we apply the steps for a hypothesis test:

1. $H_0: p_1 - p_2 \leq 0$ (there has not been a reduction in smoking) versus $H_1: p_1 - p_2 > 0$ (there has been a reduction).
2. $\alpha = .05$.
3. Test statistic:

$$Z = \frac{\hat{p}_1 - \hat{p}_2 - 0}{\text{SE}(\hat{p}_1 - \hat{p}_2)} = \frac{.51 - .43}{.071} = \frac{.08}{.071} = 1.13$$

4. Critical region: The Z distribution (Table 0.1) shows $Z > 1.64$.
5. The computed Z of 1.13 is less than the critical value of 1.64. Consequently, on the basis of the information of this sample, the official cannot reject the null hypothesis that there has not been a significant reduction in cigarette smoking 15 years after publication of the Surgeon General's Report. ■

11.6 Confidence Intervals

Although hypothesis testing is useful, we often need to go another step to learn, say, the true proportion of male smokers in 1980 or the true difference in the proportion of male smokers between 1980 and 1965. To deal with such questions, we compute confidence intervals for p and for $p_1 - p_2$ by employing a method parallel to the one used for computing confidence intervals for μ and $\mu_1 - \mu_2$.

Confidence Interval for *p*

In Chapter 8 we found the confidence interval of μ to be

$$\bar{x} \pm Z \frac{\sigma}{\sqrt{n}}$$

Similarly, the confidence interval for p is

$$\hat{p} \pm Z \sqrt{\frac{pq}{n}}$$

This expression presents a dilemma: it requires that we know p, which is unknown. The way out of this puzzle is to have a sufficiently large sample size, permitting the use of $\hat{p}$ as an estimate of p. The expression then becomes

$$\hat{p} \pm Z\sqrt{\frac{\hat{p}\hat{q}}{n}} \tag{11.13}$$

The solution for small sample sizes is known but is beyond the scope of this book.

EXAMPLE 4

■ In the previous example the public health official estimated that the proportion of male smokers in 1980 was .43. As this was only a sample estimate, the official also needed to obtain a confidence interval to bracket the true p and therefore calculated as follows:

$$95\%\text{ CI for } p = \hat{p} \pm 1.96\sqrt{\frac{\hat{p}\hat{q}}{n}}$$

$$= .43 + 1.96\sqrt{\frac{(.43)(.57)}{100}}$$

$$= .43 \pm .097$$

$$= (.33, .53)$$

The official now could have 95% confidence that the true proportion of male smokers in 1970 was between .33 and .53. ■

Confidence Interval for the Difference of $p_1 - p_2$

The confidence interval for the difference of two means is

$$\text{CI for } \mu_1 - \mu_2 = \bar{x}_1 - \bar{x}_2 \pm Z[\text{SE}(\bar{x}_1 - \bar{x}_2)]$$

The confidence interval for the difference of two proportions is similar:

$$\text{CI for } p_1 - p_2 = \hat{p}_1 - \hat{p}_2 \pm Z\sqrt{\frac{\hat{p}_1\hat{q}_1}{n_1} + \frac{\hat{p}_2\hat{q}_2}{n_2}} \tag{11.14}$$

EXAMPLE 5

■ To find the confidence interval on the true difference between male smokers in 1980 and 1965, the public health official would perform the following calculation:

$$95\%\text{ CI for } p_1 - p_2 = \hat{p}_1 - \hat{p}_2 \pm 1.96\sqrt{\frac{\hat{p}_1\hat{q}_1}{n_1} + \frac{\hat{p}_2\hat{q}_2}{n_2}}$$

$$= .51 - .43 \pm 1.96 \sqrt{\frac{.51(.49)}{100} + \frac{.43(.57)}{100}}$$

$$= .080 \pm .138$$

$$= (-.058, .218)$$

These figures would give the official 95% confidence that the change in percentage of smokers may have ranged from an increase of 5.8% to a reduction of 21.8% over the 15-year period. ■

Conclusion

The normal approximation to the binomial is a useful statistical tool. It helps answer questions regarding qualitative data involving proportions where individuals are classified into two categories. The mean and the standard deviation are, respectively, $\mu = np$ and $\sigma = \sqrt{npq}$, giving a Z score of $(x - np)/\sqrt{npq}$. With an understanding of the distribution of the binomial proportion $\hat{p}$ and of the distribution of the difference between two proportions, $\hat{p}_1 - \hat{p}_2$, we are enabled to perform tests of significance and calculate confidence intervals.

Vocabulary List

binomial proportion
Poisson distribution

Exercises

p. 22

11.1 For the Honolulu Heart Study data of Table 3.1, compute
(a) the proportion of individuals in each education category
(b) the proportion of smokers and nonsmokers
(c) the proportion for each physical activity level

11.2 Using your results from Exercise 11.1b, calculate estimates of the mean and the standard deviation of the proportion of smokers.

11.3 Given that the proportion of smokers in the United States is .31, test to see if the proportion of smokers in Honolulu is significantly different from the national proportion. Use $\alpha = .05$.

n = 100

11.4 What is the 95% confidence interval for the proportion of smokers in Honolulu for 1969? Refer to Exercise 11.1b.

11.5 In a study of hypertension and taste acuity, one variable of interest was smoking status. Of the 7 persons in the hypertensive group, 4 were smokers. The control group of 21 normotensive persons included 7 smokers. Is there a difference in the proportion of smokers in the two groups at the .05 level of significance?

11.6 Construct a 90% confidence interval for the difference in the proportions of smokers in the hypertensive and normotensive groups of Exercise 11.5.

11.7 In a study of longevity in a village in Ecuador, 29 persons in a population of 99 were age 65 or older. If it is also known that 20% of the U.S. population is 65 or over, does it appear that the proportion of Ecuadorian villagers surviving to 65 and beyond exceeds that of people in the United States? Use $\alpha = .01$.

11.8 Calculate a 99% confidence interval for the proportion of Ecuadorians (Exercise 11.7) who are age 65 or over.

11.9 Of 186 participants in a program to control heart disease, it was discovered that 102 had education beyond secondary school. Does this indicate that the program is attracting a more highly educated group of people than would be expected, given that 25% of the U.S. population has education beyond secondary school? Use $\alpha = .01$.

11.10 In a study of drug abuse among adults, 55 of 219 "abusers" and 117 of 822 "nonusers" stated they started smoking cigarettes at age 12 or younger. Do these data indicate there is a significant difference in the proportions of abusers and nonusers who took up smoking at an early age?

11.11 In a dental study of a tie between infant occlusion and feeding methods, there were 27 breast-fed and 60 bottle-fed infants. It was noted that 7 of the breast-fed babies and 26 of the bottle-fed babies developed a related open-bite gum pad in the first four months of life. Would you conclude that the bottle-fed group showed a higher proportion of the open-bite gum pad problem? Use $\alpha = .05$.

11.12 Compute the following confidence intervals for the difference in proportions, $p_1 - p_2$:

(a) 99% CI for Exercise 11.10

(b) 95% CI for Exercise 11.11

Chapter **12**

The Chi-Square Test

Chapter Outline

12.1 Rationale for the Chi-Square Test
The chi-square test is introduced as the appropriate tool for working with frequency or qualitative data.

12.2 The Basics of a Chi-Square Test
It is illustrated why the chi-square test is a popular way of testing the difference between observed and expected frequencies.

12.3 Types of Chi-Square Tests
Four types of chi-square tests are listed.

12.4 Test of Association Between Two Variables
The first type of chi-square test is illustrated with an example regarding associations between smoking and drinking during pregnancy.

12.5 Test of Homogeneity
The second type of chi-square test is illustrated with an example from the Loma Linda Fetal Alcohol Syndrome Study.

12.6 Test of Significance of the Difference Between Two Proportions
The controversy over the use of Vitamin C to prevent the common cold is used to illustrate the third type of chi-square test.

12.7 Test of Goodness of Fit
The fourth type of chi-square test, which measures the goodness of fit to a model, is described.

12.8 Two-by-Two Contingency Tables
An equation is given that directly provides a chi-square value for tables with 1 df.

12.9 Measures of Strength of Association
Two measures of the strength of association—relative risk and the phi coefficient—are described.

12.10 Limitations in the Use of Chi-Square
It is explained how certain constraints can prevent the misapplication of chi-square tests.

Learning Objectives

After studying this chapter, you should be able to

1. Indicate the kinds of data and circumstances that call for a chi-square test
2. Compute the expected value for a chi-square contingency table
3. Compute a chi-square statistic and its appropriate degrees of freedom
4. Explain the meaning of degrees of freedom
5. Indicate the type of hypothesis that can be tested with chi-square
6. Find the critical region for a chi-square test
7. Compute two different measures of the strength of association of factors reported in 2 × 2 tables

12.1 Rationale for the Chi-Square Test

Although the *t* test is popular and widely used, it may not be appropriate for certain health science problems that call for tests of significance. As the *t* test requires data that are quantitative, it is simply not applicable to qualitative data. In other chapters, whenever means or standard deviations were computed, we worked with measurement data. With such data, we were able to record a specific value for each observation. These represented quantitative variables such as height, weight, and cholesterol level. But we are often obliged to classify persons into such categories as male or female, hypertensive or normotensive, and smoker or nonsmoker, and to count the number of observations falling in each category. The result is **frequency data.** In addition, we often have to deal with **enumeration data,** because we enumerate the number of persons in each category; **categorical data,** because we count the number of persons falling into each category; and, as mentioned earlier, **qualitative data,** because we group the categories according to some quality of interest.

Categorical data are not used to quantify, for example, blood pressure levels, but to classify persons as hypertensive or normotensive. The classification table used is called a **contingency table.** Its use, though, does not permit us to determine whether there is a relationship between two variables by means of a correlation coefficient, because we don't have quantitative *x* and *y* observations for each person. Instead, we could perform a **chi-square test** to determine whether there is some association between the two variables. This chapter considers various chi-square tests to deal with such a case and related ones for frequency data.

12.2 The Basics of a Chi-Square Test

For a given phenomenon, the chi-square test compares the **observed frequencies** with the **expected frequencies.** The expected frequency is

Table 12.1 Observed and Expected Frequencies and Their Deviations for 100 Tosses of a Coin

	(1)	(2)	(3)	(4)	(5)
	O	E	O − E	$(O - E)^2$	$\frac{(O - E)^2}{E}$
H	40	50	−10	100	2
T	60	50	10	100	2
Total	100	100	0	200	4

calculated from some hypothesis. To illustrate, let's take the simple example of trying to determine whether a coin is fair.

Suppose you toss a coin 100 times and you observe that heads (H) come up 40 times and tails (T) 60 times. If you hypothesize that the coin is fair, you would expect heads and tails to occur equally, that is, 50 times each. In comparing the observed frequency (*O*) with the expected frequency (*E*), you need to determine whether the *deviations* (*O* − *E*) are significant. As you can see in Table 12.1, if you were to sum the deviations, the total would equal zero, as indicated in column 3.

To avoid this problem, you might first square each deviation, as in column 4. This approach has a problem, too: the same value is obtained for equal deviations regardless of magnitude. For instance, consider *O* − *E* for two possibilities: 60 − 50 = 10 and 510 − 500 = 10. Arithmetically, the deviations are identical, but they are far from identical in meaning; although a deviation of 10 from an expected 50 is impressive, the same deviation from an expected 500 is hardly noticeable. The best way of overcoming this problem is to look at the proportional squared deviations, $(O - E)^2/E$. Here, the two possibilities become (60 − 50)/50 = .20 and (510 − 500)/500 = .02. Now the deviations offer a more meaningful statistical perspective. From column 5 of Table 12.1 it is seen that for the coin problem, the sum of the proportional squared deviations is equal to 4.

The next question is whether the value we have just calculated,

$$\sum\frac{(O - E)^2}{E} = 4$$

can occur easily by chance or whether it is an unusual event that is unlikely to occur by chance except in rare instances, say less than 5% of the time. To resolve this question, we need to know how the quantity, designated as χ^2 (chi-square), is distributed. That is, we have to determine the probability distribution for the statistic

$$\chi^2 = \sum\frac{(O - E)^2}{E} \tag{12.1}$$

Mathematical statisticians have shown that this quantity is approximated quite well by the **chi-square distribution.** This distribution is positively skewed, beginning at zero. By figuring out the area beyond 4 on a chi-square distribution, we can determine a *p* value and either accept or reject the hypothesis.

There is, in fact, a family of chi-square distributions. The correct one to use depends, as in the *t* distribution, on the degrees of freedom. For chi-square, degrees of freedom are determined as the number of *independent* deviations (each $O - E$) in the contingency table. A two-cell table (e.g., Table 12.1) has 1 df. Wherever you can determine expected frequencies from your hypothesis, the degrees of freedom are one less than the number of categories. The coin problem has two categories, heads and tails, so there is 1 df. If you were trying to determine whether a six-sided die was unbiased, you would have $6 - 1 = 5$ df.

In Figure 12.1 you can see the shapes of several chi-square distributions. For each, the upper 5% of the area is shaded. Note that as the degrees of freedom increase, so does the critical value needed to reject a null hypothesis. Intuitively, this sounds right: since the degrees of freedom are proportional to the number of independent categories, you would well expect the critical chi-square value to increase with more categories.

Table 12.2 gives the critical values for the chi-square distribution for various degrees of freedom. Here you can see that the upper 5% chi-square value for 1 df is 3.84, for 4 df is 9.49, and for 6 df is 12.59.

Figure 12.1 The Chi-Square Distribution for Varying Degrees of Freedom

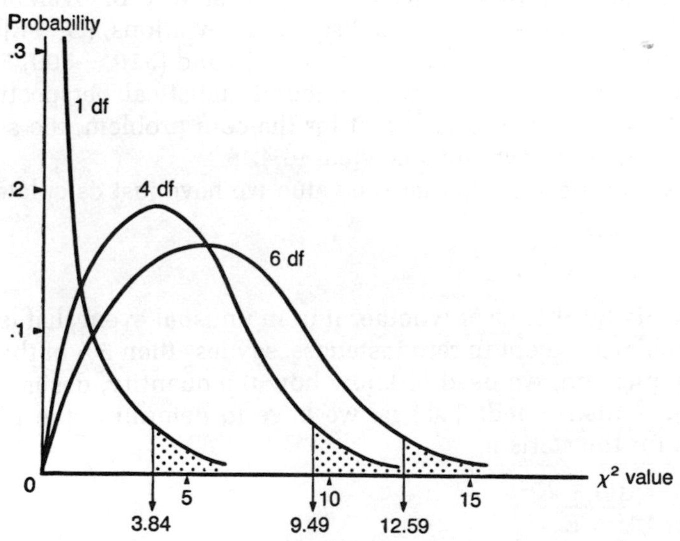

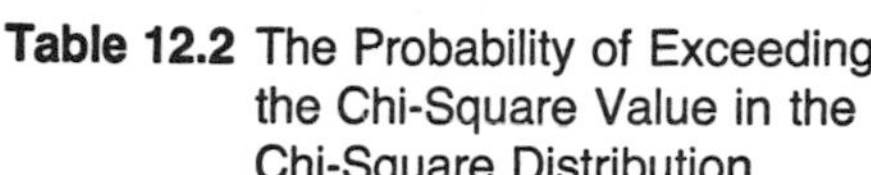
Table 12.2 The Probability of Exceeding the Chi-Square Value in the Chi-Square Distribution

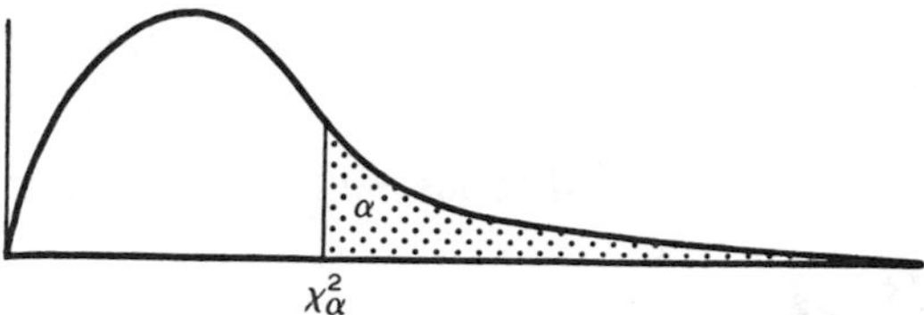

	α							
df	.99	.95	.90	.50	.10	.05	.01	.001
1	.00157	.00393	.0158	.455	2.706	3.841	6.635	10.827
2	.0201	.103	.211	1.386	4.605	5.991	9.210	13.815
3	.115	.352	.584	2.366	6.251	7.815	11.345	16.226
4	.297	.711	1.064	3.357	7.779	9.488	13.277	18.467
5	.554	1.145	1.610	4.351	9.236	11.070	15.806	20.515
6	.872	1.635	2.204	5.348	10.645	12.592	16.812	22.457
7	1.239	2.167	2.833	6.346	12.017	14.067	18.475	24.322
8	1.646	2.733	3.490	7.344	13.362	15.507	20.090	26.125
9	2.088	3.325	4.168	8.343	14.684	16.919	21.666	27.877
10	2.558	3.940	4.865	9.342	15.987	18.307	23.209	20.588
11	3.053	4.575	5.578	10.341	17.275	19.675	24.725	31.264
12	3.571	5.226	6.304	11.340	18.549	21.026	26.217	32.909
13	4.107	5.892	7.042	12.340	19.812	22.362	27.688	34.528
14	4.660	6.571	7.790	13.339	21.064	23.685	29.141	36.123
15	5.229	7.261	8.547	14.339	22.307	24.996	30.578	37.697
20	8.260	10.581	12.443	19.337	28.412	31.410	37.566	43.315
30	14.953	18.493	20.599	29.336	40.256	43.773	50.892	59.703
40	22.164	26.509	29.051	39.335	51.805	55.759	63.691	73.402
50	29.707	34.764	37.689	49.335	63.167	67.505	76.154	86.661
60	37.485	43.188	46.459	59.335	74.397	79.082	88.379	99.607

Back to our original question: "Is the coin fair?" Recall that the χ^2 sum was 4. For 1 df, this falls within the upper 5% critical region. Therefore you would reject the H_0 that the coin is fair. That is, you would not expect to observe a deviation as large as (or larger than) this to occur by chance alone. Your conclusion: the coin is probably unbalanced or loaded. A point to note is that the chi-square test, unlike some others, is a one-tailed test. The rationale for this is that we are almost always concerned only about whether the deviations are too large, seldom about whether they are too small. For example, we would worry about a dangerously high level of air pollution, but certainly not about too low a level.

12.3 Types of Chi-Square Tests

In practical applications, you will often encounter problems involving two variables. Specifically, you may employ chi-square tests to determine

1. An association (if any) between the two variables
2. Whether various subgroups are homogeneous

3. Whether there is a significant difference between two proportions
4. How well observed data fit the parameters of a specified model

We will discuss each of these tests.

12.4 Test of Association Between Two Variables

Kuzma and Kissinger (1981) published a study of the effects that maternal use of alcohol during pregnancy have on the newborn. Some of their data, regarding smoking and drinking, are shown in Table 12.3. Here you can see that 30.5% of the nondrinking women and 67.3% of the heaviest drinkers smoked during their pregnancies. We might wonder whether drinking and smoking are dependent variables and whether this relationship is explainable by chance. A way to approach this question is to test the null hypothesis that there is no relationship between smoking and drinking during pregnancy. To do this, we need to know the expected values before we can compute a χ^2 statistic. Expected values can be generated from the null hypothesis that states there is no relationship between drinking and smoking during pregnancy.

For purposes of this discussion, we set up a special notation, in which the eight cells of Table 12.3 are identified as $E_{11}, \ldots, E_{24}$, as shown in Table 12.4. The probability multiplication rule states that the probability of two independent events A and B is $P(A \text{ and } B) = P(A)P(B)$.

We are testing the hypothesis that the two variables are independent. Therefore we can apply the multiplication rule to obtain the frequencies expected if the hypothesis of independence is indeed true. That is, from the data in Table 12.4, the probability of a woman's being in the smoking group (A) *and* in the nondrinking group (B) is

$$P(A)P(B) = \left(\frac{4{,}198}{11{,}127}\right)\left(\frac{6{,}170}{11{,}127}\right) = (.377)(.555) = .2092$$

$$= \left(\frac{T_s}{T}\right)\left(\frac{T_{nd}}{T}\right)$$

Table 12.3 Alcohol Consumption and Smoking Status During Pregnancy for 11,127 Women

Smoking status	Alcohol consumption: None	Low	Medium	High	Total
Smokers	1880 (30.5%)	2048 (45.7%)	194 (53.0%)	76 (67.3%)	4,198 (37.7%)
Nonsmokers	4290 (69.5%)	2430 (54.3%)	172 (47.0%)	37 (32.7%)	6,929 (62.3%)
Total	6170 (55.5%)	4478 (40.2%)	366 (3.3%)	113 (1.0%)	11,127 (100.0%)

Table 12.4 Notation for Expected Frequencies of a Two-Variable Table

Smoking status	Alcohol consumption None	Low	Medium	High	Total
Smokers	E_{11}	E_{12}	E_{13}	E_{14}	T_s
Nonsmokers	E_{21}	E_{22}	E_{23}	E_{24}	T_{ns}
Total	T_{nd}	T_{ld}	T_{md}	T_{hd}	T

where T_s = total smokers and T_{nd} = total nondrinkers. Therefore the expected number of smokers who are also nondrinkers is

$$E_{11} = 11{,}127(.2092) = 2327.8$$

The meaning of E_{11} is what you would expect, assuming the null hypothesis to be true—that 2328 of the smokers would be nondrinkers. Continuing in a parallel fashion, we can obtain expected frequencies for all cells: for low, medium, and high alcohol consumption and for the nonsmoking categories. Thus

$$E_{12} = (.37728)(.40244)(11{,}127) = 1689.4$$

$$E_{13} = (.37728)(.03289)(11{,}127) = 138.1$$

$$E_{24} = (.62272)(.010155)(11{,}127) = 70.4$$

Although it may seem absurd to compute expected values to a fraction of a person, this is often done in order to avoid roundoff error and assure that "expected" and "observed" row totals are identical. All expected frequencies are shown in Table 12.5 (p. 148). Now we can proceed to compute the χ^2 statistic:

$$\chi^2 = \sum\frac{(O-E)^2}{E} = \frac{(1880-2327.8)^2}{2327.8} + \frac{(2048-1689.4)^2}{1689.4}$$

$$+ \frac{(194-138.1)^2}{138.1} + \frac{(76-42.7)^2}{42.7} + \frac{(4290-3842.2)^2}{3842.2}$$

$$+ \frac{(2430-2788.5)^2}{2788.5} + \frac{(172-227.9)^2}{227.9} + \frac{(37-70.4)^2}{70.4} = 338.7$$

Is a χ^2 of 338.7 significant? To find out, we check Table 12.3 for the critical value. But first, we need to know the number of degrees of freedom. In the case of our example, where we don't know the expected frequencies **a priori** (i.e., by deductive reasoning) but have obtained them from the data, the degrees of freedom are equal to $(c-1)(r-1)$ where c is the number of columns and r the number of rows. Here we have 4 columns and 2 rows; therefore df = $(4-1)(2-1) = 3$.

Table 12.5 Observed and Expected Frequency of Alcohol Consumption and Smoking During Pregnancy for 11,127 Women

	Alcohol consumption							
	None		Low		Medium		High	
Smoking status	*O*	*E*	*O*	*E*	*O*	*E*	*O*	*E*
Smokers	1880	2327.8	2048	1689.4	194	138.1	76	42.7
Nonsmokers	4290	3842.2	2430	2788.5	172	227.9	37	70.4
Total	6170		4478		366		113	

From Table 12.2 we find the critical 5% value for 3 df to be 7.8. Since the computed χ^2 of 338.7 falls well into the critical region, we reject the hypothesis of independence between drinking and smoking during pregnancy.

The preceding discussion should help you understand the meaning of degrees of freedom. Please note that the expected values for each category add up to the total observed value for that category. Note also that we could have computed expected values for only three of the eight cells, with the others obtained by subtraction. These three cells represent the three "independent" quantities; that is, the 3 df. The other five quantities are not "independent" since they can be obtained by subtracting the first three from column or row totals.

12.5 Test of Homogeneity

It is often important to determine whether the distribution of a particular characteristic is similar for various groups. To do this, we can perform a chi-square test called a test of homogeneity.

EXAMPLE 1

■ From the alcohol–pregnancy study of Kuzma and Kissinger (1981), we have data on the distribution of drinkers by ethnic group. As shown in Table 12.6, among Caucasians, 51.2% were abstainers, 43.6% light drinkers, 3.9% medium drinkers, and 1.2% heavy drinkers. The percentage distribution is fairly similar among the ethnic groups, except that the Caucasian group includes fewer abstainers and more drinkers in all categories. Is this difference real or due to chance? That is, can we assume that groups of pregnant

Table 12.6 Drinking Status During Pregnancy, by Ethnic Group

	Alcohol consumption									
	None		Light (<1.0 oz*)		Medium (1.0–2.99 oz)		Heavy (≥3.00 oz)		Total	
Ethnicity	*n*	%	*n*	%	*n*	%	*n*	%	*n*	%
Black	411	60.4	253	37.2	12	1.8	5	0.7	681	6.3
Hispanic	1459	64.0	757	33.2	53	2.3	10	0.4	2279	21.2
Caucasian	3732	51.2	3179	43.6	284	3.9	90	1.2	7285	67.7
Other	322	61.6	187	35.8	10	1.9	4	0.8	523	4.9
Total	5924	55.0	4376	40.6	359	3.3	109	1.0	10,768	100.0

*Equivalent ounces of absolute alcohol per day.

women of various ethnicity tend to have essentially the same drinking patterns?

To test for homogeneity, we again need to establish the expected frequencies, this time basing them on a somowhat different rationale than the probability argument used in Section 12.4. Nevertheless, the equations used to obtain expected frequencies are the same. For example, the expected number of abstainers among Caucasian women is computed as

$$E_{13} = \left(\frac{5924}{10{,}768}\right)\left(\frac{7285}{10{,}768}\right)(10{,}768) = 4007.8$$

The other expected frequencies are obtained similarly and are shown in parentheses in Table 12.7. Having the expected frequencies, we can now proceed with the test of significance as follows:

Table 12.7 Observed and Expected Frequencies of Alcohol Intake During Entire Pregnancy, by Ethnic Group

	Alcohol consumption								
	None		Light		Medium		Heavy		
Ethnicity	*O*	E	*O*	E	*O*	E	*O*	E	Total
Black	411	(374.7)	253	(276.8)	12	(22.7)	5	(6.9)	681
Hispanic	1,459	(1,253.8)	757	(926.2)	53	(76.0)	10	(23.1)	2,279
Caucasian	3,732	(4,007.8)	3,179	(2,960.5)	284	(242.9)	90	(73.7)	7,285
Other	322	(287.7)	187	(212.5)	10	(17.4)	4	(5.3)	523
Total	5,924		4,376		359		109		10,768

Figure 12.2 Critical Region for χ^2_9

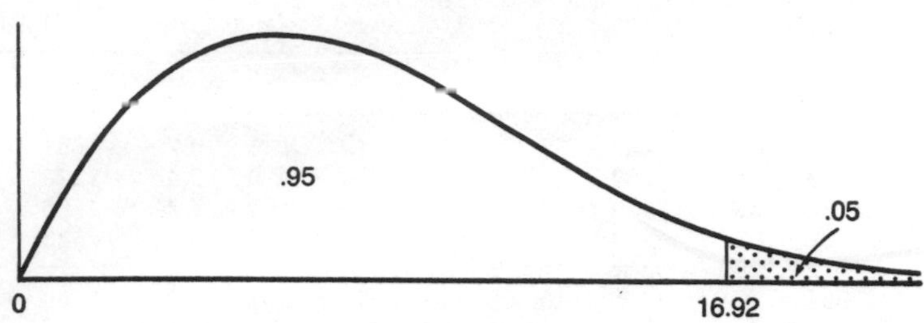

1. H_0: The several ethnic groups are homogeneous in their drinking patterns.
   H_1: The several groups are not homogeneous in their drinking patterns.
2. $\alpha = .05$.
3. Critical region: The critical region for χ^2 with $(c - 1)(r - 1) = (4 - 1)(4 - 1) = 9$ df (denoted as χ^2_9) is shown in Figure 12.2.
4. Test statistic:

$$\chi^2 = \sum \frac{(O - E)^2}{E}$$

$$= \frac{(411 - 374.7)^2}{374.7} + \frac{(253 - 276.8)^2}{276.8} + \cdots + \frac{(4 - 5.3)^2}{5.3}$$

$$= 146.3$$

5. Since the computed χ^2 of 146.3 falls in the critical region, we conclude that the deviations in drinking patterns among the various ethnic groups are not homogeneous. ■

12.6 Test of Significance of the Difference Between Two Proportions

Another application of the chi-square test is in learning whether the proportion of successes in a treated group differs significantly from the proportion in a control group.

EXAMPLE 2

■ For some years there has been a lively medical controversy over the efficacy of vitamin C in preventing the common cold. Several studies concluded that vitamin C was no more effective than a placebo. In Table 12.8, which presents some unpublished data from one such study, we find that 63% of

Table 12.8 Number and Frequencies of Children Developing Colds, by Vitamin C and Placebo Groups

Status	Vitamin C group	Placebo group	Total
Children free of colds	21 (37%)	11 (24%)	32
Children developing colds	36 (63%)	35 (76%)	71
Total	57 (100%)	46 (100%)	n = 103

the children treated with vitamin C and 76% of the placebo group caught colds. Does the number developing colds differ between the two groups?

The expected frequencies for Table 12.8 are

$$E_{11} = \frac{(32)(57)}{103} = 17.7$$

By subtraction, the remaining expected frequencies are $E_{12} = 14.3$, $E_{21} = 39.3$, and $E_{22} = 31.7$. The value of the test statistic is

$$\chi^2 = \sum \frac{(O - E)^2}{E}$$

$$= \frac{(21 - 17.7)^2}{17.7} + \frac{(11 - 14.3)^2}{14.3} + \frac{(36 - 39.3)^2}{39.3} + \frac{(35 - 31.7)^2}{31.7}$$

$$= .61 + .76 + .28 + .34$$

$$= 1.99$$

As before, there are $(c - 1)(r - 1)$ df. In this example, $(c - 1)(r - 1) = 1$. The critical χ^2 at the 5% level for 1 df is 3.84.

The resulting χ^2 of 1.99 is not within the critical region; therefore we fail to reject the hypothesis that the percentage with colds in both groups is the same. So we could logically conclude that, for this size sample, the observed difference of children free of colds between (37% − 24% = 13%) could well have occurred by chance. ■

12.7 Test of Goodness of Fit

Still another hypothesis that lends itself to the chi-square test is the determination of whether a set of data fits a particular model. For example, you might wish to know if your data follow a normal distribution or if a distribution of blood types is consistent with some predetermined standard. To find out, you obtain expected frequencies from the model, calculate the χ^2 statistic, and determine its significance, as in our examples. With a large table consisting of many cells, you can use the following computing equation to speed up the calculation:

$$\chi^2 = \sum \frac{O^2}{E} - N \tag{12.2}$$

where N is the total of all observed frequencies.

12.8 Two-by-Two Contingency Tables

Perhaps the most common chi-square analysis used in health research involves data presented in a 2 × 2 (fourfold) table in which there are two groups and two possible responses. Table 12.9 is a generalized representation of such a table. The observed frequencies are represented symbolically by the letters *a*, *b*, *c*, and *d*. With such data it is possible to compute the χ^2 statistic directly, avoiding the need to compute expected frequencies:

$$\chi^2 = \frac{n(ad - bc)^2}{(a + c)(b + d)(a + b)(c + d)} \tag{12.3}$$

This equation yields the same answer as Equation 12.2, which utilizes expected frequencies.

Thus, using the data on vitamin C in Example 2, we obtain the same result as in that example:

$$\chi^2 = \frac{103[(21)(35) - (11)(36)]^2}{(57)(46)(32)(71)} = 1.99$$

The equations we use to compute χ^2 result in approximations to the chi-square distribution. They are quite close for many degrees of freedom, not too close for few, and not so good for 1 df. As we always use discrete observations to approximate a statistic that is continuously distributed, it is desirable to apply a correction for this. A frequently used solution is the **Yates continuity correction** for chi-squares with 1 df. But it has recently been shown that, although the correction is purported to improve the approximation, it is not always appropriate and consequently should not be used.

Table 12.9 Schematic Representation for 2 × 2 Contingency Table

Response	Treatment	Control	Total
Yes	a	b	$a + b$
No	c	d	$c + d$
	$a + c$	$b + d$	$a + b + c + d = n$

Table 12.10 A 2 × 2 Table for Measuring Relative Risk

Risk factor	Disease present	Disease absent	Total
Present	a	b	$a+b$
Absent	c	d	$c+d$

12.9 Measures of Strength of Association

A popular measure of the strength of an association between two variables is relative risk (RR). Relative risk is widely used in research by clinicians and epidemiologists. This utility results largely from ease of calculation and interpretation.

We can use a generalized 2 × 2 table to represent frequencies for each of the four cells in a table (Table 12.10). Relative risk is defined as the ratio of disease rates for dichotomous exposure groups and is computed using formula 12.4:

$$\mathrm{RR} = \frac{a/(a+b)}{c/(c+d)} \tag{12.4}$$

Another commonly used measure of strength of association is the odds ratio (OR). The odds ratio, sometimes called relative odds, receives wide use in case-control studies and is defined as the ratio of a/b to c/d. Although OR is not based on disease rates, it is a valid measure of strength of association. Under certain circumstances the odds ratio offers an unbiased estimate of relative risk.

EXAMPLE 3

■ In a controversial study into the relationship of coffee consumption and pancreatic cancer, MacMahon et al. (1981) interviewed 369 cancer patients and 644 controls. Their findings, in part, showed that the patients were much more likely than the controls to have been heavy coffee drinkers. The data are shown in Table 12.11.

Table 12.11 A 2 × 2 Table for Measuring Relative Odds

Coffee drinking (cups per day)	Male pancreatic cancer patients	Male controls
≥5	60	82
0	9	32

The relative odds ratio here is computed as

$$o = \frac{ad}{bc} = \frac{(60)(32)}{(82)(9)} = 2.6$$

We would estimate from these results that habitual heavy coffee use increased the risk of pancreatic cancer in men by a factor of 2.6 relative to men who did not drink coffee. (This new finding is still to be confirmed by other studies.) ■

We use relative risk when we have two binomial variables obtained from prospective (but not retrospective) studies. Relative risk is a highly useful concept because it provides a quantitative measure relating a stimulus variable (e.g., coffee use) to an outcome variable (e.g., pancreatic cancer).

A relative risk of 2.0 would indicate that heavy coffee use is associated with a twofold (100%) increase in the risk of pancreatic cancer. So coffee may be an important etiologic factor in that type of cancer. It is thus clear why relative risk is so popular. It serves as a quantitative measure of risk, a means of drawing inferences of clinical significance, given the important proviso that statistical significance has been established.

Another measure of the strength of association between two binomial variables is the **phi (φ) coefficient.** It is obtained from the computed χ^2 as follows:

$$\phi = \frac{ad - bc}{\sqrt{(a+b)(c+d)(a+c)(b+d)}}$$

The absolute values of ϕ vary between 0 and 1. It is similar to the correlation coefficient in that values close to zero indicate a weak association. Values close to unity indicate high predictability. Its usefulness lies in providing a measure of the strength of association, particularly when one has already found that a statistically significant association exists between two variables.

EXAMPLE 4

■ Suppose we want to obtain the ϕ coefficient for the pancreatic cancer data in Example 3. First we compute χ^2 by use of Equation 12.3:

$$\chi^2 = \frac{183[(60)(32) - (82)(9)]^2}{(69)(114)(142)(41)} = 5.58$$

which shows a significant ($p < .025$) relationship between coffee consumption and pancreatic cancer. We then compute ϕ to measure the strength of the association:

$$\phi = \frac{60(32) - 82(9)}{\sqrt{(142)(41)(69)(114)}} = \frac{1182}{6767.3}$$

$$= .174$$

Though the strength of the association is low, our chi-square test indicates that it is significant. ■

12.10 Limitations in the Use of Chi-Square

We previously mentioned that the techniques suggested in this chapter produce values that follow the continuous chi-square distribution. We use discrete data to approximate a continuous distribution. The closeness of the approximation also depends on the frequency size in the various cells of the contingency table. To assure that the approximation is adequate, we follow a basic rule: the expected frequencies must not be too small. What is "small"? Its definition can vary by the type of chi-square test being performed. However, a general rule, well accepted, is that no expected frequency should be less than 1 and not more than 20% of the cells should have an expected frequency of less than 5. If a contingency table violates this rule, a good technique is to merge ("collapse") some rows or columns to increase the frequencies of some of the cells. If the expected frequencies are too small, we should use *Fisher's exact test*, described in texts such as Armitage (1971) and Rimm et al. (1980).

In performing a chi-square test we are not testing a hypothesis regarding some parameter; consequently, there are no confidence intervals. The chi-square test is very popular because it is easy to calculate. It is indeed applicable to a wide variety of applications in the health and medical sciences. But it is sometimes used so frequently that it is subject to misuse. A common misapplication is to compute a χ^2 statistic for data that do not represent independent observations. This happens when one person is included more than once, when a before-and-after experiment is involved, or when multiple responses are recorded for the same person, as in measuring the frequency of decayed or missing teeth. In the last case, there is obviously a lack of independence, because adjacent teeth in someone's mouth are more likely to be affected than are teeth from different mouths. In such a case, independence would be assured by counting the number of individuals and classifying them according to the number of decayed or missing teeth rather than by simply counting the number of teeth.

If you suspect that your data are suffering from lack of independence, a wise move would be to consult an advanced statistics textbook or obtain some help from a statistician. Advanced statistics includes a variety of appropriate methods that can solve almost any problem.

Conclusion

Qualitative data may be analyzed by use of a chi-square test. The object of the test is to determine whether the difference between observed frequencies and those expected from a hypothesis are statistically significant. The test is performed by comparing a computed test statistic, χ^2, with a one-tailed critical value found in a chi-square table. The critical value depends on the selected α and on the number of degrees of freedom, the latter reflecting the number of independent differences as computed from the data. The test statistic is computed as the sum of the ratios of squared differences to expected values. As in other tests of significance, if the computed test statistic exceeds the critical value, the null hypothesis is rejected.

Vocabulary List

a priori
categorical data
chi-square distribution
chi-square test
contingency table
enumeration data
expected frequency
frequency data
observed frequency
phi (ϕ) coefficient
relative risk (odds ratio)
Yates continuity correction

Exercises

12.1 From the Honolulu Heart Study data in Table 3.1, we can develop a number of chi-square tests of association between two factors. The contingency table for one such test is as follows:

Educational level	Smoker	Nonsmoker	Total
None	9	16	25
Primary	15	17	32
Intermediate	12	12	24
Senior high	1	8	9
Technical school	0	10	10
Total	37	63	100

(a) Using $\alpha = .05$, perform the test and determine whether there is an association between the two variables. (You may wish to use Equation 12.2.)

(b) Observe that the limitations of the test, as discussed in Section 12.9, were violated, thus invalidating the conclusion of a significant association. To correct the problem of small numbers, combine the senior high and technical school groups to make a 2×4 table and repeat the test. (Again, Equation 12.2 may be helpful.) Does collapsing the groups change the conclusion?

12.2 As in Exercise 12.1, use Table 3.1 as a source for contingency tables. Test them for associations between the two variables:

(a) Activity status (levels 1 and 2) and smoking status (smokers and nonsmokers). Use $\alpha = .01$.

(b) Activity status (levels 1 and 2) and systolic blood pressure (classify as less than 140 mmHg for group 1 and greater than or equal to 140 mmHg for group 2). Test at $\alpha = .05$. (*Hint*: Use Equation 12.3.)

12.3 A study of diet and age at menarche yielded the following information:

Age of menarche	Egg consumption			
	Never	Once/wk	2–4 times/wk	Daily
Low	5	13	8	4
Medium	4	20	14	0
High	11	18	15	0

(a) Test, at $\alpha = .05$, the hypothesis of independence of the two variables. (*Hint*: Use Equation 12.1.)

(b) Since the expected values indicate a violation of the small numbers limitation of the test, recompute by collapsing the two categories "2–4 times/wk" and "daily" into a new category: "2–7 times/wk." Does the result change your conclusion?

12.4 Perform chi-square tests for significant difference between the two proportions for the following exercises:

(a) 11.5

(b) 11.10

(c) 11.11

12.5 One of the variables considered in *Heartbeat* (a coronary risk reduction program) was age. An important question emerged: Was the age distribution of the participants different from that of the population in the standard metropolitan statistical area (SMSA) where *Heartbeat* was conducted? Perform a chi-square test to answer the question. Use the SMSA population age distribution to compute the expected values.

Age interval	Heartbeat participants	SMSA population (1970)
25–34	18	140,195
35–44	33	125,363
45–54	54	120,826
55–64	48	98,884
65 and over	35	125,884
Total	188	611,152

Chapter **13**

Correlation and Linear Regression

Chapter Outline

13.1 Relationship Between Two Variables
The devilish problem of spurious relationships between variables is introduced.

13.2 Differences Between Correlation and Regression
It is explained why correlation and regression analysis, though kindred subjects, are used to answer different questions.

13.3 The Scatter Diagram
The starting point for plotting two variables is described.

13.4 The Correlation Coefficient
A convenient method to estimate the strength of a linear relationship is presented.

13.5 Tests of Hypotheses and Confidence Belts for a Population Correlation Coefficient
It is illustrated how tests of significance of correlation coefficients can be performed like those of other statistics.

13.6 Limitations of the Correlation Coefficient
The tendency to violate some limitations necessarily imposed on the correlation coefficient is discussed.

13.7 Regression Analysis
It is explained how to determine the algebraic expression that defines the regression line.

13.8 Inferences Regarding the Slope of the Regression Line
Confidence limits and tests of significance are shown to be readily applied to the regression coefficient.

Learning Objectives

After studying this chapter, you should be able to

1. Distinguish between the basic purposes of correlation analysis and regression analysis
2. Plot a scatter diagram

3. Compute and explain the meaning of a correlation coefficient in terms of
   (a) the kind of data it may be used for
   (b) the kind of relationship it can measure
   (c) its limitations
4. Compute and interpret a regression equation
5. Perform a test of significance of a correlation coefficient and of a regression coefficient
6. Find the confidence limits for ρ and β

13.1 Relationship Between Two Variables

Some of our most intriguing scientific questions deal with the relationship between two variables. Is there a relationship between underground nuclear explosions and the increased frequency of earthquakes? Does a relationship exist between use of oral contraceptives and the incidence of thromboembolism? What is the relationship of a mother's weight to her baby's birthweight? These are typical of countless questions we pose in seeking to understand the relationship between two variables.

Whenever an unusual event occurs, people speculate as to its cause. There is an all-too-human tendency to attribute a **cause-and-effect relationship** to variables that *might* be related. Innumerable variables appear to be related to other variables but fail as plausible explanations of causal relationships. For instance, there is a significant association between a child's foot size and handwriting ability, but we would hesitate to claim that a large foot causes better handwriting. A more logical explanation is that foot size and handwriting ability both increase with age; thus the relationship is not causal but indirect and age-dependent. As another example, one investigator reported a high degree of association between increased washing machine sales and admissions to mental institutions. It would require a rather convoluted argument to demonstrate a causal relationship between these two variables.

Spurious associations between variables have so perplexed scientists that one of them, Everett Edington of the California Department of Education, composed a clever essay, "Evils of Pickle Eating" (Figure 13.1), in which he satirizes such relationships. To see how easily one might be deceived into believing that a cause-and-effect relationship, however ridiculous, exists, just exchange "milk," "candy," or "bread" for "pickle" in Edington's lampoon (p. 160).

How, then, can we demonstrate the existence of an actual causal relationship? What statistical methods are available to measure the relationship between two variables?

In previous chapters, we dealt exclusively with observations repre-

Figure 13.1 An Example of Spurious Associations Between Variables

Evils of Pickle Eating

Pickles are associated with all the major diseases of the body. Eating them breeds war and Communism. They can be related to most airline tragedies. Auto accidents are caused by pickles. There exists a positive relationship between crime waves and consumption of this fruit of the cucurbit family. For example . . .

Nearly all sick people have eaten pickles. The effects are obviously cumulative.

. . . 99.9% of all people who die from cancer have eaten pickles.
. . . 100% of all soldiers have eaten pickles.
. . . 96.8% of all Communist sympathizers have eaten pickles.
. . . 99.7% of the people involved in air and auto accidents ate pickles within 14 days preceding the accident.
. . . 93.1% of juvenile delinquents come from homes where pickles are served frequently. Evidence points to the long-term effects of pickle eating.
. . . Of the people born in 1839 who later dined on pickles, there has been a 100% mortality.

All pickle eaters born between 1849 and 1859 have wrinkled skin, have lost most of their teeth, have brittle bones and failing eyesight—if the ills of pickle eating have not already caused their death.

Even more convincing is the report of a noted team of medical specialists: rats force-fed with 20 pounds of pickles per day for 30 days developed bulging abdomens. Their appetites for WHOLESOME FOOD were destroyed.

In spite of all the evidence, pickle growers and packers continue to spread their evil. More than 120,000 acres of fertile U.S. soil are devoted to growing pickles. Our per capita consumption is nearly four pounds.

Eat orchid petal soup. Practically no one has as many problems from eating orchid petal soup as they do with eating pickles.

EVERETT D. EDINGTON

SOURCE: "Evils of Pickle Eating," by Everett D. Edington, originally printed in *Cyanograms*.

senting one variable. In this chapter we will consider the relationship of two variables, x and y, obtained for individuals or particular phenomena. Such pairs are referred to as **bivariate data.** We will discuss the methods of measuring the relationships of bivariate data, determine the strength of the relationships, and make inferences to the population from which the sample was drawn.

13.2 Differences Between Correlation and Regression

The two most common methods used to describe the relationship between two quantitative variables (x and y) are **linear correlation** and **linear regression.** The former is a statistic that measures the strength of a bivariate association; the latter is a **prediction equation** that estimates the value of y for any given x.

When should you use correlation and when regression? Your choice depends on the questions raised and the kind of assumptions you make about the data. For example, you may address questions like "Is there a relationship between IQ and grade-point average? Is there a relationship between the concentration of fluoride in drinking water and the number of cavities in children's teeth?" Such questions are approached by means of the **correlation coefficient,** which is a measure of the strength of the relationship between the two variables, providing the relationship is linear. As we will see in Section 13.4, it is appropriate to compute a correlation coefficient for such data since both x and y may be considered as random variables (i.e., variables that fluctuate in value according to their distribution).

Certain conventions apply to bivariate data. Almost universally, x refers to the **independent** (or **input**) **variable,** because its outcome is independent of the other variable; and y refers to the **dependent** (or **outcome**) **variable** because its response is dependent on the other variable. Suppose you ask, "What change will occur in the number of new cavities after the fluoride level is changed?" Here you would use the regression method, as you are interested in the *degree* of relationship between two variables. The number of cavities would be represented by y, the dependent variable; the fluoride levels by x, the independent variable. You can see from this example that the investigator may arbitrarily select the values of the independent variable and then observe the results of the experiment in terms of the dependent variable y for various levels of x.

To further illustrate the methods of correlation and regression, let's suppose you were interested in studying the relationship of the pre-pregnancy weights of a group of mothers to their infants' birthweights. "How strong," you might ask, "is the association between the mother's weight and her infant's birthweight?" The method of choice is to calculate a correlation coefficient as a measure of the strength of association between these two variables.

On the other hand, if you were to ask, "What would be an infant's predicted birthweight for a mother possessing a known prepregnancy weight?" you would employ linear regression analysis.

13.3 The Scatter Diagram

An ever-popular graphical method used to display the relationship between two variables is the **scatter diagram** (or **scattergram**). The scatter diagram plots each pair of bivariate observations (x, y) that corresponds, respectively, to the point of intersection of the vertical line through the x value on the abscissa and of the horizontal line through the y value on the ordinate. For instance, let's use data from the Loma Linda Fetal Alcohol

Table 13.1 Prepregnancy Weights of Mothers and Birthweights of Their Infants (Based on Sample Size 25)

Case number	Mother's weight (kg)	Infant's birthweight (g)
1	49.4	3515
2	63.5	3742
3	68.0	3629
4	52.2	2680
5	54.4	3006
6	70.3	4068
7	50.8	3373
8	73.9	4124
9	65.8	3572
10	54.4	3359
11	73.5	3230
12	59.0	3572
13	61.2	3062
14	52.2	3374
15	63.1	2722
16	65.8	3345
17	61.2	3714
18	55.8	2991
19	61.2	4026
20	56.7	2920
21	63.5	4152
22	59.0	2977
23	49.9	2764
24	65.8	2920
25	43.1	2693

SOURCE: Loma Linda Fetal Alcohol Syndrome study.

Figure 13.2 Scatter Diagram of Infants' Birthweights Relative to Mothers' Prepregnancy Weights

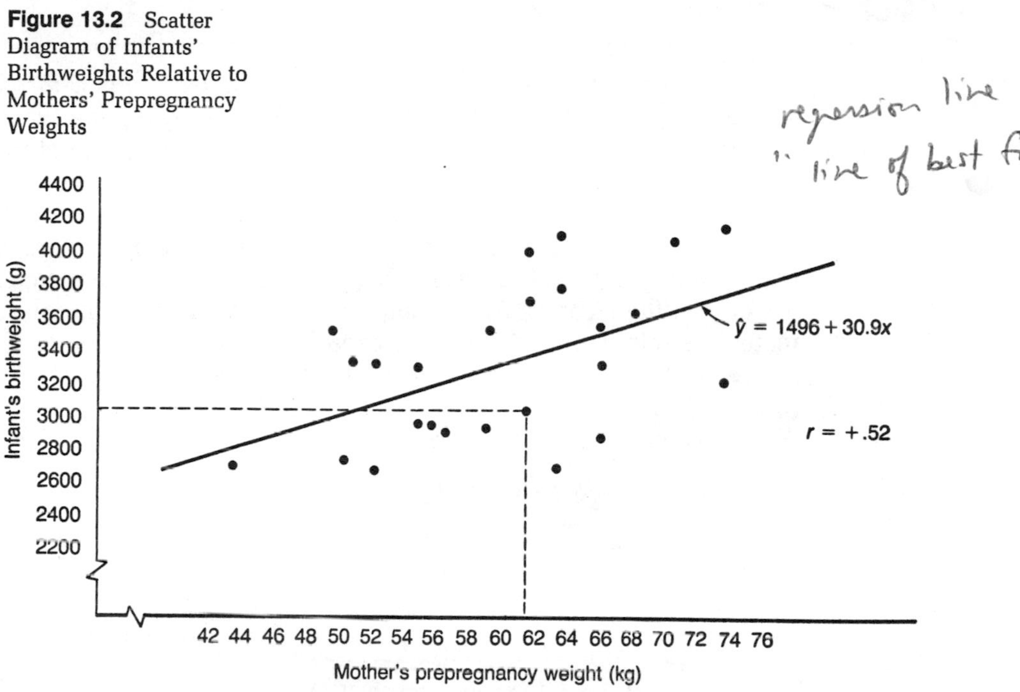

Syndrome study (Kuzma and Sokol, 1982), displayed in Table 13.1. We can make a scatter diagram of these data by plotting on a graph each point corresponding to an (x, y) value (Figure 13.2). Take case 13, for example. The mother's prepregnancy weight was 61.2 kg, and she delivered a baby weighing 3062 g. The point appears on Figure 13.2 where the lines for these values intersect. The diagonal line is called the **regression line** or, sometimes, the **line of best fit.** From this line, we expect women weighing 61.2 kg (prepregnancy) to bear babies weighing about 3400 (precisely 3387) g. But we also expect random variation—and, of course, it happens. Case 13's baby weighed 3062 g, 325 g less than would be expected solely on the basis of the mother's weight. This difference is called the **residual.** More later on the subject of regression.

In examining the data of Figure 13.2, you will notice that there is some sort of a relationship between the mother's prepregnancy weight and the infant's birthweight. Although the relationship is subtle, mothers of low prepregnancy weight are seen generally to bear infants of low birthweights, whereas mothers of high prepregnancy weight generally bear heavier infants. Is the relationship linear? An easy way to tell is to examine its scattergram to see if the trend roughly follows a straight line. How strong is the relationship? To find out, you need to compute an appropriate statistic, such as the correlation coefficient.

13.4 The Correlation Coefficient

As we noted earlier, the correlation coefficient, r, is a measure of the strength of the linear association between two variables, x and y. The correlation coefficient is often referred to as Pearson's product-moment r. It has some unique characteristics. It may take on values between −1 and +1. It is a pure number and nondimensional. That is, it has no units such as centimeters or kilograms. A correlation coefficient of zero represents no relationship between the variables. The closer the coefficient comes to either +1 or −1, the stronger is the relationship and the more nearly it approximates a straight line. A **positive correlation** implies a direct relationship between the variables; a **negative correlation** implies an inverse relationship.

The correlation coefficient is defined by

$$r = \frac{\Sigma(x - \bar{x})(y - \bar{y})}{\sqrt{[\Sigma(x - \bar{x})^2][\Sigma(y - \bar{y})^2]}} \tag{13.1}$$

In computing, we more often use

$$r = \frac{\Sigma xy - \dfrac{(\Sigma x)(\Sigma y)}{n}}{\sqrt{\left[\Sigma x^2 - \dfrac{(\Sigma x)^2}{n}\right]\left[\Sigma y^2 - \dfrac{(\Sigma y)^2}{n}\right]}} \tag{13.2}$$

Another formula, mathematically equivalent but easier to remember because it is defined in terms of the means and standard deviations of x and y, is

$$r = \frac{\Sigma xy - n\bar{x}\bar{y}}{s_x s_y} \tag{13.3}$$

Figure 13.3 illustrates six quite different sets of data and how they are summarized by r. Figure 13.3a illustrates the case of $r = +1.0$, a perfect positive correlation in which all the points fall on a straight line. It is positive because the values of y increase with an increase in x. Figure 13.3b is a perfect negative correlation of $r = -1.0$. All the points again fall on a straight line, but as x increases, y decreases.

In real life, there are always random variations in our observations; hence a perfect linear relationship is extremely rare. Some examples of positive relationships are height and weight, IQ and grade point average, cigarette consumption and heart disease risk. A negative correlation would describe the relationship between the concentration of fluoride in drinking water and the prevalence of cavities in children's teeth.

Although it is no longer 1.0, the correlation coefficient remains high when the points cluster fairly closely around a straight line (Figure 13.3c).

Figure 13.3 Examples of Various Values of r

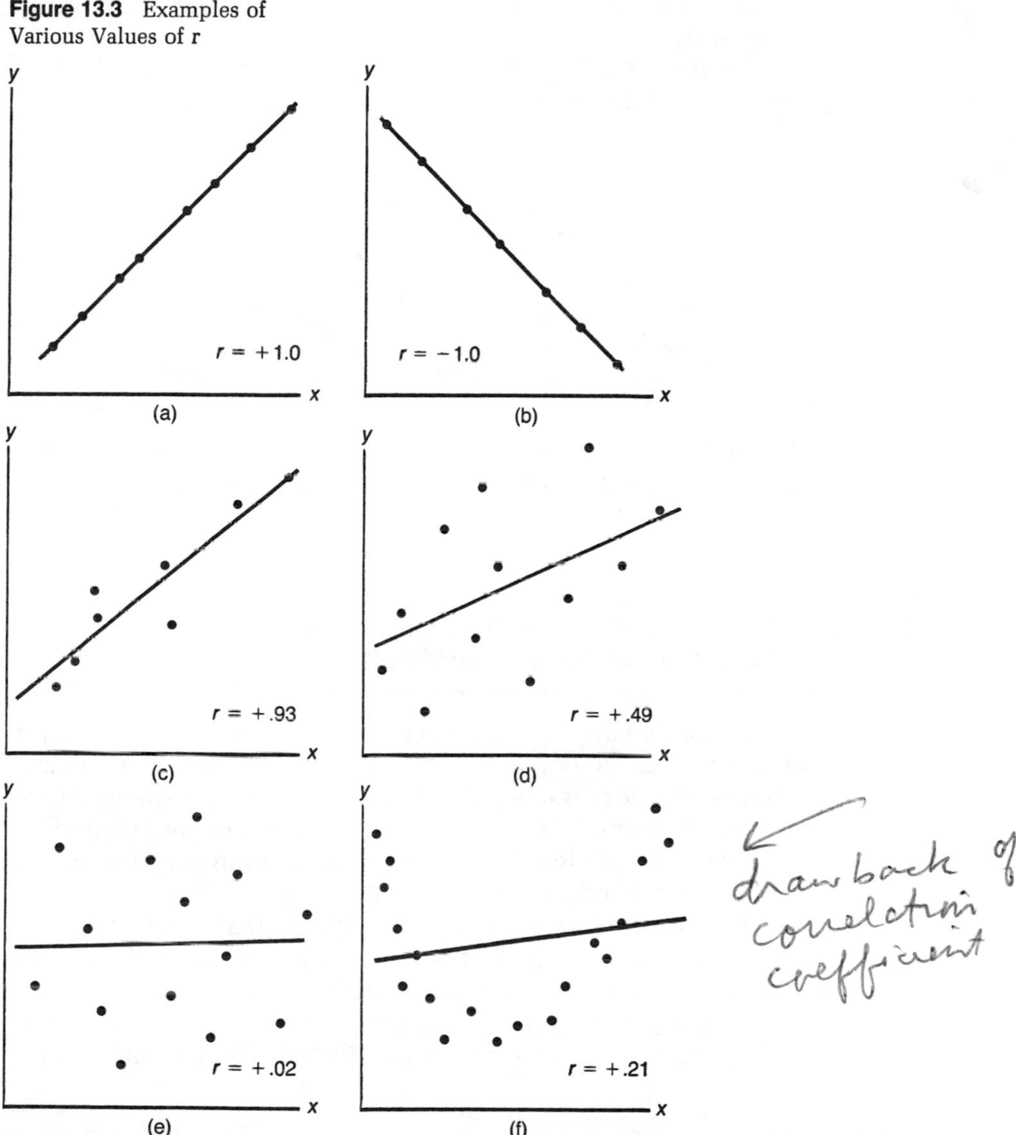

The coefficient becomes smaller and smaller as the distribution of points clusters less closely around the line (Figure 13.3d), and it becomes virtually zero (no correlation between the variables) when the distribution approximates a circle (Figure 13.3e). Figure 13.3f illustrates one drawback of the correlation coefficient: it is ineffective for measuring a relationship that is not linear. In this case we observe a neat curvilinear relationship whose linear correlation coefficient is quite low. This situation occurs because linear correlation tells its user how closely the relationship follows a straight line.

To illustrate the computation of a correlation coefficient, we can apply the data of Table 13.1. Using Equation 13.2, we obtain

$$r = \frac{\Sigma xy - \frac{(\Sigma x)(\Sigma y)}{n}}{\sqrt{\left[\Sigma x^2 - \frac{(\Sigma x)^2}{n}\right]\left[\Sigma y^2 - \frac{(\Sigma y)^2}{n}\right]}}$$

$$= \frac{5{,}036{,}414 - \frac{(1494)(83{,}530)}{25}}{\sqrt{\left[90{,}728 - \frac{(1494)^2}{25}\right]\left[284{,}266{,}104 - \frac{(83{,}530)^2}{25}\right]}} = .52$$

A correlation coefficient of .52 seems to be of moderate magnitude. But to interpret it, we need to answer two questions: What inferences can we make regarding its true value? Is the correlation statistically significant?

13.5 Tests of Hypotheses and Confidence Belts for a Population Correlation Coefficient

As you might expect, the correlation coefficient r is a sample value. It is an estimate of the population correlation coefficient ρ in the same sense that $\bar{x}$ is an estimate of the population mean μ. Since we are most often interested in drawing inferences from a sample to the general population, it is logical to perform a test of significance on the population correlation coefficient and estimate a confidence interval for it.

If you wish to test the null hypothesis that $\rho = 0$ (i.e., x and y are not correlated) against the alternative hypothesis that $\rho \neq 0$, you can use the following procedure. The only needed assumptions: the pairs of observations $(x_1, y_1), (x_2, y_2), \ldots, (x_n, y_n)$ must have been obtained randomly, and both x and y must be normally distributed. The test statistic to use is

$$t = \frac{r - 0}{\sqrt{(1 - r^2)/(n - 2)}} \qquad (13.4)$$

with $n - 2$ df, where n is the number of paired observations.

For our mother–child example,

$$t = \frac{.52}{\sqrt{[1 - (.52)^2]/(25 - 2)}} = 2.92$$

which (by reference to the t table) represents a correlation significantly

($p < .01$) different from zero. Our conclusion: there appears to be a positive association between a woman's prepregnancy weight and her infant's birthweight.

Where did the t statistic of Equation 13.4 come from? Mathematical statisticians are able to make a comparatively simple derivation from other equations, as you will see in Section 13.8.

Computing a confidence interval for ρ involves an equation much more complex than the corresponding one for the population mean. In consequence, tables giving **confidence belts** have been prepared for the convenience of the user. Figure 13.4 (p. 168) illustrates 95% confidence belts for different sample sizes. Suppose you wanted to find the 95% confidence interval for the population correlation coefficient ρ from the mother–child example ($r = .52$, $n = 25$). It's quite simple to do this by using Figure 13.4. Find the r of +.52 on the abscissa and sketch a vertical line through it. The points given by the intersection of that line and the belts for $n = 25$ give the upper and lower 95% confidence limits. Use the curves that correspond to your sample size or visually interpolate. The limits are read on the ordinate, approximately +.10 and +.75. If we can safely assume that our data for the 25 mother–child pairs (Table 13.1) are a random sample of all of the pairs in the study, then the 95% confidence interval for the true population ρ is indeed .10 to .75. Regardless of the true value of the population correlation coefficient, we can draw the inference, with 95% confidence, that it falls within the range .10–.75. Further, the test of the H_0: $\rho = 0$ at the $\alpha = .01$ level indicates that ρ is significantly different from zero because zero falls below the interval .10–.75.

13.6 Limitations of the Correlation Coefficient

As we mentioned, one limitation of the correlation coefficient is that, though it measures how closely the two variables approximate a straight line, it does not validly measure the strength of a nonlinear relationship. We also have to equivocate a bit as to the reliability of the correlation when n is small (say, fewer than about 50 pairs of observations). Further, it is always useful to plot a scattergram (e.g., Figure 13.2) to see if there are any **outliers,** that is, observations that clearly appear to be out of range of the other observations. Outliers have a marked effect on the correlation coefficient, often suggest erroneous data, and are likely to give misleading results. Perhaps the most important drawback of the correlation coefficient is that a high (or statistically significant) correlation can so easily be taken to imply a cause-and-effect relationship. Use caution: don't take it as proof of such a relationship.

With all these reservations, you may be puzzled as to how major

Figure 13.4 Confidence Belts for the Correlation Coefficient $(1 - \alpha = .95)$

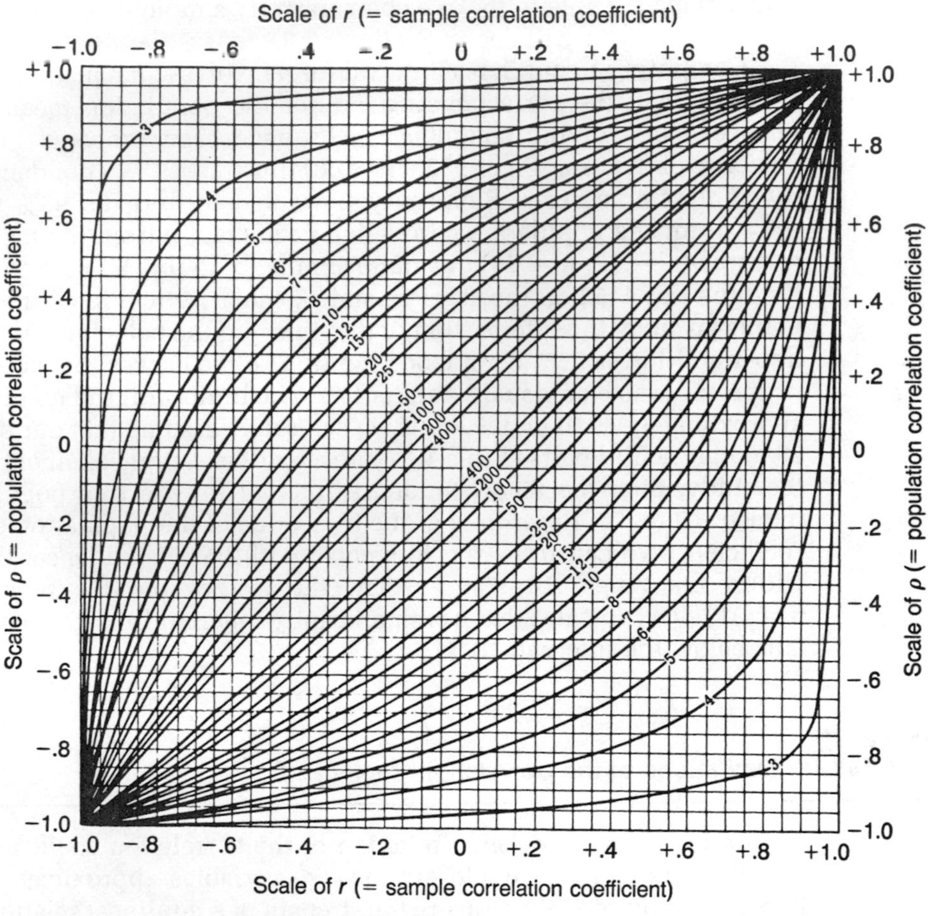

SOURCE: Reprinted with permission from *Handbook of Tables for Probability and Statistics*, ed. William H. Beyer (Boca Raton, Fl.: CRC Press, 1966). Copyright CRC Press, Inc., Boca Raton, Fl.

decisions in public policy can be based on correlation analysis. For instance, in the Surgeon General's Report (1971), we see an important public document that includes a good deal of correlation analysis and concludes that smoking causes lung cancer. In reaching their conclusions, the Surgeon General's blue-ribbon panel of experts (which included leading statisticians) relied heavily on the consistency of the results of a large number of popu-

Table 13.2 Correlation Between Increased Smoking and Increased Death Rate

No. of cigarettes smoked	Mortality ratio of smokers to nonsmokers	Excess in death rate of smokers over nonsmokers
<10	1.45	45%
10–19	1.75	75%
20–39	1.90	90%
40 or more	2.20	120%

lation and laboratory studies. In essence, their conclusion was based not on a single correlation coefficient, but on an overwhelming body of evidence, to wit:

1. The death rate for cigarette smokers was about 70% higher than for nonsmokers.
2. Death rates increased with increased smoking (Table 13.2).
3. The ratio of the death rates of heavy smokers to those of light smokers was greater than 100%.
4. The mortality ratio of cigarette smokers to nonsmokers was substantially higher for those who started to smoke under age 20 than for those who started smoking after age 25. The mortality ratio increased with more years of smoking.
5. The mortality of smokers who inhaled was higher than that of those who didn't.
6. Persons who stopped smoking had a mortality ratio 1.4 times that of persons who never smoked, while current smokers had a ratio of 1.7.
7. In prospective studies it was found that for all causes of death, smokers experienced 70% greater mortality than nonsmokers, but for respiratory system causes the excess was even higher. For lung cancer, it was 10 times higher; for bronchitis and emphysema it was 6.1 times higher.

13.7 Regression Analysis

We are indebted to Sir Francis Galton for coining the term "regression" during his study of heredity laws. He observed that physical characteristics of sons were correlated with those of their fathers. He noted particularly that the heights of sons were less extreme than those of their fathers. Specifically, he found that tall fathers tended to have shorter sons, whereas short fathers tended to have taller sons, a phenomenon he called "regression toward the mean." In plotting median heights of sons and fathers, he found that there was a positive association and that the relationship was roughly linear.

Subsequently, statisticians used means, not medians, and embraced the term **regression line** to describe a linear relationship between two variables. The regression line also indicates prediction of the value of a dependent (outcome) variable (y) from a known value of an independent variable (x), and the expected change in a dependent variable for a unit change in an independent variable. For any two variables, there is a linear equation that best represents the relationship between them. It is often useful to find an estimate of the true equation that describes the straight-line regression. Such an estimate is given by

$$\hat{y} = a + bx \tag{13.5}$$

That is, the dependent variable $\hat{y}$ can be estimated in terms of a constant, a, plus another constant, b, times the independent variable x. Note the important distinction between $\hat{y}$, the predicted value (which falls on the regression line), and y, the observed value that usually does not fall on the line. The constants a and b are estimates of the two parameters of the true regression equation that define the location of the line. Their specific meaning is illustrated in Figure 13.5. The constant a represents the point where the straight line intersects the y axis, while b is the **slope** (or **gradient**) of the line. The slope can be more precisely defined as the amount of change, Δy, in the dependent variable for a given change, Δx, in the independent variable. Thus the slope, often referred to as the **regression coefficient**, gives a good indication of the relationship between variables x and y.

Figure 13.5 Equation of a Straight Line

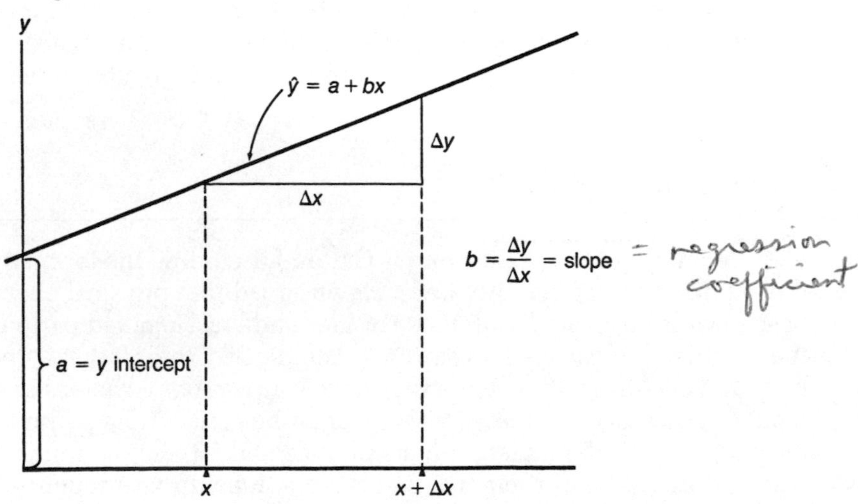

Equation 13.5 is an estimate of the following equation, which describes the population regression of y on x:

$$y = \beta_0 + \beta_1 x + \epsilon$$

where β_0 is the **y-axis intercept** and corresponds to a of Equation 13.5; β_1 is the slope of the population regression line and corresponds to b of Equation 13.5; and ϵ is the error in the observed value of y for a specified value of x. The error, the residual, is estimated by $y - \hat{y}$, the difference between the observed and the predicted value.

Certainly, you would strive to solve regression problems with some equation that provides the "best fit" to the data. But how would you do this? There is a mathematical procedure that minimizes the estimated error $(y - \hat{y})$. It is known as the **least-squares method.** This procedure utilizes equations that estimate β_0 and β_1 by the following equations for a and b. The equation for estimating β_1 is

$$\hat{\beta}_1 = b = \frac{\Sigma(x - \bar{x})(y - \bar{y})}{\Sigma(x - \bar{x})^2} = r_{xy}\frac{s_y}{s_x} \tag{13.6}$$

and the equation for estimating β_0 is

$$\hat{\beta}_0 = a = \bar{y} - b\bar{x} \tag{13.7}$$

Again using our data on mothers' and infants' weights (Table 13.1), we can now compute the slope. For convenience, we proceed using the mathematically identical computation equations:

$$b = \frac{\Sigma xy - [(\Sigma x)(\Sigma y)]/n}{\Sigma x^2 - [(\Sigma x)^2]/n} \tag{13.8}$$

$$= \frac{5{,}036{,}414 - (1{,}494)(83{,}530)/25}{90{,}728 - (1{,}494)^2/25} = 30.87$$

and

$$\begin{aligned} a &= \bar{y} - b\bar{x} \\ &= 3341 - 30.87(59.75) = 1496 \end{aligned} \tag{13.9}$$

Now that we know the values of the two constants, we can write the equation for the best-fitting line of regression:

$$\hat{y} = 1496 + 30.9x$$

Symbolically, $\hat{y}$ is the predicted value for a given value of x. It is actually the mean of all y's that could be observed for a specific value of x.

To illustrate further: Women with a prepregnancy weight of 70.3kg would be expected from the preceding equation to bear infants weighing an average of 3666 g. But case 6, a subject who weighed 70.3 kg, bore a baby weighing 4068 g. The difference, $y - \hat{y} = 4068 - 3666 = 402$ g, represents

Figure 13.6 Deviations About the Linear Regression Line for Infants' Birthweights Relative to Mothers' Prepregnancy Weights

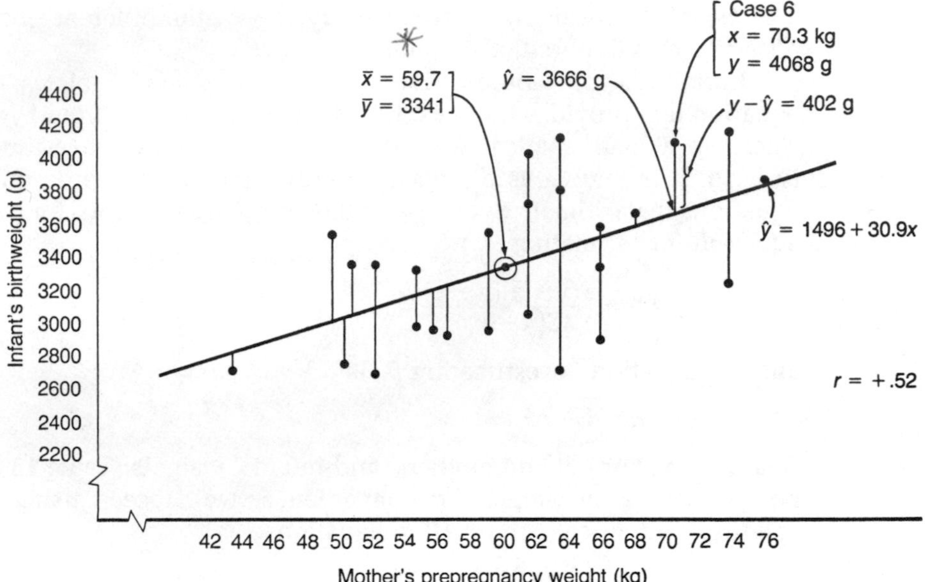

the deviation, or residual, of the observed value from the value predicted by the least-squares regression line. The residuals are shown as the vertical lines in Figure 13.6.

The regression line always passes through the means of x and y, that is, through ($x = \bar{x}$, $y = \bar{y}$). Hence it is simple to superimpose it on the scattergram. A characteristic of a least-squares regression line is that the sum of the deviations about the line is equal to zero, and the sum of the squared deviations is a minimum; that is, there is no other line for which it could be less. That is why it is referred to as the line of best fit in the sense of "least squares." Table 13.3 helps verify this. It shows that the sum of the residuals above the regression line equals the sum of those below the line; that is, $\Sigma (y - \hat{y}) = 0$ or actually −.2, which is a tiny roundoff error.

An indication of just how precisely the regression line describes the relationship between x and y is the variance of the deviations $(y - \hat{y})$ about the line. This variance is denoted $s^2_{y \cdot x}$. It is an estimate of the true error of prediction $\sigma^2_{y \cdot x}$. Underlying this estimate is an assumption of homogeneity, namely, that $\sigma^2_{y \cdot x}$ remains constant for all y's distributed about each x along the regression line.

Table 13.3 Prepregnancy Weights of Mothers and Birthweights of Their Infants—Deviations About the Linear Line of Regression

Case number	x Mother's weight (kg)	y Infant's actual birthweight (g)	$\hat{y}$ Infant's expected birthweight (g)*	$y-\hat{y}$ Residual (g)	$(y-\hat{y})^2$ Squared residual $(g)^2$
1	49.4	3515	3021.6	492.4	242,457.8
2	63.5	3742	3456.9	285.1	81,282.0
3	68.0	3629	3595.8	33.2	1,102.2
4	52.2	2680	3108.0	−428.0	183,184.0
5	54.4	3006	3175.9	−169.9	28,866.0
6	70.3	4068	3666.8	401.2	160,961.4
7	50.8	3373	3064.8	308.2	94,987.2
8	73.9	4124	3778.0	346.0	119,716.0
9	65.8	3572	3527.9	44.1	1,944.8
10	54.4	3359	3175.9	183.1	33,525.6
11	73.5	3230	3765.6	−535.6	286,867.4
12	59.0	3572	3318.0	254.0	64,516.0
13	61.2	3062	3385.9	−323.9	104,911.2
14	52.2	3374	3108.0	266.0	70,756.0
15	63.1	2722	3444.5	−722.5	522,006.3
16	65.8	3345	3527.9	−182.9	33,452.4
17	61.2	3714	3385.9	328.1	107,649.6
18	55.8	2991	3219.2	−228.2	52,075.2
19	61.2	4026	3385.9	640.1	409,728.0
20	56.7	2920	3247.0	−327.0	106,929.0
21	63.5	4152	3456.9	695.1	483,164.0
22	59.0	2977	3318.0	−341.0	116,281.0
23	49.9	2764	3037.0	−273.0	74,529.0
24	65.8	2920	3527.9	−607.9	369,542.4
25	43.1	2693	2827.1	−134.1	17,982.8
	$\bar{x} = 59.7400$	$\bar{y} = 3341.20$	—	$\Sigma(y-\hat{y}) = -2.8$	$\Sigma(y-\hat{y})^2 = 3{,}768{,}417.3$

$^*\hat{y} = 30.874x + 1496.4.$

The last column of Table 13.3 is used to compute $s^2_{y \cdot x}$, the equation being

$$s^2_{y \cdot x} = \frac{\Sigma(y-\hat{y})^2}{n-2} \tag{13.10}$$

where $n-2$ represents the degrees of freedom. From Table 13.3 we compute $s^2_{y \cdot x}$ as 3,768,417.3/23 = 163,844.2. Alternatively, the same variance can be obtained directly without computing predicted values $(\hat{y})$ by substituting $a + bx$ for y, which gives

$$s^2_{y \cdot x} = \frac{\Sigma(y-a-bx)^2}{n-2} \tag{13.11}$$

After some algebraic manipulations this can be rewritten as

$$s^2_{y \cdot x} = \frac{\Sigma y^2 - a\Sigma y - b\Sigma xy}{n-2} \tag{13.12}$$

The square root of $s^2_{y \cdot x}$ is referred to as the standard error of estimate. Once you have obtained the equation for a linear regression line, you would probably like to know how reliable the line is for predicting dependent variables. To find out, you will need to use the standard error of estimate in a test of significance or obtain confidence intervals for β_1, the slope of the population regression line.

13.8 Inferences Regarding the Slope of the Regression Line

Thus far we have assumed that (1) the means of each distribution of y's for a given x fall on a straight line, and (2) the variances, $\sigma^2_{y \cdot x}$, are homogeneous for each distribution of y's for a given x. To perform tests of significance or compute confidence intervals, we will need one more assumption: the distribution of y's is normal for each value of x.

We noted earlier that the slope, *b*, computed from sample data is an estimate of some true value, β_1, for the population regression line, which is defined by

$$y = \beta_0 + \beta_1 x + \epsilon \tag{13.13}$$

We wish to determine (1) how useful the regression line obtained from sample data is in predicting the outcome variable, and (2) whether the slope *b* differs significantly from $\beta_1 = 0$. To do this, we need to perform a hypothesis test for β much as we did for μ. The first step is to compute the standard error of *b*. Mathematical statisticians have shown that

$$\mathrm{SE}(b) = \sqrt{\frac{s^2_{y \cdot x}}{\Sigma(x - \bar{x})^2}} \tag{13.14}$$

which simplifies to

$$\mathrm{SE}(b) = \frac{s_{y \cdot x}}{s_x / \sqrt{n - 1}}$$

which for our data on mothers' weights and infants' birthweights (Table 13.3) computes to

$$\mathrm{SE}(b) = \frac{\sqrt{163{,}844.2}}{\sqrt{90{,}728 - 1494^2/25}} = \frac{404.777}{38.03} = 10.644$$

Using this value, we can now perform the following hypothesis test:

1. $H_0{:}\beta_1 = 0$ (slope of 0 means that there appears to be no relationship between x and y) versus $H_1{:}\beta_1 \neq 0$.
2. $\alpha = .05$.

3. The test statistic (with $n - 2$ df) is

$$t = \frac{b - 0}{\text{SE}(b)} \tag{13.15}$$

$$= \frac{30.874}{10.644}$$

$$= 2.90$$

4. The critical region for t with 23 df for $\alpha = .05$ is $t = 2.07$.
5. We reject H_0 because a t of 2.93 falls in the critical region.
6. We conclude that the slope differs significantly from 0; consequently, a regression line estimated from our data can, with reasonable reliability, predict dependent variables for given values of x.

From the test statistic for the regression coefficient b, it is a simple matter to describe the confidence interval for the true regression coefficient β_1:

$$\text{CI for } \beta_1 = b \pm t[\text{SE}(b)] \tag{13.16}$$

again based on $n - 2$ df.

The confidence interval corresponds to the central $(1 - \alpha)$ proportion of the area. Assuming only that our data for 25 mother–infant pairs is a random sample of all such pairs, the 95% confidence interval for β_1, the true slope, is

$$\begin{aligned} \text{CI} &= 30.874 \pm 2.07(10.644) \\ &= 30.87 \pm 22.03 \\ &= 8.84 \text{ to } 52.90 \end{aligned}$$

Therefore we can say (with 95% confidence) that β_1 is unlikely to be less than 8.84 or larger than 52.90.

It can be shown that the t statistics of Equation 13.4 can be derived from testing the null hypothesis that β, the slope of the line of regression, is zero. The equation to use is

$$t = \frac{b}{\text{SE}(b)}$$

where b represents a sample estimate of β.

Testing whether β equals zero is functionally equivalent to testing for ρ equals zero. For further details, see Armitage (1971).

Conclusion

Correlation analysis and regression analysis have different purposes. The former is used to determine whether a relationship exists between two variables and how strong that relationship is. The latter is employed to determine the equation that describes the relationship and to predict the value of y for a given x. An aid to visualizing these concepts is the scatter diagram.

A correlation coefficient (r) can take on values from −1 to +1. The closer r approaches −1 or +1, the stronger the relationship between x and y; the closer r approaches zero, the weaker the relationship. It is important to keep in mind that a high correlation merely indicates a strong association between the variables; it does not imply a cause-and-effect relationship. A correlation coefficient is valid only where a linear relationship exists between the variables. After computing the correlation coefficient r and the regression coefficient b, we are obliged to test their significance or set up confidence limits that encompass the population values they estimate.

Vocabulary List

bivariate data
cause-and-effect relationship
confidence belts
correlation coefficient
dependent variable (outcome variable)
independent variable (input variable)
least-squares method
linear correlation
linear regression
negative correlation
outlier
positive correlation
prediction equation
regression coefficient (slope, gradient)
regression line (line of best fit)
residual
scatter diagram (or scattergram)
standard error of estimate
y-axis intercept

Exercises

13.1 A correlation coefficient r consists of two parts: a sign and a numerical value.

(a) What is the range of values possible for r?

(b) What does the sign tell you about the relationship between variables x and y?

(c) What information do you derive from the value of r regarding x and y?

(d) What does r tell you about the ability of the regression line to predict values of y for a given value of x?

(e) For any given set of data, would the correlation coefficient and the regression coefficient necessarily have the same sign? The same magnitude?

13.2 For the data of Table 3.1 (Honolulu Heart Study), compute the correlation coefficient for

(a) Blood glucose (x) and serum cholesterol (y). $\Sigma x = 15{,}214$; $\Sigma y = 21{,}696$; $\Sigma x^2 = 2{,}611{,}160$; $\Sigma xy = 3{,}371{,}580$; $\Sigma y^2 = 4{,}856{,}320$.

(b) Ponderal index (x) and systolic blood pressure (y). $\Sigma x = 13{,}010$; $\Sigma y = 4{,}052$; $\Sigma x^2 = 1{,}736{,}990$; $\Sigma xy = 527{,}185$; $\Sigma y^2 = 164{,}521$. What does this correlation coefficient tell you about the scatter diagram of systolic blood pressure versus ponderal index?

13.3 In a study of systolic blood pressure (SBP) in relation to whole blood cadmium (Cd) and zinc (Zn) levels the following data were obtained:

Cd (ppm/g ash)	68	63	56	48	96	70	66	45	50	60	53	47	36	65
Zn (ppm/g ash)	127	118	78	76	181	134	122	87	80	107	116	103	64	123
SBP (mmHg)	166	162	116	120	160	120	182	134	130	116	108	134	116	96

(a) Make a scatter diagram of cadmium and systolic blood pressure, using the latter as the dependent variable.
(b) Judging from the diagram, would you be justified in using linear regression analysis to determine a line of best fit for cadmium and blood pressure? Why or why not?
(c) Compute the correlation coefficient for cadmium and blood pressure.
(d) Using zinc as the dependent variable, plot a scatter diagram of cadmium and zinc.
(e) Does the diagram of (d) provide justification for using regression analysis to determine a line of best fit? Why or why not?
(f) Calculate the equation of the line of best fit for the relationship between zinc and cadmium, and draw the line on the scatter diagram for (d).
(g) If it were determined that a patient had a whole blood cadmium level of 80, what would you expect that patient's zinc level to be?
(h) Would you be justified in stating that there is a cause-and-effect relationship between cadmium and zinc? Why or why not?

13.4 Test the correlation coefficient you calculated in Exercise 13.2(a) to determine if it is significantly different from zero.

13.5 (a) Determine the 95% confidence limits for the population correlation coefficient ρ of cadmium and blood pressure for Exercise 13.3(c).
(b) Test the hypothesis H_0: $\rho = 0$ by using the confidence interval you found in (a).

13.6 To find the equation of the regression line in Exercise 13.3(f), you had to calculate the regression coefficient β_1. Perform a significance test of the null hypothesis that the population regression coefficient is not significantly different from zero.

Chapter **14**

Nonparametric Methods

Chapter Outline

14.1 Rationale for Nonparametric Methods
The reason for the increasing popularity of nonparametric methods is explained.

14.2 Advantages and Disadvantages
Advantages and disadvantages of nonparametric methods are discussed.

14.3 Wilcoxon Rank-Sum Test
A procedure is presented that is similar to the t test for two independent samples.

14.4 Wilcoxon Signed-Rank Test
A procedure similar to the paired t test for two dependent samples is described.

14.5 Spearman Rank-Order Correlation Coefficient
The Spearman correlation coefficient, used to describe the association of two ranked variables, is discussed.

Learning Objectives

After studying this chapter, you should be able to

1. Distinguish between
   (a) parametric and nonparametric methods
   (b) rank-sum tests and signed-rank tests
   (c) Pearson and Spearman correlation coefficients
2. List the advantages and disadvantages of nonparametric methods
3. Give the equation for the sum of the first n integers
4. List the assumptions necessary to perform hypotheses tests by nonparametric methods

14.1 Rationale for Nonparametric Methods

In the preceding chapters we discussed several methods that enable us to determine whether there is a significant difference between two sample means. The most popular of these involve the normal and the *t* distributions. We also learned about the correlation coefficient that measures the amount of linear association between two variables. Underlying such test statistics were assumptions of normality, of homogeneity of variances, and linearity. Whenever we dealt with measurement data used in test statistics, we also were interested in obtaining some estimate of the population parameter, that is, μ or ρ.

All these statistical techniques are collectively referred to as **parametric methods.** In contrast to these are the **nonparametric methods,** which have been developed for conditions in which the assumptions necessary for using parametric methods cannot be made. Nonparametric methods are sometimes referred to as **distribution-free methods** because it is not necessary to assume that the observations are normally distributed. The chi-square is a distribution-free method. A nonparametric method is appropriate for dealing with data measured on a nominal or ordinal scale (discussed in Chapter 1) and whose distribution is unknown. Because of their many advantages, the use of nonparametric methods has been rapidly increasing. But, like most methods, they also have their disadvantages.

14.2 Advantages and Disadvantages

Nonparametric methods have three main advantages:

1. They do not have such restrictive assumptions as normality of the observations. In practice, data are often nonnormal or the sample size isn't large enough to gain the benefit of the central limit theorem. Consequently, nonparametric methods possess a major advantage; at most, the distribution should be somewhat symmetrical.
2. Computations can be performed speedily and easily—a prime advantage when a quick preliminary indication of results is needed.
3. They are well suited to experiments or surveys that yield outcomes that are difficult to quantify. In such cases, the parametric methods, although statistically more powerful, may yield less reliable results than the nonparametric, which tend to be less sensitive to the errors inherent in ordinal measurements.

There are three distinct disadvantages of nonparametric methods:

1. They are less efficient (i.e., they require a larger sample size to reject a false hypothesis) than comparable parametric tests.

2. Hypotheses tested with nonparametric methods are less specific than those tested comparably with parametric methods.
3. They do not take advantage of all of the special characteristics of a distribution. Consequently, these methods do not fully utilize the known information about the distribution.

In using nonparametric methods, you should be careful to view them as complementary statistical methods rather than attractive alternatives. With a knowledge of the advantages and disadvantages and some experience, you should be able easily to determine which statistical test is the most appropriate for a given application.

An inherent characteristic of nonparametric statistics is that they deal with ranks rather than values of the observations. The observations are arranged in an array, and ranks are assigned from 1 to n. Consequently, computations are simple; you deal only with positive integers: $1, 2, 3, \ldots, n$. When working with ranks we often need to compute the sum of the numbers 1 through n, which, we recall from algebra, equals $n(n + 1)/2$. For example, the sum of the first 10 integers is $10(10 + 1)/2 = 55$.

Though there are numerous nonparametric methods, we will limit ourselves to those that correspond to parametric t tests for independent samples, dependent samples, and correlation coefficients. These techniques are the Wilcoxon rank-sum test, the Wilcoxon signed-rank test, and the Spearman rank-order correlation coefficient.

14.3 Wilcoxon Rank-Sum Test

The **Wilcoxon rank-sum test** is used to test the null hypothesis that there is no difference in the distribution of two populations. Based on the ranks from two independent samples, it corresponds to the t test, except that no assumptions are necessary as to normality or equality of variances.

To carry out this test with data from Table 14.1, we proceed as follows:

1. Combine the observations from both samples and arrange them in an array from the smallest to the largest.
2. Assign ranks to each of the observations.
3. List the ranks from one sample separately from those of the other.
4. Separately sum the ranks for the first and second samples.

Given the hypothesis that the average of the ranks is approximately equal for both samples, the test statistic W_1 (the sum of the ranks of the first sample), should not differ significantly from W_e (the expected sum of the ranks). Accordingly, it can be shown that the expected sum of the ranks for

Table 14.1 Wilcoxon Rank-Sum Test for Two Independent Samples: Number of Prenatal-Care Visits for Mothers Bearing Babies of Low and of Normal Birthweight

Mothers bearing low-birthweight babies			Mothers bearing normal-birthweight babies		
No.	X (number of visits)	R (rank)	No.	X (number of visits)	R (rank)
1	3	5.5*	1	4	7.5*
2	0	1.5*	2	5	9
3	4	7.5*	3	6	10
4	0	1.5*	4	11	15
5	1	3	5	7	11
6	2	4	6	8	12
7 (= n_1)	3	5.5*	7	10	14
			8 (= n_2)	9	13
		$W_1 = 28.5$			$W_2 = 91.5$
		$\bar{R}_1 = 4.1$			$\bar{R}_2 = 11.4$

*Two-way tie.

the first sample is

$$W_e = \frac{n_1(n_1 + n_2 + 1)}{2} \tag{14.1}$$

It has been shown that if we obtain W_1's from repeated samples of lists of ranks, the standard error, σ_w, is

$$\sigma_w = \sqrt{\frac{n_1 n_2(n_1 + n_2 + 1)}{12}} \tag{14.2}$$

It has further been shown that, regardless of the shape of the population distribution, the sampling distribution for the sum of a subset of ranks is approximately normal. Consequently, we have what we need to perform a test of significance regarding the equality of the distributions, namely,

$$Z = \frac{W_1 - W_e}{\sigma_w} = \frac{W_1 - W_e}{\sqrt{n_1 n_2(n_1 + n_2 + 1)/12}} \tag{14.3}$$

Utilizing the data of Table 14.1, we can compute the Z statistic, which compares W_1, the sum of the sample ranks, to W_e, the value that would be expected if the hypothesis were true.

In attempting to rank the data in Table 14.1, we notice that we have three 2-way ties, for zero, three, and four visits. Traditionally, the procedure is to assign the average of the ranks to each tie. For example, the two zeros rank first and second, so we assign them both the average rank of 1.5.

To compute the Z statistic, we'll need the expected rank sum. To obtain it, we use Equation 14.1:

$$W_e = \frac{n_1(n_1 + n_2 + 1)}{2} = \frac{7(7 + 8 + 1)}{2} = 56 \tag{14.4}$$

To determine whether there is a significant difference between the observed sum of 28.5 and the expected value of 56, we use Equation 14.3:

$$Z = \frac{W_1 - W_e}{\sqrt{n_1 n_2 (n_1 + n_2 + 1)/12}}$$

$$= \frac{28.5 - 56}{\sqrt{7(8)(15 + 1)/12}}$$

$$= \frac{-27.5}{\sqrt{74.67}} = \frac{27.5}{8.6} = -3.2$$

From this we see that the mothers with the low-birthweight infants had a rank sum of 28.5, considerably lower than the expected rank sum of 56. In fact, the observed rank sum falls 3.2 standard errors below the mean of a normal distribution of rank sums. So our conclusion, based on rank sums, is that the mothers bearing low-birthweight infants had a significantly lower number of prenatal visits than the mothers bearing normal-birthweight infants.

We are able to perform this Z test because W is approximately normally distributed. This situation holds if we have at least six cases in each of the groups. Can we perform exact tests if we have smaller sample sizes? Yes. For such methods, with accompanying tables, see an advanced text, for example, Brown and Hollander (1977).

As mentioned earlier, the rank-sum test parallels the t test for two independent samples, but it is less powerful. Its power efficiency is greater than 92%, measured by the performance of repeated rank-sum tests, instead of t tests, on normally distributed data.

14.4 Wilcoxon Signed-Rank Test

In past pages we considered the t test for two independent samples and the paired t test for matched observations. For the latter, we will discuss a counterpart nonparametric test, the **Wilcoxon signed-rank test.** With this test we assume that we have a pair of dependent observations; we wish to test the hypothesis that the median of the first sample equals the median of the second. The procedure is to obtain the differences (d) between individual pairs of observations. Pairs yielding a difference of zero are eliminated from the computation; the sample size is reduced accordingly.

To perform the test, we rank the absolute differences by assigning ranks of 1 for the smallest to n for the largest. If ties are encountered, they are treated as before. The signs of the original differences are restored to each rank. We obtain the sum of the positive ranks, W_1, which serves as the test statistic. If the null hypothesis is true, we would expect to have about an

Table 14.2 Wilcoxon Signed-Rank Test: Number of Cigarettes Usually Smoked per Day—Before and After Pregnancy

	Number of cigarettes smoked per day				
Subject	x_b: Before pregnancy	x_a: After pregnancy	$d = x_a - x_b$	$\lvert d \rvert$	r_d
1	8	5	−3	3	3(−)
2	13	15	+2	2	2(+)
3	24	11	−13	13	9(−)
4	15	19	+4	4	4(+)
5	7	0	−7	7	7(−)
6	11	12	+1	1	1(+)
7	20	15	−5	5	5(−)
8	22	0	−22	22	10(−)
9	6	0	−6	6	6(−)
10	15	6	−9	9	8(−)
11	20	20	0	—	—

$\Sigma r_d = \frac{n(n+1)}{2} = \frac{10(11)}{2} = 55$ $\Sigma r_{d(+)} = W_1 = 7$

$W_e = \frac{\Sigma r_d}{2} = \frac{55}{2} = 27.5$ $\Sigma r_{d(-)} = W_2 = 48$

equal mixture of positive and negative ranks. Viewing it another way, we would expect the sum of the positive ranks to equal that of the negative ranks.

Using the data in Table 14.2 on pregnancy and smoking, we see that, since each pair of observations is on the same woman, we have **dependent** samples; therefore the Wilcoxon signed-rank test is the appropriate one to perform. The column denoted by d represents differences (before and after pregnancy); the column labeled r_d is the rank by size of the absolute difference. Rank 1 is assigned to the smallest and n (here, 10) to the largest. Now we can obtain W_1 and W_2, the sums, respectively, of the positive and negative ranks. Recall that the sum of all ranks is $n(n + 1)/2$. Under the null hypothesis we assume that the sum of the ranks of the positive d's is equal to the sum of the ranks of the negative d's. That is, each will be half of the total sum of the ranks, or, algebraically, the expected sum of the ranks will be

$$W_e = \left(\frac{1}{2}\right)\frac{n(n+1)}{2} \tag{14.5}$$

which, for the data of Table 14.2, is $10(11)/2 = 27.5$

Since W_1 is approximately normally distributed with a mean of W_e and a standard deviation of σ_w, we are able to perform a Z test for the difference between the sums of the matched ranks by utilizing the following equation:

$$\begin{aligned} Z &= \frac{W_1 - W_e}{\sigma_W} \\ &= \frac{W_1 - W_e}{\sqrt{(2n+1)W_e/6}} \\ &= \frac{7 - 27.5}{\sqrt{[2(10)+1]27.5/6}} \\ &= \frac{-20.5}{\sqrt{96.25}} \\ &= \frac{20.5}{9.81} = -2.09 \end{aligned} \tag{14.6}$$

This result indicates that the difference between the observed and expected rank sums is significant ($p < .05$). The implication: there is a significant reduction in the smoking habit consequent to pregnancy.

The Wilcoxon signed-rank test has a power efficiency of 92% as compared with paired t tests that satisfy the assumption of normality. Note that this technique is somewhat less sensitive than the parametric one in that the ranks do not directly describe the amount of reduction in smoking.

The assumption of normality for the sum of the signed-rank test is appropriate, providing you have at least eight pairs. For a smaller sample size, you will need an exact test. Tables for such a test are available in more advanced textbooks, such as Brown and Hollander (1977), which also includes confidence intervals for the Wilcoxon tests.

A natural question arises here: Does a nonparametric procedure exist for making comparisons of more than two groups? That is, is there a parallel nonparametric ANOVA test? There is; it is called the **Kruskal–Wallis test.** For a discussion, see a text such as Steel and Torrie (1980).

14.5 Spearman Rank-Order Correlation Coefficient

In Chapter 13 we discussed in detail the Pearson correlation coefficient, which describes the association between measurement variables x and y. In this section we discuss an association between two ranked variables. With the **Spearman rank-order correlation coefficient,** we obtain perfect correlation (±1) if the ranks for variables x and y are equal for each individual. Conversely, lack of association is measured by examining the differences in the ordered ranks, $d_i = x_i - y_i$. The Spearman rank-order correlation coefficient n can be derived from the Pearson correlation coefficient r. The symbol for the Spearman coefficient is r_s (the s is for Spearman), and the equation is

$$r_s = 1 - \frac{6\Sigma d_i^2}{n(n^2 - 1)} \tag{14.7}$$

where d_i is the difference between the paired ranks and n is the number of pairs. Like the Pearson correlation coefficient, the Spearman rank-order correlation coefficient may take on values from −1 to +1. Values close to ±1 indicate a high correlation; values close to zero indicate a lack of association. The minus or plus signs indicate whether the correlation coefficient is negative or positive.

To illustrate the use of the Spearman rank-order correlation coefficient, let's consider a situation that is all too familiar to any college student. The work of 12 students is observed independently by two faculty evaluators who rank their performance from 1 to 12 (Table 14.3). As before, ties in rank are handled by averaging the ranks. Note that observer C had a three-way tie for first place. The x and y columns of Table 14.3 are the ranks, the d_i column is the difference between the ranks, and the final column is d_i^2. Using Equation 14.7, we obtain

$$r_s = 1 - \frac{6\Sigma d_i^2}{n(n^2 - 1)}$$

$$= 1 - \frac{6(55.50)}{12(14401)} = .81$$

Table 14.3 Ranking of Students' Performance by Two Independent Observers

Student no.	Observer B: Rank order (x)	Observer C: Rank order (y)	$d_i = x_i - y_i$	$d_i^2 = (x_i - y_i)^2$
1	2.5*	5	−2.5	6.25
2	2.5*	2†	0.5	0.25
3	9	8	1.0	1.00
4	5.5*	7	−1.5	2.25
5	12	12	0	0
6	7.5*	11	−3.5	12.25
7	1	2†	−1.0	1.00
8	10	6	4.0	16.00
9	4	2†	2.0	4.00
10	5.5*	4	1.5	2.25
11	7.5*	10	−2.5	6.25
12	11	9	2.0	4.00
				$\Sigma d_i^2 = 55.50$

*Two-way tie.
†Three-way tie.

To determine whether this coefficient significantly differs from zero, we need to assume that x and y represent randomly selected and independent pairs of ranks. We can use the same test procedure as for the Pearson r. It provides a good approximation if the sample size is at least 10. The equation for the test statistic is

$$t - \frac{r_s\sqrt{n-2}}{\sqrt{1-r_s^2}} \tag{14.8}$$

with $n - 2$ df. Using the data from Table 14.3, we find that

$$t = \frac{.81\sqrt{10}}{\sqrt{1-.66}} = \frac{(.81)(3.16)}{.58} = 4.41$$

Since the computed t of 4.41 is greater than the critical $t_{.95}$ of 1.81 for 10 df, we reject H_0 and conclude that the correlation differs significantly from zero.

Whenever you are able to meet the assumptions for computing a Pearson r, use it. It is preferable to the Spearman r_s because the power of the latter is not as great as that of r. For samples having 10 or fewer observations, see advanced textbooks such as Dixon and Massey (1969) and Brown and Hollander (1977), which also give tabulations for critical values of r_s.

Conclusion

There are nonparametric methods that correspond to such parametric methods as the t test, paired t test, and correlation coefficient. The primary advantage of these methods is that they do not involve such restrictive assumptions as those of normality and homogeneity of variance. Their major disadvantage is that they are less efficient than the corresponding parametric methods. The three methods described here are the nonparametric methods used most frequently in the health sciences.

Vocabulary List

Kruskal–Wallis test
nonparametric methods (distribution-free methods)
parametric methods
Spearman rank-order correlation coefficient
Wilcoxon rank-sum test
Wilcoxon signed-rank test

Exercises

14.1 To learn if babies who were breast-fed had a better dental record than those who were not, 13 children were picked at random to see at what age they acquired their first cavities. The results are as follows:

Subject	Breast-fed—yes/no	Age at first cavity
1	No	9
2	No	10
3	Yes	14
4	No	8
5	Yes	15
6	No	6
7	No	10
8	Yes	12
9	No	12
10	Yes	13
11	No	6
12	No	20
13	Yes	19

(a) State the null hypothesis.
(b) State the alternative hypothesis.
(c) Do a Wilcoxon rank-sum test.

14.2 Refer to Table 2.2. Compute a Wilcoxon rank-sum test to determine whether there is a significant difference in diastolic blood pressure between
(a) vegetarian males and nonvegetarian males
(b) vegetarian males and vegetarian females

14.3 Two communities are to be compared to see which has a better dental record. Town A has fluoride in the water; Town B does not. Ten persons are randomly picked from each town and their dental cavities are counted and reported. The data are as follows:

	Person									
	1	2	3	4	5	6	7	8	9	10
Town A	0	1	3	1	1	2	1	2	3	1
Town B	3	2	2	3	4	3	2	3	4	3

(a) State the null hypothesis.
(b) State the alternative hypothesis.
(c) Do a Wilcoxon rank-sum test.

14.4 There are two methods of counting heartbeats: (1) by counting the pulse at the wrist and (2) by counting the pulse on the neck. An investigator wishes to know the degree of correlation between the two methods. The data are as follows:

	Person									
	1	2	3	4	5	6	7	8	9	10
Neck pulse	73	99	77	63	50	80	83	73	66	82
Wrist pulse	74	103	77	61	51	81	82	74	66	83

(a) State the null hypothesis.
(b) State the alternative hypothesis.
(c) Do a Spearman rank-order correlation coefficient. (*Hint:* Rank the neck pulse from highest to lowest; do the same for the wrist pulse.)

14.5 Two health inspectors rate 11 hospitals on cleanliness, as shown in the tabulation below. Determine if their rankings are comparable:

	Hospital										
	1	2	3	4	5	6	7	8	9	10	11
Inspector 1	2	3	2	3	1	4	5	3	1	3	4
Inspector 2	1	3	3	2	2	5	4	2	1	4	3

(a) State the null hypothesis.
(b) State the alternative hypothesis.
(c) Perform the appropriate test.

Chapter **15**

Vital Statistics and Demographic Methods

Chapter Outline

15.1 Introduction
The importance of vital statistics and demographics is pointed out.

15.2 Sources of Vital Statistics and Demographic Data
Three sources of data—census data, registration of births and deaths, and morbidity data—are discussed as the building blocks for computing vital rates, ratios, and proportions.

15.3 Vital Statistics Rates, Ratios, and Proportions
Concepts of rates, ratios, and proportions are introduced within the context of vital statistics.

15.4 Measures of Mortality
A variety of measures are presented, each being a means of measuring the frequency of deaths in a community.

15.5 Measures of Fertility
Two key methods for quantifying fertility are shown to be indispensable in making population estimates.

15.6 Measures of Morbidity
Of the many measures of illness that exist, three are described.

15.7 Adjustment of Rates
How to make reasonable comparisons between noncomparable populations is explained.

Learning Objectives

After studying this chapter, you should be able to

1. Distinguish among
   (a) rates, ratios, and proportions
   (b) measures of morbidity, mortality, and fertility
2. Compute and understand the meaning of various vital measures
3. State the reasons why measures are adjusted
4. Compute an adjusted rate by the direct method

15.1 Introduction

Decision-making in the health sciences is continually becoming more quantitative. Demographic data and **vital statistics** have emerged as indispensable tools for researchers, health planners, and other health professionals. To determine the health status of a community, to decide how best to provide a health service, to plan a public health program, or to evaluate a program's effectiveness, it is essential to use these tools knowledgeably.

Demographic variables describe a population's characteristics: for instance, its size and how that changes over time; its composition by age, sex, income, occupation, and utilization of health services; its geographic location and density. Once you possess demographic data and information about **vital events** (births, deaths, marriages, and divorces), you can tackle a remarkable variety of problems regarding a community's status at a particular time or its trends over a period. Together with measures of illness and disease, demographic data are invaluable in program planning and disease control. Such data also go a long way toward providing research clues as to the often unexpected associations between a population's health practices and its disease experience.

A wide array of methodological tools is available to deal with such data. In this chapter we consider *vital rates, ratios, proportions, measures of fertility* and *morbidity*, and *adjustment of rates*. But first, we will discuss some of the sources of demographic data and vital statistics.

15.2 Sources of Vital Statistics and Demographic Data

The three main sources of demographic data, vital statistics, and morbidity data are the census, registration of vital events, and morbidity surveys.

The Census

The United States has conducted a **decennial census** of the population since 1790. In a census, each household and resident is enumerated. Information obtained on each person includes his or her sex, age, race, marital status, place of residence, and relationship to or position as the head of household. A systematic sample of households then provides more information, such as income, housing, number of children born, education, employment status, means of transportation to work, and occupation. Census tables are published for the entire United States, for each state, for **Standard Metropolitan Statistical Areas (SMSAs)**, for counties, and for cities, neighborhoods (census tracts), and city blocks. The SMSAs are urbanized areas. An area qualifies as an SMSA if it has one or more cities of at least 50,000 residents and there is a social and economic integration of the cities with the surrounding rural areas. In the 1980 census, there were 323 SMSAs (including 5 in Puerto Rico).

Census results are published in the *Decennial Census of the United States* about two years after the census is taken. They are also made available on magnetic tape for computerized analysis. A good deal of census information is summarized annually in the *Statistical Abstract of the United States*. The importance of census data is universally recognized. More than four-fifths of the world's population is counted in some kind of census.

Annual Registration of Vital Events

As noted earlier, vital events are births, deaths, marriages, and divorces. State laws require that all vital events be registered. Registration is now quite complete and reliable. Birth certificates serve as proof of citizenship, age, birthplace, and parentage; death certificates are required as burial documents and in the settlement of estates and insurance claims. In the United States, **death registration** began in Massachusetts in 1857, was extended to 10 states, the District of Columbia, and several other cities by 1900, and has been nationwide since 1933. **Birth registration** began in 1915, encompassing 10 states and the District of Columbia. By 1933, all states had been admitted to the nationwide birth and death registration system. A great deal of information is recorded on birth and death certificates. Some of the key elements are as follows:

Birth certificate	Death certificate
Name	Name
Sex	Date and time of death
Date and time of birth	Race
Weight and length at birth	Age
Race of parents	Place of birth
Age of parents	Names of decedent's parents
Birth order	Name and address of survivor (or informant)
Occupation of father	Marital status
Place of birth	Occupation
Residence of mother	Place of residence
Physician's (or attendant's) certification	Cause(s) of death
	Place of death
	Burial data
	If death due to injury: accident, suicide, or homicide
	Physician's (or coroner's) certification

The National Center for Health Statistics collects a systematic sample of 10% of the births and deaths in each state. From this, it publishes the monthly *Vital Statistics Report*. Annually, it issues the four-volume set *Vital Statistics of the United States*, which includes many detailed tables on vital events for all sorts of demographic characteristics and for major geographical subdivisions. Data on marriages and divorces are similarly collected and published in a separate volume of *Vital Statistics of the United States*.

All states are now compiling computerized death certificate data, or "death tapes," which are computer-readable extracts of the most important data appearing on death certificates. Since 1979, the National Center for Health Statistics has prepared the National Death Index, a nationwide, computerized index of death records compiled from tapes submitted by the vital statistics offices of each state. These tapes contain a standard set of identifying data for each decedent. The index (National Center for Health Statistics, 1981) permits researchers to determine if persons in their studies have died; for each such case, the death certificate number is available, along with the identity of the state where the death occurred and the date of death. Given these **mortality data,** the researcher can order a copy of the death certificate from the state's vital statistics office. Confidentiality of data is guaranteed by law.

Morbidity Surveys

Morbidity data (i.e., data on the prevalence of disease) are far more difficult to gather and interpret than are mortality data. Whereas death registration is now estimated to be 99% complete, cases of communicable disease are all too often underreported.

Reporting of communicable diseases is a time-honored, if flawed, method of gathering morbidity data. In 1876, Massachusetts tried voluntary case reporting; the first compulsory reporting began in Michigan in 1883 (Winslow et al., 1952). But even now, a century later, there are wide gaps in the data. California, for example, has 52 reportable diseases. Various surveys have concluded that the more serious diseases are well reported. But whereas virtually every case of cholera, plague, yellow fever, rabies, and paralytic polio is promptly brought to the attention of health authorities, the common childhood diseases are notoriously underreported.

Each local health department tallies the number of cases of reportable communicable disease within its area and forwards its count to the state health department, where a cumulative total is made and sent to the Centers for Disease Control in Atlanta for publication in *Morbidity and Mortality Weekly Reports* (*MMWR*).

Because of the chronic underreporting, a number of novel systems have been developed to make better estimates of morbidity data. In the following partial list of these systems, note that many of them go far beyond communicable-disease reporting to include data on noninfectious, occupational, and chronic diseases.

1. Reportable diseases
2. National Health Survey
3. Hospital records data
4. Industrial hygiene records
5. School nurse records
6. Medical care subgroups (most often: prepaid medical plans)
7. Chronic-disease registries (most often: tumor registries)
8. Insurance industry data

The **National Health Survey** is worthy of special note. Originated by an Act of Congress in 1956, it provides for an annual nationwide survey of a representative sample of 40,000 persons. A number of subprograms are included, the most notable of which are the National Health Interview Survey, National Health and Nutrition Examination Survey (HANES), National Hospital Discharge Survey, National Ambulatory Medical Care Survey, and National Nursing Home Survey. The results are published in *Vital and Health Statistics*, sometimes referred to (from its colorful covers) as the "rainbow series." Published results encompass a vast spectrum of medical care data, including incidence or prevalence rates for many diseases, length of hospital stays, hospitalizations by cause, number of days of disability, and patterns of ambulatory care service.

Hospital records are a fair source of morbidity data. However, except for prepaid medical plans, the population served by a hospital is hard to define. The Professional Activity Study of Battle Creek, Michigan, provides a uniform reporting system that is used by over 2000 hospitals nationwide. Researchers use this system to make morbidity estimates for population studies. Hospital administrators find this and other resources to be invaluable for planning strategies of health care delivery.

Chronic-disease registries are rapidly taking on a major role in the understanding of morbidity data. Most such registries are cancer-oriented (and are therefore termed cancer, or tumor, registries), although some are specialized for such diseases as cardiovascular disease, tuberculosis, diabetes, and psychiatric disease. A cancer registry is defined as a "facility for the collection, storage, analysis, and interpretation of data on persons with cancer." Some such registries are hospital-based; that is, they work within the walls of a hospital or group of hospitals. Others are population-based, in that they serve a population of defined composition and size. Among the best-known of the latter are the tumor registries of Connecticut and Iowa, each serving the entire state (Muir and Nectoux, 1977).

Although we have focused on data for the United States, similar data are available for most of the developed world. You can find them in the annual *Demographic Yearbook* (United Nations, 1983).

15.3 Vital Statistics Rates, Ratios, and Proportions

The field of vital statistics makes some special applications of rates, ratios, and proportions. A **rate** is an expression of the form

$$\left[\frac{a}{(a+b)t}\right]c \tag{15.1}$$

where a = the number of persons experiencing a particular event during a given period

$a + b$ = the number of persons who are at risk of experiencing the particular event during the same period

t = total time at risk

c = a multiplier, such as 100, 1000, 10,000, or 100,000

The purpose of the multiplier, also referred to as the **base,** is to avoid the inconvenience of working with minute decimal fractions; it therefore helps users to comprehend the meaning of a given rate. We usually choose c to give a rate that is in the tens or hundreds.

Three kinds of rates are commonly used in vital statistics: crude, specific, and adjusted rates. **Crude rates** are computed for an entire population. They disregard differences that usually exist by age, sex, race, or some category of disease. **Specific rates** consider the differences among subgroups and are computed by age, race, sex, or other variables. **Adjusted** (or **standardized**) **rates** are used to make valid summary comparisons between two or more groups possessing different age (or other) distributions.

A **ratio** is a computation of the form

$$\left(\frac{a}{d}\right)c \tag{15.2}$$

where a and c are defined as for rates, and d is the number of individuals experiencing some event different from event a during the same period. Quite commonly used is the sex ratio; by convention, it places males in the numerator and females in the denominator. A ratio of 1.0 would describe a population with an equal number of males and females.

A **proportion** is an expression of the form

$$\left(\frac{a}{a+b}\right)c \tag{15.3}$$

where a, $a + b$, and c are defined as for rates.

15.4 Measures of Mortality

A wide variety of rates, ratios, and proportions are based on numbers of deaths. Each rate is a measure of the relative frequency of deaths that occurred in a given population over a specific period. If we know the population and **time at risk,** we can compute a mortality rate. Unfortunately, these figures are sometimes difficult to obtain. A convention is used to define population size: the population at midyear (July 1). The figure obtained serves as a reasonable estimate of the **population at risk** $(a + b)$ over the time (t) of one year. If this convention cannot be met, the calculation should preferably be termed a "proportion" rather than a "rate."

In the health sciences the fine distinctions among rates, ratios, and proportions are often ignored. Consequently, you may find that some sources erroneously term certain ratios as "rates"; the most common of these are starred (*) in the discussion that follows. Some proportions are similarly misnamed "rates"; these also are starred.

Annual Crude Death Rate

The annual crude death rate is defined as the number of deaths in a calendar year, divided by the population on July 1 of that year, the quotient being multiplied by 1000.

EXAMPLE 1

■ California, 1980—population: 23,060,000; deaths: 190,247.

$$\text{Crude death rate} = \frac{190{,}247}{23{,}060{,}000} \times 1000$$

$$= 8.3 \text{ deaths per 1000 population per year}$$ ■

The annual crude death rate is universally used. It is indeed crude—a generalized indicator of the health of a population. In our example, the rate of 8.2 deaths per 1000 is a bit less than the overall U.S. death rate of 8.9. But it is often incautious to make such a comparison, especially when the two populations are known to differ on an important characteristic such as age, race, or sex. More appropriate comparisons are made by use of adjusted rates. The process of adjustment is a bit involved; we deal with it later. In the meantime, there is another way of making fair comparisons between groups—by use of *specific* rates. Death rates may be specific for age, for sex, or for some particular cause of death.

Age-Specific Death Rate

The age-specific death rate is defined as the number of deaths in a specific age group in a calendar year, divided by the population of the same age group on July 1 of that year, the quotient being multiplied by 1000.

EXAMPLE 2

■ United States, 1980—age group: 25–34 years; population: 36,130,000; deaths: 50,840.

$$\text{Age-specific death rate} = \frac{50{,}840}{36{,}130{,}000} \times 1000$$

$$= 1.4 \text{ deaths per 1000 population per year for age group 25–34}$$ ■

Cause-Specific Death Rate

The cause-specific death rate is defined as the number of deaths assigned to a specific cause in a calendar year, divided by the population on July 1 of that year, the quotient being multiplied by 100,000.

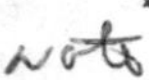

EXAMPLE 3

■ United States, 1980—cause: accidents; population: 222,400,000; deaths: 106,550.

$$\text{Cause-specific death rate} = \frac{106{,}550}{222{,}400{,}000} \times 100{,}000$$

$$= 47.9 \text{ accidental deaths per 100,000 population per year}$$ ■

Cause-Race–Specific Death Rate

The cause-race–specific death rate is one of many possible examples of how the idea of specific death rates may be extended simultaneously to cover two characteristics.

EXAMPLE 4

■ United States, 1977—white male population, 91,429,000; nonwhite male population, 13,811,000.

The full data for this example are given in Table 15.1. Note the striking difference in the death rate between the two racial groups. But the under-

Table 15.1 Cause-Race–Specific Death Rate, United States, 1977

	White males	Nonwhite males
Population	91,429,000	13,811,000
Deaths assigned to accidents	90,798	20,670
Cause-race–specific death rate per 100,000	99.3	149.7

lying explanation for the difference may be something other than race. What other factor might explain the difference? ■

*Proportional Mortality

Proportional mortality is defined as the number of deaths assigned to a specific cause in a calendar year, divided by the total number of deaths in that year, the quotient being multiplied by 100.

EXAMPLE 5

■ United States, 1980—total deaths from all causes: 1,986,000; deaths assigned to malignant neoplasms: 414,320.

$$\text{Proportional mortality} = \frac{414{,}320}{1{,}986{,}000} \times 100$$

$$= 20.9\% \text{ of total deaths per year from malignant neoplasms}$$ ■

EXAMPLE 6

■ United States, 1979—persons 15–24 years old: 41,393,000; persons age 65 or over: 24,658,000.

From the full data for this example in Table 15.2, you can see that this proportion is useful as a measure of the relative importance of a specific cause of death. But though it is quite simple to compute, it should be used with caution because it is quite easy to misinterpret. For instance, the proportional mortality for accidental death here is much greater for young adults than for elderly persons. Nevertheless, the death rate from accidents is higher for the elderly. This apparent dilemma disappears when you realize the numerical impact of the large number of deaths from all causes among the elderly.

Table 15.2 Cause-Specific Death Rate, United States, 1979

	Persons ages 15–24	Persons age 65 and over
Population	41,393,000	24,658,000
Deaths—all causes		
Number	48,719	1,271,656
Death rate per 100,000	117.7	5,157.2
Deaths—accidental causes		
Number	26,574	24,032
Death rate per 100,000	64.2	97.5
Proportional mortality—accidental causes (%)	54.5%	1.9%

Proportional mortality is particularly useful in occupational studies as a measure of the relative importance of a specific cause of death. It suffers from not having a population base in the denominator. Although it does not provide a reliable population estimate as does the cause-specific death rate, it is valuable in making preliminary assessments when denominator data are not available. ■

The next five measures are concerned with events involved in pregnancy, birth, and infancy. Most are based on the number of live births.

*Maternal Mortality Ratio

The **maternal mortality ratio** is defined as the number of deaths assigned to puerperal causes (i.e., those related to childbearing) in a calendar year, divided by the number of live births in that year, the quotient being multiplied by 100,000.

EXAMPLE 7

■ United States, 1980—deaths assigned to puerperal causes: 250; live births: 3,598,000.

$$\text{Maternal mortality ratio} = \frac{250}{3{,}598{,}000} \times 100{,}000$$

$$= 6.9 \text{ maternal deaths per 100,000 live births per year}$$

Note that this ratio has an inherent problem: it includes maternal deaths in the numerator but only live births in the denominator. Fetal deaths are not represented. Consequently, this practice has a tendency to inflate the ratio slightly. A second problem derives from multiple births. They inflate the denominator but do not affect the numerator. As such events are comparatively rare, the net effect would be a minor change to a ratio based on an otherwise large population. ■

Infant Mortality Rate

The **infant mortality rate** is defined as the number of deaths of persons of age zero to one in a calendar year, divided by the number of live births in that year, the quotient being multiplied by 1000.

EXAMPLE 8

■ California, 1980—live births: 401,581; infant deaths: 4593.

$$\text{Infant mortality rate} = \frac{4593}{401{,}581} \times 1000$$

$$= 11.4 \text{ infant deaths per 1000 live births per year}$$ ■

This rate has an inherent problem in those populations that are experiencing rapidly changing birthrates. As you can see from our example, the numerator includes some infants who died in 1980 but were born in 1979; and some of the infants born in 1980 would die in 1981. In a population with a stable birthrate (e.g., that of the United States or Western Europe), such differences are likely to cancel out; this is not the case in a population undergoing a sharp change in its birthrate.

Neonatal Mortality Proportion

The **neonatal mortality proportion** is defined as the number of deaths of neonates (infants less than 28 days of age) that occurred in a calendar year, divided by the number of live births in that year, the quotient being multiplied by 1000.

EXAMPLE 9

■ California, 1977—deaths at age less than 1 year: 4186; deaths at age less than 28 days: 2743; live births: 347,000.

$$\text{Neonatal mortality proportion} = \frac{2743}{347{,}000} \times 1000$$

$$= 7.9 \text{ neonatal deaths per 1000 live births per year}$$

As this example shows that 65.53% of all infant deaths were neonatal, it underscores the importance of neonatal mortality: the great bulk of infant deaths occur in a relatively short period following birth. ■

Fetal Death Ratio

A fetal death is defined as the delivery of a fetus that shows no evidence of life (no heart action, breathing, or movement of voluntary muscles) if the 20th week of gestation has been completed or if the period of gestation was unstated.

The **fetal death ratio** is defined as the number of fetal deaths in a calendar year, divided by the number of live births in that year, the quotient being multiplied by 1000. Note that this ratio applies only to fetal deaths that occur in the second half of pregnancy. There is no reporting required for early miscarriages.

EXAMPLE 10

■ California, 1977—fetal deaths: 2911; live births: 347,000

$$\text{Fetal death ratio} = \frac{2911}{347{,}000} \times 1000$$

$$= 8.4 \text{ fetal deaths per 1000 live births per year}$$ ■

Regrettably, fetal deaths tend to be grossly underreported, so every fetal death ratio is an underestimate (McMillen, 1979).

Perinatal Mortality Proportion

The **perinatal mortality proportion** is defined as the number of fetal plus neonatal deaths, divided by the number of live births plus fetal deaths, the quotient being multiplied by 1000.

EXAMPLE 11

■ California, 1977—fetal deaths: 2911; neonatal deaths: 2743; live births: 347,000.

$$\text{Perinatal mortality proportion} = \frac{2911 + 2743}{2911 + 347{,}000} \times 1000$$

= 16.2 perinatal deaths per 1000 fetal deaths plus live births per year ■

15.5 Measures of Fertility

Measures of fertility are indispensable when approaching population control problems. They are particularly useful in the planning of maternal and child health services. These measures also help school boards in planning their future needs for facilities and teachers. The two most common measures of fertility are the *crude birthrate* and the *general fertility rate.*

Crude Birthrate

The **crude birthrate** is defined as the number of live births in a calendar year, divided by the population on July 1 of that year, the quotient being multiplied by 1000.

EXAMPLE 12

■ California, 1980—live births: 401,581; population: 23,060,000.

$$\text{Crude birthrate} = \frac{401{,}581}{23{,}060{,}000} \times 1000$$

= 17.4 live births per 1000 population per year ■

The crude birthrate, although quite commonly used, is a none-too-sensitive measure of fertility because its denominator includes both men and women. Strictly speaking, this measure cannot be a rate because only a fraction of the population is capable of bearing children. A more sensitive measure is the general fertility rate.

General Fertility Rate

The **general fertility rate** is defined as the number of live births in a calendar year, divided by the number of women ages 15–44 at midyear, the quotient being multiplied by 1000.

EXAMPLE 13

■ United States, 1980—live births: 3,598,000; number of women ages 15–44: 51,990,000.

$$\text{General fertility rate} = \frac{3{,}598{,}000}{51{,}990{,}000} \times 1000$$

$$= 69.2 \text{ live births per 1000 women ages 15–44 per year} \quad ■$$

This rate is more sensitive than the crude birthrate because its denominator includes only women of child-bearing age.

Other measures of fertility are *age-specific fertility rates* and *age-adjusted fertility rates*. Both can be used to make valid comparisons between different population groups.

15.6 Measures of Morbidity

At best, mortality data provide indirect means of assessing the health of a community. The **underlying cause of death** hardly provides an adequate picture of the countless illnesses and other health problems that exist in any community. Since morbidity is less precisely recorded than mortality, such data are difficult to analyze, but they are nonetheless useful in program planning and evaluation. Many measures exist. We will discuss here three that deal with the frequency, prevalence, and seriousness of disease.

Incidence Rate

The **incidence rate** is defined as the number of newly reported cases of a given disease in a calendar year, divided by the population on July 1 of that year, the quotient being multiplied by a convenient factor, usually 1000, 100,000, or 1,000,000.

EXAMPLE 14

■ California, 1979—new cases of gonorrhea reported to the State Health Department: 132,376; population: 22,694,000.

$$\text{Incidence rate} = \frac{132{,}376}{22{,}694{,}000} \times 100{,}000$$

= 583 new cases of gonorrhea per 100,000 population per year ■

*Prevalence Proportion

The **prevalence proportion** is defined as the number of existing cases of a given disease at a given time, divided by the population at that time, the quotient being multiplied by 1000, 100,000, or 1,000,000.

EXAMPLE 15

■ United States, 1971—number of men alive with history of prostate cancer: 201,000; population: 99,700,000 men.

$$\text{Prevalence proportion} = \frac{201{,}000}{99{,}700{,}000} \times 1000$$

= 2.02 prostate cancer cases per 1000 men per year ■

*Case-Fatality Proportion

The **case-fatality proportion** is defined as the number of deaths assigned to a given cause in a certain period, divided by the number of cases of the disease reported during the same period, the quotient being multiplied by 100.

EXAMPLE 16

■ United States, 1978—reported cases of infectious hepatitis (hepatitis A): 29,500; deaths from the disease: 508.

$$\text{Case-fatality proportion} = \frac{508}{29{,}500} \times 100$$

= 1.7% mortality among reported cases of hepatitis A per year ■

This proportion uses the relative number of deaths as an indicator of the seriousness of a disease. It is often used as a means of showing the relative effectiveness of various methods of treatment.

15.7 Adjustment of Rates

Crude rates can be used to make approximate comparisons between different populations. But the comparisons are invalid if the populations are

Table 15.3 Population Distributions and Age-Specific Death Rates for Alaska and Florida, 1977

	Alaska				Florida			
		Population				Population		
Age group	Number of deaths	Persons	%	Deaths per 100,000 persons	Number of deaths	Persons	%	Deaths per 100,000 persons
0–4	162	40,000	9.83	405.0	2,049	546,000	6.46	375.3
5–19	107	128,000	31.45	83.6	1,195	1,982,000	23.44	60.3
20–44	449	172,000	42.26	261.0	5,097	2,676,000	31.65	190.5
45–64	451	58,000	14.25	777.6	19,904	1,807,000	21.37	1101.5
65+	444	9,000	2.21	4933.3	63,505	1,444,000	17.08	4397.9
Total	1615	407,000	100.00	396.8	91,760	8,455,000	100.00	1085.3

SOURCE: National Center for Health Statistics, 1977, pp. 1–47.

dissimilar with respect to an important characteristic such as age, sex, or race. As we know so well, many diseases have quite different impacts on different groups: on men and women, on old and young persons, on blacks and whites. We would therefore hesitate to compare the death rate for Alaska, with its young population, to that of Florida, with its relatively old population. We can see in Table 15.3 that the crude death rate for Alaska is much lower than that for Florida. The real explanation for this is that Alaska has many more young people than does Florida, and the death rate for a younger group is low. A good way to handle the comparison is to examine the corresponding age-specific death rates for the two states. In this example, Alaska had higher death rates than Florida for five of the six age groups. However, comparing a long series of age-specific rates is often quite cumbersome, especially if more than two populations are involved. To solve this, an *adjusted, or standardized,* rate is used to make the comparison valid. Statistically, the adjustment removes the difference in composition with respect to age.

There are two methods of adjustment—direct and indirect. The type of data available dictates the method to be used. But keep in mind that an adjusted rate is artificial in that it is a rate applied to a population with a hypothetical distribution. Such rates do not at all reflect the actual rates of a population. They have real meaning only as relative comparisons. The numerical values of the adjusted rates depend in large part on the choice of the standard population.

The Direct Method

The **direct method of adjustment** applies a standard population distribution to the death rates of two comparison groups. The sum of the expected deaths for the two groups is then used in computing the adjusted death rate (dividing the expected deaths by the total of the standard population). For the direct method it is essential to have both the age-specific death rates for the populations being adjusted and the distribution of the standard population by age (or by whatever other factor is being adjusted).

EXAMPLE 17

■ In Table 15.3, we see that the 1977 crude death rate per 100,000 population for Alaska was 396.8, and for Florida, 1085.7. But a close look at the age distribution discloses that Alaska had a higher percentage of its population in the younger age groups. This finding makes it essential to adjust the death rates of the two states in order to make a valid comparison. With the direct method, we can figure out what the death rate would be for each state if the age distributions of both populations were identical. A neat way to make this calculation is to apply the U.S. standard population to both states and then compute the expected number of deaths for each state as if its population distribution were indeed the same as for the U.S. standard.

To carry out this method, we use the **U.S. standard million.** It is a population of 1 million persons that identically follows the age distribution for the entire United States, as shown in column 1 of Table 15.4.

The specific steps involved in calculating the age-adjusted rate are as follows:

1. Compute the expected number of deaths for the standard population by applying the age-specific death rates of the state. For Alaska, multiply column 1 by column 2, divide the product by 1,000,000, and enter the result in column 3. For Florida, multiply column 1 by column 4, divide the product by 1,000,000, and enter the result in column 5.
2. Total the expected deaths in columns 3 and 5. You can see that if Alaska's population were distributed the same as the standard million, the expected number of deaths (given Alaska's known age-specific death rates) would be 788.6. Similarly, the expected number of deaths for Florida would be 770.5.

Table 15.4 Age-Adjusted Death Rates per 100,000 Population for Alaska and Florida (1977) Using the Direct Method and Based on the 1970 U.S. Standard Million

Age group	(1) 1970 U.S. standard million	(2) Alaska age-specific death rates	(3) Alaska expected deaths with U.S. standard million	(4) Florida age-specific death rates	(5) Florida expected deaths with U.S. standard million
0–4	84,416	405.0	34.2	375.3	31.7
5–19	294,353	83.6	24.6	60.3	17.7
20–44	316,744	261.0	82.7	190.5	60.3
45–64	205,745	777.6	160.0	1101.5	226.6
65+	98,742	4933.3	487.1	4397.9	434.3
Total	1,000,000		788.6		770.6

3. Compute the age-adjusted death rate per 1000 by dividing the total expected deaths by 100. For Alaska the adjusted rate is 7.89, and for Florida it is 7.71. Remember the crude death rates (Table 15.3) were 3.97 for Alaska and 10.86 for Florida.

The striking result: Florida's crude death rate was much higher than Alaska's. However, where based on a comparable population, the age-adjusted death rate proved higher for Alaska! ■

The choice of the standard population affects the values of the adjusted rates. Therefore, in comparing adjusted rates between different states or countries, you should know which standard population was used.

The Indirect Method

The **indirect method of adjustment** is somewhat different from the direct method. It is utilized when age-specific death rates are not available for the populations being adjusted. But the age-specific death rates for the standard population must be known. With this method, we compute a **standard mortality ratio** (SMR) (observed deaths divided by expected deaths) and use it as a standardizing factor to adjust the crude death rates of the given populations. The SMR increases or decreases a crude rate in relation to the excess or deficit of the group's composition as compared to the standard population. A detailed treatment appears in several textbooks. See, for instance, Remington and Schork (1970) or Lilienfeld, Pedersen, and Dowd (1967). Both this method and the direct method are as applicable to ratios and proportions as to rates.

Conclusion

Public health decision-making is a quantitative matter. The health of a population is assessed by use of its vital statistics and demographic data. Information about demographic characteristics is obtainable from census data, registration of vital events, and morbidity surveys. Such data are used to calculate vital rates and other statistics that are used to indicate the magnitude of health problems.

Vital rates, ratios, and proportions are classified into measures of mortality (death), fertility (birth), and morbidity (illness). These measures may be crude or specific, the latter referring to calculations for subgroups selected for a common characteristic such as age, sex, race, or disease experience. Comparisons of vital rates, ratios, or proportions among different populations should be made with care and be validated by use of specific or adjusted measures. Choice of the adjustment method depends on the type of data available.

Vocabulary List

adjusted rate (standardized rate)
base
birth registration
case-fatality proportion
crude birth rate
crude rate
death registration
decennial census
demographic variables
direct method of adjustment
fetal death rate
general fertility ratio
incidence rate
indirect method of adjustment
infant mortality rate
maternal mortality ratio
morbidity data
mortality data
National Health Survey
neonatal mortality proportion
perinatal mortality proportion
population at risk
prevalence proportion
proportion
proportional mortality rate
ratio
specific rate
Standard Metropolitan Statistical Area (SMSA)
standard mortality ratio
time at risk
underlying cause of death
U.S. standard million
vital events
vital statistics

Exercises

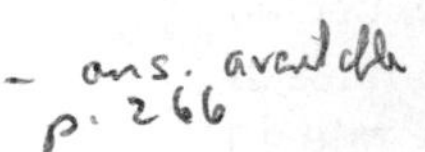

Note: For all these exercises, use as appropriate the sources referred to in Section 15.2.

15.1 Find the size of the U.S. population (including those in the armed forces) for 1970, 1980, and 1990 (conservative estimate).

15.2 What was the population of New York State in 1970? In 1980?

15.3 In 1982 how many Iowans were
(a) under 5 years old?
(b) 65 or more years old?

15.4 What was the percentage of blacks living in 1980 in Minnesota? In Georgia?

15.5 In 1980 what were the birth and death rates for Alaska? For Kansas?

15.6 For the United States during 1980, what were the five leading causes of death?

15.7 What were the maternal mortality ratios for U.S. whites and nonwhites in 1950? In 1980?

15.8 What were the death rates from cirrhosis of the liver by sex and race (white and nonwhite) for the United States in 1978?

15.9 What were the numbers of total deaths, infant deaths, and neonatal deaths, by place of residence, for two California counties, Riverside and San Bernardino, in 1978?

15.10 (a) For 1980 compute the crude birthrates for Alaska and for Arizona.
(b) What do you observe about the birthrates of these two states? What are some possible explanations?

Chapter

16

Life Tables

Chapter Outline

16.1 Introduction
Life tables, used by demographers and researchers to describe the mortality or longevity of a population, are discussed.
16.2 Current Life Tables
A current life table is dissected.
16.3 Follow-up Life Tables
A neat technique is described for tracking survival of patients with chronic diseases.

Learning Objectives

After studying this chapter, you should be able to

1. Distinguish among the three types of life tables
2. Identity and be able to compute the components of a current life table
3. Compute measures of mortality and longevity from a life table
4. Construct a follow-up life table

16.1 Introduction

Life tables have been in use for centuries. The first systematic, if inexact, life table was developed by British astronomer Edmund Halley (of Halley's comet fame) to describe the longevity of residents of seventeenth-century Breslau. In 1815, Joshua Milne published the first mathematically accurate life table, which described the mortality experience of a city in northern England (Shyrock and Siegel, 1973).

Life tables are now in general use and have many important applications. For instance, they are used by demographers to measure and analyze the mortality or longevity of a population or one of its segments; by insurance companies to compute premiums; and by research workers to determine whether the differences in mortality or longevity of two groups are significant. They are employed to predict survival or the likelihood of death at any time. A life table analysis can be fundamental to the solution of many public health and medical problems.

Three types of life tables are in general use. They are the *current* life table, the *cohort*, or *generation*, life table, and the *follow-up*, or *modified*, life table. Current and follow-up life tables are the most common and will be discussed in some detail.

The **current life table** illustrates how age-specific death rates affect a population. Such a table considers mortality rates for the entire population for a given period. For instance, a 1979–1981 life table considers the mortality of the various age groups over three years. It does not follow the mortality experience of a single age group throughout its life. Three years are used in preference to one year because this span tends to stabilize the death rates, which otherwise would be unduly sensitive to year-by-year fluctuations.

By contrast, the **cohort life table** follows a defined group (**cohort**) from birth (or some other measurable point in time) until the last person in the group has died, which is why it is also known as a **generation life table.** The key difference between the current life table and the cohort life table is that the former generates a fictitious pattern of mortality, whereas the latter presents the historical record of what actually occurred.

Since there are usually major differences in the patterns of mortality among various subgroups of a population, life tables are quite commonly constructed for specific groups: by race, sex, occupation, or specific diseases.

An interesting extension of the life-table idea has come into general use in recent years. Life tables may be employed for studies wherein the outcome variable is an event other than death. For example, an outcome could be recurrence of coronary heart disease, a contraceptive failure, or time from driver's license application to first reported accident. An illustration of the recurrence of cancer as an outcome variable appears in Kuzma and Dixon (1966).

16.2 Current Life Tables

To demonstrate the many applications of a current life table, we will use an **abridged life table** for the 1980 U.S. population. Table 16.1 illustrates what would have happened to a hypothetical population of 100,000 persons

Table 16.1 Abridged Life Table for the Total U.S. Population, 1980

Age interval	Proportion dying: Uncorrected	Proportion dying: Correction term	Proportion dying: Corrected	Of 100,000 born alive		Person-years lived		Average remaining lifetime
Period of life between two exact ages stated	Average annual age-specific death rate*	Fraction of last age interval lived	Proportion dying during age interval	Number living at beginning of age interval	Number dying during age interval	In the age interval	In this and all subsequent age intervals	Average number of years of life remaining at beginning of age interval
x to (x + n)	${}_nm_x$	${}_na_x$	${}_n\hat{q}_x$	l_x	${}_nd_x$	L_x	T_x	e_x
<1	.0127445	.10	.0126000	100,000	1,260	98,866	7,361,560	73.62
2–4	.0006510	.39	.0025999	98,740	257	394,334	7,262,690	73.55
5–9	.0003403	.46	.0016999	98,483	167	491,964	6,868,360	69.74
10–14	.0003002	.56	.0015000	98,316	147	491,255	6,376,390	64.86
15–19	.0010222	.57	.0050998	98,168	501	489,766	5,885,140	59.95
20–24	.0013647	.49	.0067998	97,668	664	486,645	5,395,370	55.24
25–29	.0013646	.50	.0067998	97,004	660	483,369	4,908,730	50.60
30–34	.0014651	.52	.0072998	96,344	703	480,032	4,425,360	45.93
35–39	.0017873	.54	.0088999	95,641	851	476,246	3,945,330	41.25
40–44	.0028181	.54	.0139998	94,790	1,327	470,896	3,469,080	36.60
45–49	.0045062	.54	.0222999	93,463	2,084	462,519	2,998,180	32.08
50–54	.0072412	.53	.0356002	91,378	3,253	449,247	2,535,660	27.75
55–59	.0111928	.52	.0545000	88,125	4,803	429,099	2,086,420	23.68
60–64	.0169420	.52	.0814002	83,322	6,782	400,334	1,657,320	19.89
65–69	.0246352	.52	.1163000	76,540	8,902	361,336	1,256,980	16.42
70–74	.0363293	.51	.1668000	67,638	11,282	310,551	895,649	13.24
75–79	.0608562	.51	.2648000	56,356	14,923	245,220	585,098	10.38
80–84	.0894622	.48	.3629000	41,433	15,036	168,072	339,878	8.20
85+	.1536440	—	1.0000000	26,397	26,397	171,806	171,806	6.51

SOURCE: *Monthly Vital Statistics Report* (National Center for Health Statistics) 29(13):13, 1981.

*As the final death counts were not available at time of publication, these rates are estimates.

as it passed through time; that is, how many persons would have died and how many would have survived in each particular age group. The table also indicates the probability of dying during any age interval, the probability of surviving to a particular age, and the average life expectancy. The table is *abridged* for convenience, most of the age intervals covering five-year periods. A **complete life table** would have a separate entry for each year.

By systematically dissecting a life table, we can gain some valuable insights into what it means and how it works. We will begin by discussing the several columns of Table 16.1.

Age Interval [x to $(x + n)$]

The **age interval** is the period between the two exact ages stated. For example, 35–40 means the five-year span between the 35th birthday and the 40th.

Age-Specific Death Rate ($_nm_x$)

The symbol $_nm_x$ denotes the average annual age-specific death rate for the age interval stated. The numerator for this rate is the average number of deaths per year in a three-year period (1979–1981), divided by the July 1 average population for 1979, 1980, and 1981. For example, the age-specific death rate for age group 35–40, $_5m_{35}$, is .0017873, or about 1.8 per 1000.

Correction Term ($_na_x$)

We need a correction term for a very simple reason. Among tiny infants most deaths occur early in the first year, whereas among adults deaths are fairly uniformly distributed throughout the year. The correction term defines and corrects for the maldistribution. The $_na_x$ column shows the average fraction of the age interval lived by persons who die during that interval. Notice that $_5a_{35}$ is .54, a shade more than half a year. Values for $_na_x$ are computed by use of a complex equation discussed in advanced treatments of this topic.

Corrected Death Rate ($_n\hat{q}_x$)

The symbol $_n\hat{q}_x$ denotes the proportion of those persons who are alive at the beginning of the age interval but die during that interval. For example, the probability that a 35-year-old will die before reaching 40 is $_5\hat{q}_{35} = .0089$.

Number Living at Beginning of Age Interval (l_x)

We use l_x to indicate the number of persons, starting with the original cohort of 100,000 live births, who survive to the exact age marking the beginning of each interval. Each l_x value is computed by subtracting the $_nd_x$ (number dying during interval) for the previous age interval from the l_x for that interval; that is,

$$l_{x+n} = l_x - d_x \qquad (16.1)$$

Thus

$$l_{35} = l_{30} - {}_5d_{30} = 96{,}353 - 704 = 95{,}649$$

Number Dying During Age Interval (${}_nd_x$)

The number of persons of the original 100,000 who die during each successive age interval is denoted by ${}_nd_x$. It is calculated by applying the proportion dying (${}_n\hat{q}_x$) during the interval to the number alive (l_x) at the beginning of the interval.

$${}_nd_x = (l_x)({}_n\hat{q}_x) \qquad (16.2)$$

For example,

$${}_5d_{30} = (l_{30})({}_5\hat{q}_{30}) = 96{,}353(.0073) = 704$$

Person-Years Lived in Interval (${}_nL_x$)

The symbol ${}_nL_x$ designates the totality of years lived by the survivors of the original 100,000 (the l_x) between the ages x and (x + n). For example, ${}_5L_{30} = 480{,}075$ is the number of **person-years** lived by the 96,353 (l_{30}) alive at the beginning of the 30th year. It is computed by the equation

$${}_nL_x = n[l_{x+n} + ({}_na_x)({}_nd_x)] \qquad (16.3)$$

for all intervals except the last, for which

$${}_nL_x = \frac{{}_nd_x}{{}_nm_x} \qquad (16.4)$$

So

$$\begin{aligned} {}_5L_{30} &= 5[l_{35} + ({}_5a_{30})({}_5d_{30})] \\ &= 5[95{,}649 + (.52)(704)] \\ &= 480{,}075 \end{aligned}$$

Sometimes ${}_nL_x$ is termed the **stationary population.** Given the hypothetical assumption that the number of births and deaths remains constant each year, the number of person-years would in fact be unchanging. Hence the term. This idea is useful in certain applications to studies of population structure.

Total Number of Person-Years (T_x)

The symbol T_x denotes the total number of person-years lived by the l_x survivors from year 0 to x. It is obtained by cumulating the person-years lived in the intervals (${}_nL_x$):

$$T_0 = {}_1L_0 + {}_4L_1 + {}_5L_5 + \cdots + {}_5L_{80} + {}_5L_{85} = 7{,}361{,}891$$

Expectation of Life ($\hat{e}_x$)

Because of its general usefulness, $\hat{e}_x$ may be the most valuable feature of the life table. It denotes **life expectation,** the average number of years of life remaining to those who survive to the beginning of the age interval. It is calculated by dividing the number of person-years lived after a given age (T_x) by the number who reached that same age (l_x):

$$\hat{e}_x = \frac{T_x}{l_x} \tag{16.5}$$

The future life expectancy for a 35-year-old, for example, is calculated by $\hat{e}_{35} = T_{35}/l_{35} = 3{,}945{,}433/95{,}649 = 41.2$ years. That is, on average, persons reaching age 35 may expect to live to 76.2.

A life table enables us to compute some special measures of mortality that are real improvements over the use of general rates. One of these measures is the *expectation of life at age 1*, which removes the considerable impact that infant mortality has on life expectation from birth. Another is the *expectation of life at age 65*, which zeros in on the mortality of the older ages when most deaths occur. Still another is the *probability of surviving from birth to age 65*, which is defined as

$$_{65}P_0 = \frac{l_{65}}{l_0}$$

An interesting measure is the **median age at death,** which is the age to which precisely half of the cohort survives. It corresponds to the age x at which $l_x = 50{,}000$ in a life table based on a cohort of 100,000 persons. By interpolation from Table 16.1, we would estimate the median age at death as 77.1 years.

A commonly used survival rate in population studies is

$$_np_x = \frac{l_{x+n}}{l_x} \tag{16.7}$$

the probability of surviving from year x to year x + *n*. For example, using Table 16.1, we can calculate the proportion of newborn babies who will reach their tenth birthday:

$$_{10}p_0 = \frac{l_{10}}{l_0} = \frac{98{,}323}{100{,}000} = .98323$$

Similarly, the proportion of newborns who will reach their first birthday is

$$_1p_0 = \frac{l_1}{l_0} = \frac{98{,}743}{100{,}000} = .98743$$

and the probability that a 25-year-old will survive 10 more years is

$$_{10}p_{25} = \frac{l_{35}}{l_{25}} = \frac{95{,}649}{97{,}011} = .98596$$

Not surprisingly, we can follow the same pattern to compute probabilities of death. The probability that a 25-year-old will die before reaching age 30 is

$$_5q_{25} = \frac{_5d_{25}}{l_{25}} = \frac{658}{97{,}011} = .00678$$

Note that l_x may be thought of as a cumulation of the *age-specific death rates up to (but not including) age* x. In other words, it shows the net effect of all death rates up to that age, whereas life expectation, $\hat{e}_x$, shows the effect of the age-specific death rates after that age.

We already mentioned that the current life table considers a hypothetical cohort. The assumption is that the cohort is subject throughout its existence to those age-specific mortality rates that were observed for one particular period. However, specific rates actually vary with time. Although little variation occurs from one year to the next, significant changes are common over long periods. Table 16.2 illustrates the point for U.S. white males for the years 1900–1980. Note that most of the improvement in longevity has occurred under age 65, and especially in the first year of life. 

Demographers make an important distinction between **life span** and *life expectation*. A life span of "four score years and ten" has been well known from time immemorial. Although inexact, life span is that age which persons are likely to reach, given optimum conditions. Life span could be defined as that age reached by the longest-lived 0.1% of the population, which would currently be quite close to 100 years (Shyrock and Siegel, 1973). Life expectation has increased not so much by virtue of a longer life span as by reduction of infant mortality, and thus an increase in the average years of life.

Table 16.2 Changes in the Mortality of White Males in the United States According to Various Life Table Measures, 1900–1980

	Base period for life table*						
Measure	1900	1910	1920	1930	1940	1950	1980
Expectation of life at birth	48.2	50.2	56.3	59.1	62.8	66.3	73.6
Expectation of life at age 1	54.6	56.3	60.2	62.0	65.0	67.1	73.6
Expectation of life at age 65	11.5	11.3	12.2	11.8	12.1	12.8	16.4
Probability of surviving from birth to age 65	.39	.41	.51	.53	.58	.64	.77
Median age at death of initial cohort	57.2	59.3	65.4	66.4	68.7	70.7	77.1

*Life tables for periods before 1929–1931 relate to those states that required death registration.

16.3 Follow-up Life Tables

"How long do I have?" is often the first question a patient asks the physician when told that he or she is suffering from a life-threatening chronic disease. The **follow-up life table** (or **modified life table**) provides a basis for answering this difficult question. Chronic-disease registries, especially cancer registries, make regular use of the follow-up table to track the survival of patients over time. In this connection, life tables are often used to evaluate the relative effectiveness of alternative modes of treatment by computing the probability of survival of patients treated by each mode.

The follow-up table is particularly useful because it utilizes the experience of each person for the entire time he or she was in the study. That is, the method considers the period of exposure in terms of person-years or other appropriate units.

Life tables may be calculated for a cohort in which all the members start the study at the same time or for one in which the members are admitted to the study at different times over a period of years. In either case, the data are handled identically, providing that (1) death rates do not change materially over time, and (2) exposure to the disease prior to treatment is not increasing with time.

Construction of a Follow-up Life Table

To construct a follow-up life table, you will need to know the period of follow-up after some event, such as a heart attack, diagnosis of cancer, or surgery. To ensure accuracy, you need well-defined starting and end points. Given a known period of observation for each patient, you can then tally how many survive, how many die, and how many are lost to follow-up during the first and subsequent years of the study.

The construction of such a table is illustrated in Table 16.3 with data from a cancer follow-up study. A total of 356 (l_0) patients began the study.

Table 16.3 Follow-up Life Table: Classification of Cases and Survival Rates of Cancer Patients

Interval in years x to (x + 1)	Alive at beginning of interval l_x	Died during interval d_x	Lost to follow-up f_x	Withdrawn alive w_x	Effective no. exposed to risk of dying l'_x	Proportion dying $\hat{q}_x$	Proportion surviving $\hat{p}_x$	Survival rate P_{0x}
0–1	356	60	0	0	356	0.1685	.8315	.8315
1–2	296	47	1	0	295.5	0.1591	.8408	.6992
2–3	248	29	5	0	245.5	0.1181	.8818	.6166
3–4	214	24	20	25	191.5	0.1253	.8746	.5393
4–5	145	11	13	50	113.5	0.0969	.9032	.4871
5–6	71	4	0	57	42.5	0.0941	.9057	.4412

During the first year of follow-up, 60 (d_0) patients died. Thus the probability of surviving the first year was $\hat{p}_1 = (356 - 60)/356 = .8315$. During the second year, of the 296 patients remaining, 47 died; 1 was lost to follow-up. By convention, it is assumed that a person who is lost to follow-up (f_x) or who withdraws from the study alive (w_x) lives through half the interval. Consequently, the effective number exposed to the risk of dying is here estimated as $l'_x = 296 - .5 = 295.5$. The probability of surviving the second year of follow-up is then estimated as

$$\hat{p}_2 = \frac{l'_2 - d_2}{l'_2} = \frac{295.5 - 47}{295.5} = .8408 \tag{16.8}$$

The probabilities of surviving successive years are computed similarly. The equation for the effective number exposed to the risk of dying may be summarized as

$$l'_x = l_x - .5(w_x + f_x) \tag{16.9}$$

Having found the probabilities of survival for each individual year, we can now easily compute the probability of surviving several years. For example, the probability of surviving the first two years is $P_{02} = (p_1)(p_2)$, and the first five years is $P_{05} = (p_1)(p_2)(p_3)(p_4)(p_5)$.

The **five-year survival rate** is commonly used in cancer research as a measure of a treatment's effectiveness. Differences between survival rates of two groups are tested by means of a t test, which implies the need to know standard errors. For a detailed discussion of two different methods of preparing a life table, see Kuzma (1967).

Some special problems in calculating survival rates occur when persons are lost to follow-up or withdraw alive (i.e., persons are known to be alive at the beginning of the time interval, but their fate is unknown at the end). Numerous suggestions have been offered on how to handle these problems. For instance, if the proportion of such cases is small, the assumption is made that each case was lost or withdrew at the middle of the last known interval. Thus the convention is that such cases are considered to be alive for half of the last interval during which they were observed.

Clinical trials frequently utilize life tables to estimate survival rates. It is often necessary to determine whether there is a statistically significant difference between p'_x, the xth year survival rate of a treatment group, and p_x, the xth year survival rate of a control group. The equation used is

$$Z = \frac{p'_x - p_x}{\sqrt{SE(p'_x)^2 + SE(p_x)^2}} \tag{16.10}$$

where $SE(p'_x)$ and $SE(p_x)$ are standard errors for the two groups and Z is the normal deviate.

A rigorous justification for the standard-error equation is beyond the scope of this work. However, an approximation suggested by M. Greenwood as described in Cutler and Ederer (1958) is as follows:

$$SE(p_x) = \sqrt{\frac{d_x}{(l_x - \frac{1}{2}w_x)(l_x - d_x - \frac{1}{2}w_x)}} \tag{16.11}$$

Conclusion

Life tables provide excellent means for measuring mortality and longevity. The current life table shows the effects of age-specific death rates on a group. From this table, measures of mortality and life expectation can be computed. Whereas the current life table presents a hypothetical picture of the effects of present mortality rates, the cohort life table is an actual historical record of the mortality of a group followed through life. The follow-up life table considers the experience of persons from event to event during the period of a study.

Vocabulary List

abridged life table
age interval
cohort
cohort life table
complete life table
current life table
five-year survival rate
follow-up life table
(modified life table)
(generation life table)
life expectation
life span
life table
median age at death
person-years
stationary population

Exercises

16.1 Table 16.4 is an incomplete abridged life table for the U.S. population (1971). Complete the table by filling in the blanks.

16.2 A distinguished citizen is celebrating his 75th birthday. Use Table 16.1 to compute the probability that he will live to celebrate his 80th.

In Exercises 16.3 through 16.9 use your completed life table from Exercise 16.1.

16.3 Calculate the probability at birth of living to be 80.

16.4 Compute the following proportions:
(a) All persons dying between birth and the first birthday
(b) All persons dying between birth and the fifth birthday
(c) Babies born alive dying between birth and the fifth birthday

16.5 Find the proportion of
(a) all persons dying between the ages of 35 and 45
(b) 35-year-olds dying between the ages of 35 and 45

Table 16.4 Abridged Life Table for Total U.S. Population, 1971

Age interval	Proportion dying			Of 100,000 born alive		Stationary population		Average remaining lifetime
	Uncorrected	Correction term	Corrected					
Period of life between two exact ages stated	Average annual age-specific death rate	Fraction of last age interval lived	Proportion dying during age interval	Number living at beginning of age interval	Number dying during age interval	In the age interval	In this and all subsequent age intervals	Average number of years of life remaining at beginning of age interval
x to (x + n)	${}_n m_x$	${}_n a_x$	${}_n \hat{q}_x$	l_x	${}_n d_x$	${}_n L_x$	T_x	$\hat{e}_x$
0–1	.0193306	.10	.0190	100,000	1,902	98,288	7,102,496	71.02
1–5	.0003016	.39	.0032	98,098	314	391,626	7,004,208	71.40
5–10	.0004004	.46	.0020	97,784	196	488,391	6,612,582	67.62
10–15	.0004004	.56	.0020	97,588	195	487,511	6,124,191	62.76
15–20	.0011227	.57	.0056	97,393	545	485,793	5,636,680	57.83
20–25	.0014453	.49	.0072	96,848	697	482,463	5,150,887	53.19
25–30	.0014251	.50	.0071	96,151	683	479,048	4,668,424	48.55
30–35	.0017070	.52	.0085	95,468	811	475,394	4,189,376	43.88
35–40	.0024538	.54	.0122	94,657	1,155	470,628	3,713,982	39.24
40–45	.0037114	.54	.0184	93,502	1,720	463,554	3,243,354	34.69
45–50	.0056320	.54	.0278	91,782	2,552	453,040	2,779,800	30.29
50–55	.0086732	.53	.0425	89,230	3,792	437,239	2,326,760	26.08
55–60	.0131418	.52	.0637	85,438	5,442	414,129	1,889,521	22.12
60–65	.0201055	.52	.0959	79,996	7,672	381,567	1,475,392	18.44
65–70	.0201225	.52	.1361	72,324	9,843	337,997	1,093,825	15.12
70–75	.0449120	.51	.2023					
75–80	.0660900	.51	.2844					
80–85	.0961178	.48	.3845					
85+	.1872383	—	1.0000	21,952	21,952	117,241	117,241	5.34

16.6 What is the probability that a person aged 20 will survive until age 65?

16.7 Find the expectation of life at birth, at 1 year, at 35 years, and at 75 years of age.

16.8 Find the proportion of 70-year-olds dying between the ages of 70 and 75. Compare this figure with that found in Exercise 16.4c and explain the difference.

16.9 Why are the results of (b) and (c) of Exercise 16.4 the same and the results of (a) and (b) of Exercise 16.5 different?

Chapter **17**

The Health Survey and the Research Report

Chapter Outline

17.1 Planning a Health Survey
An outline for a survey is presented with a brief discussion of the steps involved.
17.2 Evaluation of a Research Report
Steps for evaluating a medical report are listed and discussed.

Learning Objectives

After studying this chapter, you should be able to

1. Prepare an outline for a health survey
2. Be prepared to critically evaluate a medical report

17.1 Planning a Health Survey

So far in this book we have discussed the kinds of statistical topics generally covered by most introductory statistics textbooks. In this section we will consider the survey, one of two research tools that are indispensable to persons who deal with data and statistics. In the next section we will discuss the second tool, the evaluation of research articles. The coverage of both topics is all too brief since each could itself be the subject of a good-sized book.

Health surveys are conducted for a number of reasons, but most often they are undertaken to determine the health needs of a community. Subjects of a health survey are members of the general public, all of whom are, to some degree, users of health services. In the same sense that people consume gasoline, stockings, and corn flakes, they are regarded as **consumers** of health services.

What constitutes a health survey? Many things. For instance, health surveys may entail inquiries into the consumer's knowledge, attitudes, and practices, his or her utilization of health services, disease experience in the past, and satisfaction (or dissatisfaction) with health service delivery; or they involve research directed ultimately toward elucidating the etiology of a disease or evaluation of a program's success. All these points are generally focused in one direction: toward aiding the decision-making process of health service (or public health) managers.

The goal of most researchers is to be able to conduct a survey that clearly and accurately describes some health-related phenomenon. But caution is advised; a health survey can be a tricky business. Unless it follows a prescribed stepwise procedure (like the one we will outline here), a survey could produce faulty information leading to unfortunate (possibly grave) consequences.

Immediately after the following outline, each step will be briefly described.

*Outline for Planning a Health Survey**

1. Make a written statement of the purpose of the survey.
2. Write out the objectives and hypotheses.
3. Specify the target population.
4. List the variables to be measured.
5. Review existing pertinent data.
6. Outline the methods of data collection.
7. Establish the time frame.
8. Design the questionnaire.
9. Pretest the questionnaire.
10. Select subjects for the sample.
11. Collect the data.
12. Edit, code, and enter the data on a computer and verify the data entry.
13. Analyze the data.
14. Report the findings.

Step 1: Making a Written Statement of the Purpose

The purpose of your survey should be well thought out, carefully defined, and clearly stated in two or three sentences. This step will aid your

*Credit for this outline goes to Dr. David Abbey, a survey statistician who developed it for a course on Health Survey Methods.

own thinking and will assist you in carrying out the subsequent steps. Without it, a survey is doomed to failure.

Step 2: Formulating Objectives and Hypotheses

A descriptive survey seeks to estimate one or more characteristics of a population. That, quite simply, is its specific objective. An analytical survey seeks to examine relationships among some specified characteristics. To carry it out, you need to define the hypotheses to be tested.

Step 3: Specifying the Target Population

The **target population** is that group of people from whom inferences are to be drawn. This population may well be restricted to one from which the investigator may feasibly draw a sample. To test your research hypothesis, it is essential to estimate certain key characteristics of individual members of the target population. In statistical sampling, an individual member of a population is often referred to as an **element.** But in health surveys the element may be a person, a mother–child pair, or some logical group of persons such as a household. Measurements are taken on the element. The population can be defined as the collection of all elements.

Once your target population is defined and elements are identified, list the variables that are to be assessed on each element. For example, a target population might be all the students enrolled in a college course who successfully stopped smoking during the last 12 months. The element would be each member of the class possessing that characteristic; variables measured might be age, sex, amount of smoking, and number of years of smoking before quitting.

Step 4: Listing the Variables

There is a endless list of potential variables that you may wish to measure. In general, the researcher focuses on personal characteristics of individual members of the target population. Such characteristics could be a person's weight, blood pressure, age, race, smoking status, and so on. The variables considered should be potentially measurable on each person. In a health survey, one usually desires to collect information both on outcome variables and on concomitant variables. The latter are those covariables that, although themselves uncontrollable, may well affect the outcome. All variables should be clearly defined during the planning stages.

Step 5: Reviewing Existing Data

It is important to review current literature on the topic being surveyed so that you can determine the state of the art, current hypotheses, those variables regarded as pertinent, and the likely success of your chosen strategy. It is often advisable to utilize standardized questions for which ample documentation exists regarding validity and reliability. And by using the standard wording of standardized questions, you will be able to compare results with those of well-known studies.

Step 6: Deciding How to Collect Data

In collecting data, there are numerous methods to choose from, each of which has certain advantages and disadvantages. The **person-to-person interview** is often regarded as the industry standard because of the high response rate. The interviewer, being at the scene, can make additional observations regarding subtle aspects of the interviewee's behavior; these may be used to help validate the interview. But this approach is costly; an alternative is the **telephone interview,** which can be performed at approximately half the cost and produce essentially similar results. But telephoning introduces a new potential bias in that it excludes approximately 10% of the households—those that do not have a telephone or have an unlisted number. Still another approach is the **mailed questionnaire.** This costs less than person-to-person or telephone inteviews and may be done anonymously. Mailed questionnaires rule out the problem of **interviewer bias;** the respondent is less likely to be defensive about answering socially sensitive questions. But this approach does have a serious drawback: poor response rates. It usually requires at least two follow-up mailings to obtain a satisfactory number of responses. Other problems include uncertainty as to whether the intended person actually completed the questionnaire, plus nagging doubts as to whether the respondents are truly representative of the target population.

Step 7: Establishing the Time Frame

It is necessary to establish a time frame to realistically schedule survey events. The schedule should not be so tight as to jeopardize succeeding steps in case of a delay in preceding events. Plan for backup procedures and personnel to avoid major delays. It is a good idea to have some trained interviewers on call.

Step 8: Designing the Questionnaire

Questions need to be carefully worded so as not to confuse the respondent or arouse extraneous attitudes. The questions should provide a clear understanding of the information sought. Be precise; avoid ambiguity and wording that might be perceived to elicit a specific response. Questions may be open-ended, multiple choice, completion, or a variation of these. You should studiously avoid overly complex questions. The key principles to keep in mind while constructing a questionnaire are that it should (1) be easy for the respondent to read, understand, and answer; (2) motivate the respondent to answer; (3) be designed for efficient data processing; (4) have a well-designed professional appearance; and (5) be designed to minimize missing data.

Step 9: Pretesting the Questionnaire

It is never possible to anticipate in advance all the potential problems that may occur when you administer a questionnaire. So it is important to **pretest** it. A pretest will identify questions that respondents tend to misinterpret, omit, or answer inappropriately. It should be done on a handful of individuals similar to, but not included in, the target population and should utilize the same methodology that will be used in the actual survey.

Step 10: Selecting the Sample

You should select the sample in such a way that valid statistical inferences can be drawn regarding the target population. You wish to obtain a representative sample, one that minimizes **sampling bias** and is designed for economy in operation. A variety of sampling designs are available: simple random, systematic random, stratified random, and multistage sampling. To determine the most appropriate design for a complex survey, consult a survey statistician.

Step 11: Collecting the Data

With a completed and pretested questionnaire, you are ready for data collection. This step requires careful planning and supervision to ensure data of good quality. You want to attain the following objectives: maximize the response rate by minimizing nonresponses, keep track of the nonrespondents, avoid duplication, avoid failing to contact part of the sample, protect confidentiality of the data, provide anonymity, and maintain a cooperative spirit in the target population. Interviewers should be well-trained and coached in regard to how to approach the respondents, how to conduct the interview, how to handle various answers, and how to inform respondents about what is expected of them during the inteview.

Step 12: Editing and Coding the Data

Editing of data is analogous to editing newspaper copy. The editor's job is to make sure that the text meets certain standards and that errors are corrected. The editor checks for missing data, for inconsistencies, and for problems that can be remedied. Editing of data should be done as soon as possible after data collection.

To permit computerized analysis of data, it is essential that the variables be reduced to a form in which a numerical value may be assigned to each possible choice. This process is referred to as **coding.** It is carried out simultaneously with editing. Coding may be done either by use of an ad hoc coding system specifically developed for your own data base or by use of a standard coding system. A well-accepted technique for the coding of diseases or causes of death is the International Classification of Diseases (World Health Organization, 1977). This flexible system can provide either a broad categorization of disease groups or quite detailed coding of specific entities.

For years, the standard procedure was to use punch cards for computer entry. The current method of choice is to enter data directly via an interactive terminal. In this way, a validation program is able to inform the key-entry operator immediately about possibly invalid data. To maintain accuracy, it is essential that, by program or otherwise, the data entry be verified.

Step 13: Analyzing the Data

After data have been collected, edited, coded, and key-entered, they are soon ready for analysis. But a preliminary step is needed: some advance data analysis to ferret out possible outliers, look at the distribution of the various variables, provide an item analysis for the variables of special interest, and assess the amount of missing data. Once this analysis is completed, you are ready to perform the major analysis of data, a task dictated by the specific objectives of the survey.

Step 14: Reporting the Findings

The report should begin with background information that provides a rationale for the study. It should indicate the specific objectives that the survey seeks to accomplish. A "methods" section should describe the target population, the test instruments, and the sampling design. The "results" section should discuss the findings and possible future implications.

17.2 Evaluation of a Research Report

It is quite unlikely that all the users of this book will become regular producers of research literature. But, almost without exception, everyone will be a consumer of such literature. Research literature comes in many forms: books, journal articles, monographs, administrative documents, program evaluations, and the like.

A valuable skill to develop is the ability to critically read and evaluate research literature. Without this, a person is unable to differentiate between a pedestrian report and one of quality. A top-grade report stands unshaken under the critical process of **peer review.** In a sense, every user of literature, by doing a critical analysis, is carrying peer review to its ultimate step.

It is a well-known, if regrettable, fact that some research literature is of poor quality. After wading through a mire of jargon, inconsistencies, poor grammar, tangles of qualifications, and some muddy logic, the user is expected to draw a brilliantly clear scientific conclusion. This problem is chronic in much scientific writing. A full discussion is well beyond the scope of this book. See one of the several excellent treatments of the subject (for example, Flesch, 1974; Sheen, 1982).

A parallel problem exists when dealing with the quantitative aspects of a report. It is hoped that by reading this section you will gain at least a glimmer of how to be critical, analytical, and discriminating in your use of research literature.

Researchers, being human, must exercise constant vigilance to avoid bias while working toward a prized objective. As mentioned briefly in Chapter 1, bias may well creep in—usually inadvertently, perhaps subconsciously, and often as a consequence of some aspect of the research design. Although the best researchers are carefully trained in its avoidance, bias assumes so many forms that it is difficult to recognize and avoid them all. By examining a few of these, we should be more capable of effectively evaluating a research report. For a comprehensive catalogue of research bias, see Sackett (1979).

Observer Bias

When the observer (or interviewer) is fully aware that the person being interviewed has a certain disease, the observer may subconsciously attribute certain characteristics to the subject. The result of this **observer bias** is that those characteristics are more likely to be recorded for cases than for controls. The solution of choice is to "blind" the observer as to whether the subject is a case or a control.

Sampling Bias

Bias may enter whenever samples are chosen in a nonrandom fashion. **Convenience sampling** (choosing only subjects who are easy to find) leads almost invariably to biased results. **Systematic sampling** (choosing every nth person from a list) carries the potential of subtle error, especially if the list has some cyclical pattern. Telephone and household sampling have their own potentials for bias. What if no one answers the phone or comes to the door? Should the interviewer skip that household? On the contrary. The interviewer should try again (and again), realizing that a household where no one is at home in the daytime is quite different from one where someone is nearly always present.

Selection Bias

Were the cases and controls drawn from the same population? This question, which sounds simple, has profound implications. **Selection bias** may lead to a false association between a disease and some factor because of different probabilities of selecting persons with and without the disease and with and without the variable of interest. This problem was first quantified by Berkson (1946) and is sometimes called **Berksonian bias,** or hospital selection bias.

Response Bias

When participation in a study is voluntary, **response bias** (sometimes called **non-respondent bias** or **self-selection bias**) is a matter of importance.

Owing to their psychological makeup, internal motivation, concern for their own health, educational background, and many other reasons, persons who choose voluntarily to participate are known to differ from those who decline. Nevertheless, many important research studies (e.g., the Framingham Study) depend in part on volunteers. A way to control for response bias is to compare characteristics of volunteer subgroups with those of randomly chosen subgroups.

Dropout Bias

Dropout bias is the mirror image of response bias. In long-term studies, a certain proportion of participants, for reasons of their own, choose to drop out. These persons are likely to differ from those who continue.

Memory Bias

There are several well-known aspects of **memory bias** (also known as **subjective bias**). Memory for recent events is much more accurate than for remote events. Hence persons interviewed concerning past illnesses tend to report a greater prevalence in the recent past than in the distant past (Stocks, 1944). A perhaps more profound form of memory bias is the tendency of persons with a disease to overemphasize the importance of events they may consider to be predisposing causes (e.g., breast cancer patients who trace their disease to traumatic breast injury).

Participant Bias

Participant bias is an interesting form of bias that derives from the participant's knowledge of being a member of the experimental or control group and his or her perception of the research objectives. For example, a member of a heart disease intervention study may report and exaggerate minor symptoms actually unrelated to the disease under study.

Lead-Time Bias

Does early detection of chronic disease actually result in improved survival or does it merely provide a longer period between first detection and death? This fascinating question of **lead-time bias** is fully considered in Cole and Morrison (1980).

Keys to a Systematic Approach

Awareness of the potential for bias underlies a critical reading of any research report. But bias is not the only issue to keep in mind. A great deal may be learned by using a systematic approach toward a critique of any research literature. Here are some of the most important questions that should be considered:

1. *Research objectives.* Does the research report clearly state its objectives? Do the conclusions address the same objectives?
2. *Study design.* What type of study was it? Was sample selection random

and appropriate to the study design? Were cases and controls comparable and drawn from the same reference group?

3. *Data collection.* Were criteria for diagnosis precisely defined? Were end points (or outcome criteria) clearly stated? Were research instruments (whether mechanical or electronic devices, or printed questionnaires) standardized? Can the study be independently replicated?
4. *Discussion of results.* Are results presented clearly and quantitatively? Do tables and figures agree with the text? Are various tables consistent with one another?
5. *Data analysis.* Does the report address the statistical significance of its results? If not, are you able to draw a reasonable inference of significance (or nonsignificance) from the data as presented? Were the statistical tests appropriate to the data? Does the report discuss alternative explanations for what might be spurious statistical significance?
6. *Conclusions.* Are the findings justified by the data? Do the findings relate appropriately to the research objectives originally set forth?

Serious users of research literature have found this step-by-step approach extremely helpful. For a more thorough discussion, see the excellent treatment in Colton (1974).

Conclusion

Two fundamental research tools, the health survey and the research report, are inseparable parts of the same process: that of aiding scientists, managers, and public officials in their decision-making. Health surveys need careful planning; a systematic stepwise procedure is the best means of avoiding error in their use. Research reports are read by nearly everyone in the health sciences. It is important to develop a critical eye to distinguish between ordinary reports and those of quality. Especially when dealing with human populations, the researcher is susceptible to many sources of bias. An understanding of the origins of bias, and of the means to avoid bias in whatever form, helps the user assess the quality of any research report.

Vocabulary List

coding
consumer
convenience sampling
dropout bias
editing
element
interviewer bias
lead-time bias
mailed questionnaire
memory bias (subjective bias)
observer bias
participant bias
peer review
person-to-person interview
pretest
response bias (nonrespondent bias; self-selection bias)
sampling bias
selection bias (Berksonian bias)
systematic sampling
target population
telephone interview

Exercises

17.1 Prepare an outline for a health survey on a subject of special interest to yourself.

17.2 Locate a completed health survey. Is it constructed in keeping with the guidelines of this chapter? In what ways is it imperfectly planned? What would you do to improve it?

17.3 Choose a scientific article that reports on research in your own field. Subject it to the evaluation process suggested in this chapter.

17.4 Using the survey of Exercise 17.2, the article for Exercise 17.3, or any health survey report, discuss how the authors handled potential bias. What steps did they take to minimize it? What types of bias may have crept in? How could these have been avoided?

Chapter **18**

Computers: An Introduction

Chapter Outline

18.1 Introduction
A few comments are made about computers and their applications in the health sciences, including uses and misuses.

18.2 Hardware
The principal components of electronic computers are described.

18.3 Software
The programs and compilers that provide the instructions computers use to do their jobs are discussed.

18.4 Computer Programs
A step-by-step example is presented of a simple program, together with some discussion of popular packaged programs and the terminology used with them.

18.5 Computerized Data Entry: An Example
An example from the Honolulu Heart Study illustrates a typical method of statistical data entry.

18.6 Computerized Data Output: An Example
The example of Section 18.5 is extended to provide a glimpse at the end result of a computer's work.

18.7 Microcomputers
The role of microcomputers in data analysis is discussed.

Learning Objectives

After studying this chapter, you should be able to

1. State some of the principal applications of computers to the health sciences
2. Distinguish between hardware and software
3. Identify the principal components of a computer system, including types of input and output devices
4. Appreciate the importance of accuracy in data coding and entry
5. Recognize a typical computer program and the elements of a computerized data output

18.1 Introduction

Computers have been among the greatest technological developments of our time. Their impact is felt daily in countless areas of human life. The applications of computers to the health sciences are continually proliferating. Health agencies use computers for administrative tasks: to maintain patients' records, personnel files, accounts, and billing. Patient-care systems are now computerized. Computers monitor medication regimens, keep track of clinical laboratory values, monitor patients' vital functions, and control sophisticated diagnostic equipment. Computers aid in teaching by providing preprogrammed instructions for teaching new procedures or by simulating real-life situations. The computer permits researchers to process and analyze enormous quantities of data. Consequently, the validity of various scientific hypotheses may now be tested at a speed and accuracy heretofore unknown.

Most unfortunately, the accessibility of computers with their powerful packaged programs has led to a *misuse* of both the computers and their statistical methods. The computer is a marvelous machine that follows instructions precisely; it cannot discriminate on its own as to whether the data are accurate or the statistical methods to be used are appropriate. So it is not uncommon that the results obtained turn out to be erroneous. Obviously, the mistakes are not the computer's fault; the responsibility rests with the person who may not have sufficient experience in processing and analyzing computerized data. Because of the relative frequency of this problem, it has been named the **GIGO** syndrome: "garbage in, garbage out." To minimize the problem and to provide students with some insight into computers—what they are and what they can do—this chapter is offered as a simplified introduction to this broad subject.

18.2 Hardware

A computer is an electronic device that is able, at the speed of light, to perform a series of tasks such as adding, subtracting, and comparing by means of a list of detailed instructions called a **program.** Programs are referred to as **software;** the computer and its peripheral equipment are referred to as **hardware.** The main component of the computer is the **central processing unit (CPU).** As shown in Figure 18.1, the CPU receives data through an **input device,** executes specific instructions contained in the program, and sends out results in an organized, readable fashion through an **output device.** Input devices include teletypes, punch-card readers, magnetic disks, optical scanners, and magnetic tape units. Output devices include typewriters, **cathode-ray terminals (CRTs),** magnetic tape units, disks, card punchers

Figure 18.1 Major Components of a Computer

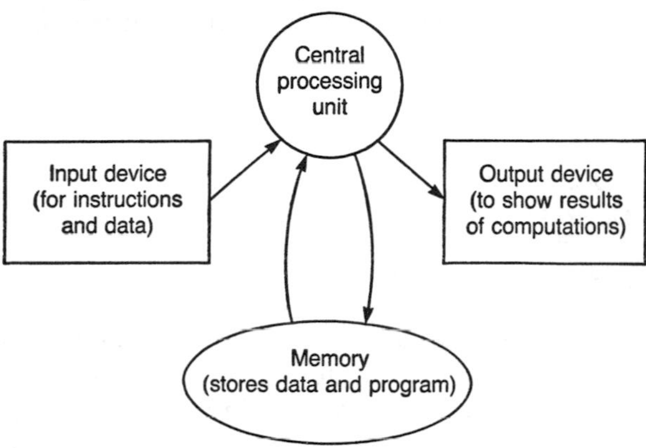

and printer-plotters. Some devices double as input-output units. These include teletypes, typewriter terminals, and CRTs. Linked to the CPU are **memory units** that store data and program instructions. Computer memories are made of building blocks, the most fundamental of which is the **bit,** a binary digit that indicates whether a specific electronic path is "on" or "off." Eight bits constitute a **byte,** while two or more bytes constitute a **word.** Like humans, computers communicate with words.

Digital computers represent information by means of electronic signals that are binary numbers: 0 or 1. The software converts these binary representations into a more readable form. Programming a computer by use of binary arithmetic codes would be an insuperable task. Fortunately, convenient **languages** are available (e.g., FORTRAN and BASIC) that automatically convert common decimal arithmetic into binary form.

18.3 Software

The computer performs specific tasks by explicitly following the instructions contained in the program. Computer programmers, proficient in the use of languages such as BASIC, FORTRAN, COBOL, PASCAL, and PL/1, are able to prepare programs specific to the needs of any computation or series of computations. The computer is able to respond to instructions represented by binary codes. Consequently, instructions written in a computer language must be translated into the machine language of binary codes by a program referred to as a **compiler.** Compilers and other programs are parts of the software. They are stored, ready for use, in the computer's memory.

18.4 Computer Programs

To gain some insight into how a program is written, let's consider a simple program in BASIC for computing the arithmetic mean.

1. INPUT X1
2. INPUT X2
3. INPUT X3
4. SUMX = X1 + X2 + X3
5. XBAR = SUMX ÷ 3
6. PRINT XBAR
7. END

In this program, statements 1, 2, and 3 instruct the computer to read the values of X1, X2, and X3 from the input device. Statement 4 instructs the computer to add ("SUM") the values of X1, X2, and X3. Statement 5 instructs the computer to divide the sum by 3 and store it in memory as $\bar{X}$ ("XBAR"). Statement 6 tells the computer to print the value of $\bar{X}$. And statement 7 instructs the computer that it is the end of the program. This is a simple program. Before attempting to write a complicated program, a programmer usually prepares a **flowchart** that schematically illustrates each step necessary to accomplish the specific task. The programmer uses the flowchart as a guide while he or she writes detailed program instructions. More often than not, a complex program when first written will fail because of "bugs" in it. The process of correcting erroneous instructions is called "debugging."

Writing a complicated statistical program consumes real time and effort. For this reason, many packaged programs have been developed for application to a large number of different computers. Among the well-known statistical programs are SPSS, BMD, and SAS. These packages include a variety of features that enable them to accept data in a standard fashion and produce results in a number of options. The packages contain programs for nearly all the standard statistical analyses; they make it possible to utilize powerful statistical tools economically with the knowledge that the programs have been validated in advance as capable of giving reliable results.

The user may submit jobs to use packaged programs either in a *batch* mode or an *interactive* mode. In **batch processing,** the user prepares **job cards,** which direct the computer to use the programs, and submits them along with data cards or via a CRT. The jobs are then processed; the user obtains the results some time later. In **interactive processing,** the user's data is processed in real time, i.e., interactively, or "while you wait." By using this approach, the user is able to see the intermediate steps of the analysis and guide it to the desired end. Because of the lightning speed of computers, waiting time is usually imperceptible to the user. In fact, several users may simultaneously share the computer, a feature called **time-sharing.** SCSS and MINITAB are examples of interactive type package programs.

18.5 Computerized Data Entry: An Example

Using the data on the sample of 100 persons selected from the Honolulu Heart Study (Table 3.1), let's see how typical data might be processed and submitted for analysis by use of an SPSS program.

Figure 18.2 (p. 234) is part of a questionnaire that could have been used to obtain the information of Table 3.1. The questionnaire is **precoded** so that data may easily be transferred from the questionnaire to a punch card or directly into the computer memory fields that correspond to those on the punch card. Precoding involves the assignment of small numbers that identify various choices in the answers to each question. We see in the figure that the columns describing the width of the field for a specific variable are defined by large numbers in the left-hand margin or beneath the entry blanks. This scheme allows the responses to be automatically coded, and the precoded values are entered into the computer. The width of any field depends on the number of digits to be used for coding the response. Thus, for education, the field is one column in width; for height, the field is three columns wide. Fields corresponding to the various questions are designated on the card and are shown in Figure 18.3 (p. 235). We have coded 10 variables that use the first 33 columns. Forty-seven columns are unused; they could be used for additional variables. Note that we utilize one case per card, and each case is identified by a unique ID number. We have here allocated three columns as the ID. The case illustrated is no. 1 (in computer lingo, case 001), which is entered in column 3. The ID field is three columns wide; it can handle up to 999 cases. Education is coded in column 6; the person answering the questionnaire entered code 2, representing completion of the primary grades. His weight was 70 kg (columns 0–9). He was a smoker (column 19), and his systolic blood pressure was 102 mmHg (columns 31–33). The complete set of data for case 001 is a **record**; the sequential listing of records for all cases is a computer **file.**

To avoid entering "garbage" and to ensure reliable data for analysis, the user must adhere precisely to the basic data processing principles. One way to do this is to provide numerical (not alphabetic) codes. It is important to code missing data in some way other than entering zeros, because zero is a legitimate value for most data. Other sound steps are to edit returned questionnaires for completeness, assign correct codes for open-ended responses, and assign ID numbers to the various cases.

Once fields are defined for the several variables, the designated codes need to be entered accurately into computer memory. The user must be especially careful that data are entered in their designated columns and that decimal places are entered correctly. Data for variables having a field width greater than 1 must be right-justified (punched as far to the right as possible in the field).

When key-entry has been completed, the user proceeds with **verifi-**

Figure 18.2 Sample of a Coded Questionnaire That Could Be Used to Obtain the Data from the Honolulu Heart Study

______ ______ ______ ID#
1 2 3

1. Please indicate the educational level that you have attained.
   1[ ] None
   2[ ] Primary (1–8)
6 3[ ] Intermediate (9–10)
   4[ ] Senior High (11–12)
   5[ ] Technical School
   6[ ] Some college or college graduate
2. What is your weight without shoes?
   ______ ______ kg
   8 9
3. What is your height without shoes?
   ______ ______ ______ cm
   12 13 14
4. What is your present age?
   ______ ______
   16 17
5. Are you currently a smoker?
   0[ ] No
19 1[ ] Yes
6. Which of these categories describe your physical activity on a typical work day?
   1[ ] Mostly sitting
21 2[ ] Moderate activity
   3[ ] Much activity
7. Blood glucose level
   ______ ______ ______ (mg %)
   23 24 25
8. Serum cholesterol
   ______ ______ ______ (mg %)
   27 28 29
9. Systolic blood pressure
   ______ ______ ______ (mmHg)
   31 32 33

Figure 18.3 Sample of Punched Card for Data from Questionnaire Shown in Figure 18.2

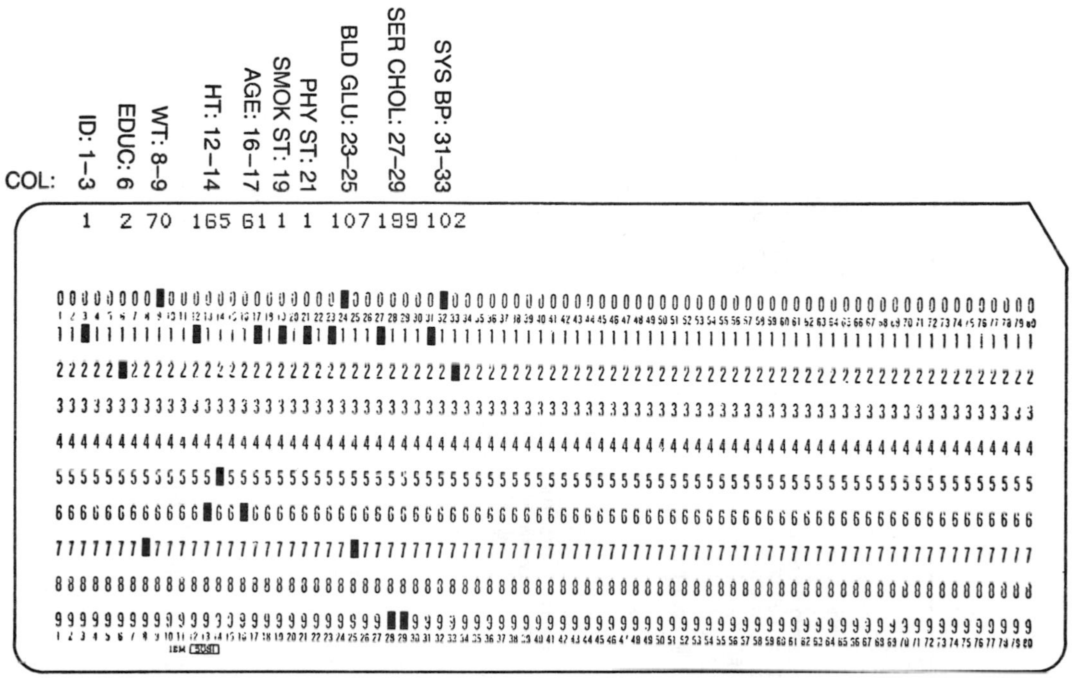

COL: ID: 1–3 EDUC: 6 WT: 8–9 HT: 12–14 AGE: 16–17 SMOK ST: 19 PHY ST: 21 BLD GLU: 23–25 SER CHOL: 27–29 SYS BP: 31–33

1 2 70 165 61 1 1 107 199 102

Code for variables:

Education: 1—none, 2—primary, 3—intermediate, 4—senior high, 5—technical school, 6—university
Weight: in kilograms
Height: in centimeters
Smoking: 0—no, 1—yes
Physical activity: 1—mostly sitting, 2—moderate, 3—much
Blood glucose: in milligrams %
Serum cholesterol: in milligrams %
Systolic blood pressure: in millimeters of mercury

cation, which consists of a careful check of input data for possible errors. This can be done by proofreading the data against a printed file or by independently reentering the data (utilizing a different person) and having a computer program identify any differences.

After the data have been verified and corrected, they are ready for analysis, which initially usually consists of a simple frequency distribution that will show whether there are any codes that are out of range.

Figure 18.4 Sample Job Card for Initiating a "Frequencies" Program

```
RUN NAME        HONOLULU HEART STUDY SAMPLE
DATA LIST       FIXED (1)/1 ID 1-3 EDUC 6 WT 8-9 HT 12-14 AGE 16-17
                SMOKST 19 PHYS 21 BLDGLU 23-25 SCHOL 27-29 SYSBP 31-33
OTHER DATA LIST PROVIDES FOR 10 VARIABLES AND  1 RECORDS ('CARDS') PER CASE. A MAXIMUM OF   33 COLUMNS ARE USED ON A RECORD.

 LIST OF THE CONSTRUCTED FORMAT STATEMENT..
        (F3.0,2X,F1.0,1X,F2.0,2X,F3.0,1X,F2.0,1X,F1.0,1X,F1.0,1X,F3.0,1X,F3.0,1X
        ,F3.0)

INPUT MEDIUM    CRT
N OF CASES      100
RECODE          ALL(BLANK=-1)
MISSING VALUES  ID TO SYSBP(-1)
RECODE          SYSBP(LO THRU 119=120)(120 THRU 160=160)(161 THRU HI=161)
VALUE LABELS    SYSBP(120) LESS THAN 120MM HG (160) 120-160MM HG
                         (161) GREATER THAN 160MM HG/
COMMENT         RUN FREQUENCIES FOR SMOK. & NON SMOK.
*SELECT IF      (SMOKST EQ 1)
FREQUENCIES     GENERAL=SYSBP
STATISTICS      ALL
```

The user next selects an appropriate software package program to conduct a specific analysis. Suppose we wish to obtain a frequency count and some descriptive statistics for our data. We can obtain these by using the SPSS package program called "Frequencies." The information needed for the job card is listed in Figure 18.4. Item 1 is the name for the computer run. Item 2 identifies variables. Item 3 lists **format statements** that indicate the width of each field and the location of the decimal point for each variable. Item 4 indicates that the data were entered by means of a CRT. Item 5 shows that there were 100 cases. Item 6 shows that all blank responses were coded as −1. Item 7 shows that the program treats all −1's as missing values and therefore excludes those cases from analysis. Item 8 indicates that the values of systolic blood pressure are categorized into three categories—less than 120, 120–160, and greater than 160. Items 9–10 indicate the labels of these three categories. Item 11 indicates that analyses are to be performed separately for smokers and nonsmokers. Item 12 is a reminder that the smoking and nonsmoking groups are to be selected for this analysis. Item 13 instructs the "Frequencies" program to be run for systolic blood pressure values. Item 14 indicates that all statistics are to be printed. Items 15–17 (not shown) repeat the last three steps for the nonsmokers.

18.6 Computerized Data Output: An Example

Figure 18.5 (p. 238) is a copy of the computer output. Item 1 is a frequency table listing the absolute, relative, and cumulative frequencies for smokers. Item 2 shows the descriptive statistics for the 37 smokers. The corresponding information for nonsmokers is shown in items 3 and 4. Specifically, we can see that the mean systolic blood pressure was 131.9 for smokers and 129.0 for nonsmokers. From the frequency tables we can see that 13.5% of smokers and 6.3% of nonsmokers had a blood pressure greater than 160. This output contains other information useful in checking data entry; for example, it gives minimum and maximum values and indicates whether any of the records had missing values. Other descriptive statistics such as the mean, median, mode, and standard deviation are computed and listed. The frequency tables show cumulative frequencies. An impressive sidelight: all these computations were performed in 5.93 seconds. The output is simple and easy to follow, particularly with the aid of an instruction manual for the software package in use. Such manuals provide full instructions on how to set up job cards, submit data, and interpret results.

Although our example is a quite simple program, more involved and elaborate outputs are common. They result from more complex analyses.

Figure 18.5 Sample Computer Output for Frequencies and Descriptive Statistics of Systolic Blood Pressure for Smokers and Nonsmokers for the Honolulu Heart Study Sample

```
    SYSBP     SYSTOLIC BLOOD PRESSURE  (SMOKERS)
  -                                                 RELATIVE  ADJUSTED    CUM
                                          ABSOLUTE    FREQ      FREQ      FREQ
1  CATEGORY LABEL               CODE        FREQ     (PCT)     (PCT)     (PCT)
  LESS THAN 120MM HG            <120.         15      40.5      40.5      40.5
  120-160MM HG               120-160.         17      45.9      45.9      86.5
  GREATER THAN 160MM HG         >160.          5      13.5      13.5     100.0
                                           ------    ------    ------
                               TOTAL          37     100.0     100.0

   MEAN          131.892     STD ERR          4.156       MEDIAN        125.500
   MODE          116.000     STD DEV         25.280       VARIANCE      639.099
2  KURTOSIS        1.484     SKEWNESS         1.244       RANGE         110.000
   MINIMUM        98.000     MAXIMUM        208.000

   VALID CASES        37     MISSING CASES        0

                  15 *SELECT IF        (SMOKST EQ 0)
                  16 FREQUENCIES       GENERAL=SYSBP
                  17 STATISTICS        ALL

    SYSBP     SYSTOLIC BLOOD PRESSURE  (NONSMOKERS)
  -                                                 RELATIVE  ADJUSTED    CUM
                                          ABSOLUTE    FREQ      FREQ      FREQ
3  CATEGORY LABEL               CODE        FREQ     (PCT)     (PCT)     (PCT)
  LESS THAN 120MM HG            <120.         19      30.2      30.2      30.2
  120-160MM HG                120-160.        40      63.5      63.5      93.7
   GREATER THAN 161MM HG        >161.          4       6.3       6.3     100.0
                                           ------    ------    ------
                               TOTAL          63     100.0     100.0


   MEAN          129.048     STD ERR          2.337       MEDIAN        128.375
   MODE          128.000     STD DEV         18.547       VARIANCE      343.982
4  KURTOSIS       -0.251     SKEWNESS         0.201       RANGE          80.000
   MINIMUM        92.000     MAXIMUM        172.000

   VALID CASES        63     MISSING CASES        0
                  18 FINISH
  1           NORMAL END OF SPSS RUN.
                18 COMMAND RECORDS READ
                 0 ERRORS DETECTED

  0******JOB EXITED ON 28 SEP 82 10:45:32     ******
  0******CPU TIME=       0MINS     5.93SECS   ******
  0******CONNECT TIME=     0MINS    29SECS    ******
```

18.7 Microcomputers

The computer revolution may well be unparalleled in history. It certainly will rank with the industrial revolution as a point of departure in world events. The industrial revolution had its cotton gin and steam engine; the computer revolution has its micro (or personal) computer.

So many things are possible with microcomputers: composing and editing texts (word processing); solving all sorts of quantitative problems—personal, business, or scientific; preparing graphic layouts, sensing and recognizing patterns, automatically controlling equipment or processes;

communicating with persons near or far; and playing games of skill or chance.

In dealing with scientific material, the microcomputer enables you to interact directly with your data. Until quite recently, this was hard to do, because large-scale computers either did not have this feature or provided it only at enormous cost. With the advent of the personal computer, quite adequate interactive statistical programs have become available and affordable to many. Good-quality statistical software is readily available for many microcomputers, such as the Apple IIe, TRS-80, Kaypro II, Commodore 64, Hewlett-Packard, Victor 9000, and IBM Personal Computer.

Are you on the verge of buying a personal computer? The market is saturated with a bewildering variety of products, some of which may nicely meet your needs. Before investing in a personal computer, you would be well advised to refer to an authoritative introduction to the subject, such as Willis and Miller (1983) or McWilliams (1982). These books discuss the characteristics of microcomputers, your software and hardware options, and guidelines for selecting the micro appropriate to your particular needs. Other books of special interest include Frenzel (1980), Savage (1981), and Billings and Moursund (1979).

Conclusion

Computers are marvelous devices that permit statisticians and health scientists to do their work faster and more accurately than previously thought possible. However, computers indiscriminately do precisely as they are told; inexperience or poor judgment can lead to their misuse. The computer field has a colorful vocabulary and special terminology. Special languages have been devised for communicating with computers. A number of packaged programs have been written in these languages so that computers can carry out statistical manipulations. The entry of data is a particularly critical step, in which extraordinary precautions should be taken to ensure accuracy.

Vocabulary

batch processing
bit
byte
cathode-ray terminal (CRT)
central processing unit (CPU)
compiler
file
flowchart
format statement
GIGO
hardware
input device
interactive processing
job card
language
memory unit
output device
precoding
program
record
software
time-sharing
verification
word

Exercises

18.1 Refer to the data of Table 2.2.

(a) Prepare a code for key-entering the data.

(b) Using an existing computer program available to you, key-enter the data of Table 2.2 and obtain the mean and the standard deviation for the diastolic blood pressure separately for the male vegetarians and the male nonvegetarians.

(c) Using an existing computer program available to you, obtain the frequency distribution of the number of vegetarians and nonvegetarians by sex.

18.2 (a) Complete the following table by using data from the computer output shown in Figure 18.5.

Systolic blood pressure	Smokers		Nonsmokers	
	No.	%	No.	%
<120 mmHg	____	____	____	____
120–160 mmHg	____	____	____	____
>160 mmHg	____	____	____	____

(b) Using the data from the completed table in Exercise 18.2a test the following null hypothesis at the $\alpha = .05$ level.

H_0: Smokers and nonsmokers are homogeneous in the distribution of their systolic blood pressures.

Epilogue

It is hoped that the techniques and methods presented in this book will provide you with some useful tools that can be used to separate fact from fiction, to determine the significance of experimental results, and ultimately to assist your search for truth. The road to truth is seldom an easy one, but a great deal of satisfaction can be attained while traversing it. This is particularly true when one is able to establish the significance of a new finding, to learn that a commonly accepted approach is not really valid, or to gain the kind of insight that begins to shed new light on the process of discovery. The journey may be rough, but it is surely worthwhile. Godspeed!

Appendix A

Binomial Probability Table

n	x	.01	.05	.10	.15	.20	.25	.30	1/3	.35	.40	.45	.50
1	0	.9900	.9500	.9000	.8500	.8000	.7500	.7000	.6667	.6500	.6000	.5500	.5000
	1	.0100	.0500	.1000	.1500	.2000	.2500	.3000	.3333	.3500	.4000	.4500	.5000
2	0	.9801	.9025	.8100	.7225	.6400	.5625	.4900	.4444	.4225	.3600	.3025	.2500
	1	.0198	.0950	.1800	.2550	.3200	.3750	.4200	.4444	.4550	.4800	.4950	.5000
	2	.0001	.0025	.0100	.0225	.0400	.0625	.0900	.1111	.1225	.1600	.2025	.2500
3	0	.9703	.8574	.7290	.6141	.5120	.4219	.3430	.2963	.2746	.2160	.1664	.1250
	1	.0294	.1354	.2430	.3251	.3840	.4219	.4410	.4444	.4436	.4320	.4084	.3750
	2	.0003	.0071	.0270	.0574	.0960	.1406	.1890	.2222	.2389	.2880	.3341	.3750
	3	.0000	.0001	.0010	.0034	.0080	.0156	.0270	.0370	.0429	.0640	.0911	.1250
4	0	.9606	.8145	.6561	.5220	.4096	.3164	.2401	.1975	.1785	.1296	.0915	.0625
	1	.0388	.1715	.2916	.3685	.4096	.4219	.4116	.3951	.3845	.3456	.2995	.2500
	2	.0006	.0135	.0486	.0975	.1536	.2109	.2646	.2963	.3105	.3456	.3675	.3750
	3	.0000	.0005	.0036	.0115	.0256	.0469	.0756	.0988	.1115	.1536	.2005	.2500
	4	.0000	.0000	.0001	.0005	.0016	.0039	.0081	.0123	.0150	.0256	.0410	.0625
5	0	.9510	.7738	.5905	.4437	.3277	.2373	.1681	.1317	.1160	.0778	.0503	.0312
	1	.0480	.2036	.3280	.3915	.4096	.3955	.3601	.3292	.3124	.2592	.2059	.1563
	2	.0010	.0214	.0729	.1382	.2048	.2637	.3087	.3292	.3364	.3456	.3369	.3125
	3	.0000	.0012	.0081	.0244	.0512	.0879	.1323	.1646	.1812	.2304	.2757	.3125
	4	.0000	.0000	.0005	.0021	.0064	.0146	.0284	.0412	.0487	.0768	.1127	.1563
	5	.0000	.0000	.0000	.0001	.0003	.0010	.0024	.0041	.0053	.0102	.0185	.0312
6	0	.9415	.7351	.5314	.3771	.2621	.1780	.1176	.0878	.0754	.0467	.0277	.0156
	1	.0570	.2321	.3543	.3994	.3932	.3559	.3026	.2634	.2437	.1866	.1359	.0938
	2	.0015	.0306	.0984	.1762	.2458	.2967	.3241	.3292	.3280	.3110	.2779	.2344
	3	.0000	.0021	.0146	.0414	.0819	.1318	.1852	.2195	.2355	.2765	.3032	.3125
	4	.0000	.0001	.0012	.0055	.0154	.0330	.0596	.0823	.0951	.1382	.1861	.2344
	5	.0000	.0000	.0001	.0004	.0015	.0044	.0102	.0165	.0205	.0369	.0609	.0938
	6	.0000	.0000	.0000	.0000	.0001	.0002	.0007	.0014	.0018	.0041	.0083	.0156

		p											
n	x	.01	.05	.10	.15	.20	.25	.30	1/3	.35	.40	.45	.50
	0	.9321	.6983	.4783	.3206	.2097	.1335	.0824	.0585	.0490	.0280	.0152	.0078
	1	.0659	.2573	.3720	.3960	.3670	.3114	.2470	.2048	.1848	.1306	.0872	.0547
	2	.0020	.0406	.1240	.2096	.2753	.3115	.3177	.3073	.2985	.2613	.2140	.1641
7	3	.0000	.0036	.0230	.0617	.1147	.1730	.2269	.2561	.2679	.2903	.2919	.2734
	4	.0000	.0002	.0025	.0109	.0286	.0577	.0972	.1280	.1442	.1935	.2388	.2734
	5	.0000	.0000	.0002	.0011	.0043	.0116	.0250	.0384	.0466	.0775	.1172	.1641
	6	.0000	.0000	.0000	.0001	.0004	.0012	.0036	.0064	.0084	.0172	.0320	.0547
	7	.0000	.0000	.0000	.0000	.0000	.0001	.0002	.0005	.0006	.0016	.0037	.0078
	0	.9227	.6634	.4305	.2725	.1678	.1001	.0576	.0390	.0319	.0168	.0084	.0039
	1	.0746	.2794	.3826	.3847	.3355	.2670	.1977	.1561	.1372	.0896	.0548	.0313
	2	.0026	.0514	.1488	.2376	.2936	.3114	.2965	.2731	.2587	.2090	.1570	.1093
	3	.0001	.0054	.0331	.0838	.1468	.2077	.2541	.2731	.2786	.2787	.2569	.2188
8	4	.0000	.0004	.0046	.0185	.0459	.0865	.1361	.1707	.1875	.2322	.2626	.2734
	5	.0000	.0000	.0004	.0027	.0092	.0231	.0467	.0683	.0808	.1239	.1718	.2188
	6	.0000	.0000	.0000	.0002	.0011	.0038	.0100	.0171	.0217	.0413	.0704	.1093
	7	.0000	.0000	.0000	.0000	.0001	.0004	.0012	.0024	.0034	.0078	.0164	.0313
	8	.0000	.0000	.0000	.0000	.0000	.0000	.0001	.0002	.0002	.0007	.0017	.0039
	0	.9135	.6302	.3874	.2316	.1342	.0751	.0404	.0260	.0207	.0101	.0046	.0020
	1	.0831	.2986	.3874	.3678	.3020	.2252	.1556	.1171	.1004	.0604	.0339	.0175
	2	.0033	.0628	.1722	.2597	.3020	.3004	.2668	.2341	.2162	.1613	.1110	.0703
	3	.0001	.0078	.0447	.1070	.1762	.2336	.2669	.2731	.2716	.2508	.2119	.1641
9	4	.0000	.0006	.0074	.0283	.0660	.1168	.1715	.2048	.2194	.2508	.2600	.2461
	5	.0000	.0000	.0008	.0050	.0165	.0389	.0735	.1024	.1181	.1672	.2128	.2461
	6	.0000	.0000	.0001	.0006	.0028	.0087	.0210	.0341	.0424	.0744	.1160	.1641
	7	.0000	.0000	.0000	.0000	.0003	.0012	.0039	.0073	.0098	.0212	.0407	.0703
	8	.0000	.0000	.0000	.0000	.0000	.0001	.0004	.0009	.0013	.0035	.0083	.0175
	9	.0000	.0000	.0000	.0000	.0000	.0000	.0000	.0001	.0001	.0003	.0008	.0020
	0	.9044	.5987	.3487	.1969	.1074	.0563	.0282	.0173	.0135	.0060	.0025	.0010
	1	.0913	.3152	.3874	.3474	.2684	.1877	.1211	.0867	.0725	.0404	.0208	.0097
	2	.0042	.0746	.1937	.2759	.3020	.2816	.2335	.1951	.1756	.1209	.0763	.0440
	3	.0001	.0105	.0574	.1298	.2013	.2503	.2668	.2601	.2522	.2150	.1664	.1172
	4	.0000	.0009	.0112	.0401	.0881	.1460	.2001	.2276	.2377	.2508	.2384	.2051
10	5	.0000	.0001	.0015	.0085	.0264	.0584	.1030	.1366	.1536	.2007	.2340	.2460
	6	.0000	.0000	.0001	.0013	.0055	.0162	.0367	.0569	.0689	.1114	.1596	.2051
	7			.0000	.0001	.0008	.0031	.0090	.0163	.0212	.0425	.0746	.1172
	8				.0000	.0001	.0004	.0015	.0030	.0043	.0106	.0229	.0440
	9				.0000	.0000	.0000	.0001	.0003	.0005	.0016	.0042	.0097
	10	.0000	.0000	.0000	.0000	.0000	.0000	.0000	.0000	.0000	.0001	.0003	.0010
	0	.8953	.5688	.3138	.1673	.0859	.0422	.0198	.0116	.0088	.0036	.0014	.0005
	1	.0995	.3293	.3836	.3249	.2362	.1549	.0932	.0636	.0518	.0266	.0125	.0054
	2	.0050	.0867	.2130	.2866	.2953	.2581	.1998	.1590	.1395	.0887	.0513	.0268
	3	.0002	.0136	.0711	.1518	.2215	.2581	.2568	.2384	.2255	.1774	.1259	.0806
	4	.0000	.0015	.0157	.0535	.1107	.1721	.2201	.2384	.2427	.2365	.2060	.1611
11	5		.0001	.0025	.0132	.0387	.0803	.1321	.1669	.1830	.2207	.2360	.2256
	6		.0000	.0003	.0024	.0097	.0267	.0566	.0835	.0986	.1471	.1931	.2256
	7			.0000	.0003	.0018	.0064	.0173	.0298	.0379	.0701	.1128	.1611
	8				.0000	.0002	.0011	.0037	.0075	.0102	.0234	.0462	.0806
	9					.0000	.0001	.0006	.0012	.0018	.0052	.0126	.0268
	10						.0000	.0000	.0001	.0002	.0007	.0020	.0054
	11	.0000	.0000	.0000	.0000	.0000	.0000	.0000	.0000	.0000	.0000	.0002	.0005

n	x	p .01	.05	.10	.15	.20	.25	.30	1/3	.35	.40	.45	.50
	0	.8864	.5404	.2824	.1422	.0687	.0317	.0138	.0077	.0057	.0022	.0008	.0002
	1	.1074	.3412	.3766	.3013	.2062	.1267	.0712	.0462	.0367	.0174	.0075	.0030
	2	.0060	.0988	.2301	.2923	.2834	.2323	.1678	.1272	.1089	.0638	.0338	.0161
	3	.0002	.0174	.0853	.1720	.2363	.2581	.2397	.2120	.1954	.1419	.0924	.0537
	4	.0000	.0020	.0213	.0683	.1328	.1936	.2312	.2384	.2366	.2129	.1700	.1208
	5		.0002	.0038	.0193	.0532	.1032	.1585	.1908	.2040	.2270	.2225	.1934
12	6		.0000	.0004	.0039	.0155	.0401	.0792	.1113	.1281	.1766	.2124	.2256
	7			.0001	.0006	.0033	.0115	.0291	.0477	.0591	.1009	.1489	.1934
	8			.0000	.0001	.0005	.0024	.0078	.0149	.0199	.0420	.0761	.1208
	9				.0000	.0001	.0004	.0015	.0033	.0048	.0125	.0277	.0537
	10					.0000	.0000	.0002	.0005	.0007	.0025	.0068	.0161
	11						.0000	.0000	.0000	.0001	.0003	.0010	.0030
	12	.0000	.0000	.0000	.0000	.0000	.0000	.0000	.0000	.0000	.0000	.0001	.0002
	0	.8601	.4633	.2059	.0874	.0352	.0134	.0047	.0023	.0016	.0005	.0001	.0000
	1	.1301	.3667	.3431	.2312	.1319	.0668	.0306	.0171	.0126	.0047	.0016	.0005
	2	.0092	.1348	.2669	.2856	.2309	.1559	.0915	.0599	.0475	.0219	.0090	.0032
	3	.0004	.0307	.1285	.2185	.2502	.2252	.1701	.1299	.1110	.0634	.0317	.0139
	4	.0000	.0049	.0429	.1156	.1876	.2252	.2186	.1948	.1792	.1268	.0780	.0416
	5		.0005	.0105	.0449	.1031	.1651	.2061	.2143	.2124	.1859	.1404	.0917
15	6		.0001	.0019	.0132	.0430	.0916	.1473	.1786	.1906	.2066	.1914	.1527
	7		.0000	.0003	.0030	.0139	.0393	.0811	.1148	.1320	.1771	.2013	.1964
	8			.0000	.0005	.0034	.0131	.0348	.0574	.0710	.1181	.1657	.1964
	9				.0001	.0007	.0034	.0115	.0223	.0298	.0612	.1049	.1527
	10				.0000	.0001	.0007	.0030	.0067	.0096	.0245	.0514	.0917
	11					.0000	.0001	.0006	.0015	.0023	.0074	.0192	.0416
	12						.0000	.0001	.0003	.0004	.0016	.0052	.0139
	13							.0000	.0000	.0001	.0003	.0010	.0032
	14							.0000	.0000	.0000	.0000	.0001	.0005
	15	.0000	.0000	.0000	.0000	.0000	.0000	.0000	.0000	.0000	.0000	.0000	.0000
	0	.8179	.3583	.1216	.0388	.0115	.0032	.0008	.0003	.0002	.0000	.0000	.0000
	1	.1652	.3773	.2701	.1368	.0577	.0211	.0068	.0030	.0019	.0005	.0001	.0000
	2	.0159	.1887	.2852	.2293	.1369	.0670	.0279	.0143	.0100	.0031	.0008	.0002
	3	.0010	.0596	.1901	.2428	.2053	.1339	.0716	.0429	.0323	.0124	.0040	.0011
	4	.0000	.0133	.0898	.1821	.2182	.1896	.1304	.0911	.0738	.0350	.0140	.0046
	5		.0023	.0319	.1029	.1746	.2024	.1789	.1457	.1272	.0746	.0364	.0148
	6		.0003	.0089	.0454	.1091	.1686	.1916	.1821	.1714	.1244	.0746	.0370
	7		.0000	.0020	.0160	.0546	.1124	.1643	.1821	.1844	.1659	.1221	.0739
	8			.0003	.0046	.0221	.0609	.1144	.1480	.1614	.1797	.1623	.1201
20	9			.0001	.0011	.0074	.0270	.0653	.0987	.1158	.1597	.1771	.1602
	10			.0000	.0002	.0020	.0100	.0309	.0543	.0686	.1172	.1593	.1762
	11				.0000	.0005	.0030	.0120	.0247	.0336	.0710	.1185	.1602
	12					.0001	.0007	.0038	.0092	.0136	.0355	.0728	.1201
	13					.0000	.0002	.0010	.0028	.0045	.0145	.0366	.0739
	14						.0000	.0003	.0007	.0012	.0049	.0150	.0370
	15							.0000	.0001	.0003	.0013	.0049	.0148
	16								.0000	.0000	.0003	.0012	.0046
	17										.0000	.0003	.0011
	18											.0000	.0002
	19											.0000	.0000
	20	.0000	.0000	.0000	.0000	.0000	.0000	.0000	.0000	.0000	.0000	.0000	.0000

Appendix **B**

Percentiles of the *F* Distribution

$F_{.95}$ (use with $\alpha = .05$)

f_2 \ f_1	1	2	3	4	5	6	7	8	9
1	161.4	199.5	215.7	224.6	230.2	234.0	236.8	238.9	240.5
2	18.51	19.00	19.16	19.25	19.30	19.33	19.35	19.37	19.38
3	10.13	9.55	9.28	9.12	9.01	8.94	8.89	8.85	8.81
4	7.71	6.94	6.59	6.39	6.26	6.16	6.09	6.04	6.00
5	6.61	5.79	5.41	5.19	5.05	4.95	4.88	4.82	4.77
6	5.99	5.14	4.76	4.53	4.39	4.28	4.21	4.15	4.10
7	5.59	4.74	4.35	4.12	3.97	3.87	3.79	3.73	3.68
8	5.32	4.46	4.07	3.84	3.69	3.58	3.50	3.44	3.39
9	5.12	4.26	3.86	3.63	3.48	3.37	3.29	3.23	3.18
10	4.96	4.10	3.71	3.48	3.33	3.22	3.14	3.07	3.02
11	4.84	3.98	3.59	3.36	3.20	3.09	3.01	2.95	2.90
12	4.75	3.89	3.49	3.26	3.11	3.00	2.91	2.85	2.80
13	4.67	3.81	3.41	3.18	3.03	2.92	2.83	2.77	2.71
14	4.60	3.74	3.34	3.11	2.96	2.85	2.76	2.70	2.65
15	4.54	3.68	3.29	3.06	2.90	2.79	2.71	2.64	2.59
16	4.49	3.63	3.24	3.01	2.85	2.74	2.66	2.59	2.54
17	4.45	3.59	3.20	2.96	2.81	2.70	2.61	2.55	2.49
18	4.41	3.55	3.16	2.93	2.77	2.66	2.58	2.51	2.46
19	4.38	3.52	3.13	2.90	2.74	2.63	2.54	2.48	2.42
20	4.35	3.49	3.10	2.87	2.71	2.60	2.51	2.45	2.39
21	4.32	3.47	3.07	2.84	2.68	2.57	2.49	2.42	2.37
22	4.30	3.44	3.05	2.82	2.66	2.55	2.46	2.40	2.34
23	4.28	3.42	3.03	2.80	2.64	2.53	2.44	2.37	2.32
24	4.26	3.40	3.01	2.78	2.62	2.51	2.42	2.36	2.30
25	4.24	3.39	2.99	2.76	2.60	2.49	2.40	2.34	2.28
26	4.23	3.37	2.98	2.74	2.59	2.47	2.39	2.32	2.27
27	4.21	3.35	2.96	2.73	2.57	2.46	2.37	2.31	2.25
28	4.20	3.34	2.95	2.71	2.56	2.45	2.36	2.29	2.24
29	4.18	3.33	2.93	2.70	2.55	2.43	2.35	2.28	2.22
30	4.17	3.32	2.92	2.69	2.53	2.42	2.33	2.27	2.21
40	4.08	3.23	2.84	2.61	2.45	2.34	2.25	2.18	2.12
60	4.00	3.15	2.76	2.53	2.37	2.25	2.17	2.10	2.04
120	3.92	3.07	2.68	2.45	2.29	2.17	2.09	2.02	1.96
∞	3.84	3.00	2.60	2.37	2.21	2.10	2.01	1.94	1.88

SOURCE: Reprinted with permission from *Handbook of Tables for Probability and Statistics*, ed. William H. Beyer (Boca Raton, Fl.: CRC Press, 1966). Copyright CRC Press, Inc., Boca Raton, Fl.

Note: f_1 is the number of degrees of freedom in the numerator; f_2 is the number of degrees of freedom in the denominator.

$F_{.95}$ (use with $\alpha = .05$)

f_1 / f_2	10	12	15	20	24	30	40	60	120	∞
1	241.9	243.9	245.9	248.0	249.1	250.1	251.1	252.2	255.3	254.3
2	19.40	19.41	19.43	19.45	19.45	19.46	19.47	19.48	19.49	19.50
3	8.79	8.74	8.70	8.66	8.64	8.62	8.59	8.57	8.55	8.53
4	5.96	5.91	5.86	5.80	5.77	5.75	5.72	5.69	5.66	5.63
5	4.74	4.68	4.62	4.56	4.53	4.50	4.46	4.43	4.40	4.36
6	4.06	4.00	3.94	3.87	3.84	3.81	3.77	3.74	3.70	3.67
7	3.64	3.57	3.51	3.44	3.41	3.38	3.34	3.30	3.27	3.23
8	3.35	3.28	3.22	3.15	3.12	3.08	3.04	3.01	2.97	2.93
9	3.14	3.07	3.01	2.94	2.90	2.86	2.83	2.79	2.75	2.71
10	2.98	2.91	2.85	2.77	2.74	2.70	2.66	2.62	2.58	2.54
11	2.85	2.79	2.72	2.65	2.61	2.57	2.53	2.49	2.45	2.40
12	2.75	2.69	2.62	2.54	2.51	2.47	2.43	2.38	2.34	2.30
13	2.67	2.60	2.53	2.46	2.42	2.38	2.34	2.30	2.25	2.21
14	2.60	2.53	2.46	2.39	2.35	2.31	2.27	2.22	2.18	2.13
15	2.54	2.48	2.40	2.33	2.29	2.25	2.20	2.16	2.11	2.07
16	2.49	2.42	2.35	2.28	2.24	2.19	2.15	2.11	2.06	2.01
17	2.45	2.38	2.31	2.23	2.19	2.15	2.10	2.06	2.01	1.96
18	2.41	2.34	2.27	2.19	2.15	2.11	2.06	2.02	1.97	1.92
19	2.38	2.31	2.23	2.16	2.11	2.07	2.03	1.98	1.93	1.88
20	2.35	2.28	2.20	2.12	2.08	2.04	1.99	1.95	1.90	1.84
21	2.32	2.25	2.18	2.10	2.05	2.01	1.96	1.92	1.87	1.81
22	2.30	2.23	2.15	2.07	2.03	1.98	1.94	1.89	1.84	1.78
23	2.27	2.20	2.13	2.05	2.01	1.96	1.91	1.86	1.81	1.76
24	2.25	2.18	2.11	2.03	1.98	1.94	1.89	1.84	1.79	1.73
25	2.24	2.16	2.09	2.01	1.96	1.92	1.87	1.82	1.77	1.71
26	2.22	2.15	2.07	1.99	1.95	1.90	1.85	1.80	1.75	1.69
27	2.20	2.13	2.06	1.97	1.93	1.88	1.84	1.79	1.73	1.67
28	2.19	2.12	2.04	1.96	1.91	1.87	1.82	1.77	1.71	1.65
29	2.18	2.10	2.03	1.94	1.90	1.85	1.81	1.75	1.70	1.64
30	2.16	2.09	2.01	1.93	1.89	1.84	1.79	1.74	1.68	1.62
40	2.08	2.00	1.92	1.84	1.79	1.74	1.69	1.64	1.58	1.51
60	1.99	1.92	1.84	1.75	1.70	1.65	1.59	1.53	1.47	1.39
120	1.91	1.83	1.75	1.66	1.61	1.55	1.50	1.43	1.35	1.25
∞	1.83	1.75	1.67	1.57	1.52	1.46	1.39	1.32	1.22	1.00

$F_{.99}$ (use with $\alpha = .01$)

f_2 \ f_1	1	2	3	4	5	6	7	8	9
1	4052	4999.5	5403	5625	5764	5859	5928	5981	6022
2	98.50	99.00	99.17	99.25	99.30	99.33	99.36	99.37	99.39
3	34.12	30.82	29.46	28.71	28.24	27.91	27.67	27.49	27.35
4	21.20	18.00	16.69	15.98	15.52	15.21	14.98	14.80	14.55
5	16.26	13.27	12.06	11.39	10.97	10.67	10.46	10.29	10.16
6	13.75	10.92	9.78	9.15	8.75	8.47	8.26	8.10	7.98
7	12.25	9.55	8.45	7.85	7.46	7.19	6.99	6.84	6.72
8	11.26	8.65	7.59	7.01	6.63	6.37	6.18	6.03	5.91
9	10.56	8.02	6.99	6.42	6.06	5.80	5.61	5.47	5.35
10	10.04	7.56	6.55	5.99	5.64	5.39	5.20	5.06	4.94
11	9.65	7.21	6.22	5.67	5.32	5.07	4.89	4.74	4.63
12	9.33	6.93	5.95	5.41	5.06	4.82	4.64	4.50	4.39
13	9.07	6.70	5.74	5.21	4.86	4.62	4.44	4.30	4.19
14	8.86	6.51	5.56	5.04	4.69	4.46	4.28	4.14	4.03
15	8.68	6.36	5.42	4.89	4.56	4.32	4.14	4.00	3.89
16	8.53	6.23	5.29	4.77	4.44	4.20	4.03	3.89	3.78
17	8.40	6.11	5.18	4.67	4.34	4.10	3.93	3.79	3.68
18	8.29	6.01	5.09	4.58	4.25	4.01	3.84	3.71	3.60
19	8.18	5.93	5.01	4.50	4.17	3.94	3.77	3.63	3.52
20	8.10	5.85	4.94	4.43	4.10	3.87	3.70	3.56	3.46
21	8.02	5.78	4.87	4.37	4.04	3.81	3.64	3.51	3.40
22	7.95	5.72	4.82	4.31	3.99	3.76	3.59	3.45	3.35
23	7.88	5.66	4.76	4.26	3.94	3.71	3.54	3.41	3.30
24	7.82	5.61	4.79	4.22	3.90	3.67	3.50	3.36	3.26
25	7.77	5.57	4.68	4.18	3.85	3.63	3.46	3.32	3.22
26	7.72	5.53	4.64	4.14	3.82	3.59	3.42	3.29	3.18
27	7.68	5.49	4.60	4.11	3.78	3.56	3.39	3.26	3.15
28	7.64	5.45	4.57	4.07	3.75	3.53	3.36	3.23	3.12
29	7.60	5.42	4.54	4.04	3.73	3.50	3.33	3.20	3.09
30	7.56	5.39	4.51	4.02	3.70	3.47	3.30	3.17	3.07
40	7.31	5.18	4.31	3.83	3.51	3.29	3.12	2.99	2.89
60	7.08	4.98	4.13	3.65	3.34	3.12	2.95	2.82	2.72
120	6.85	4.79	3.95	3.48	3.17	2.96	2.79	2.66	2.56
∞	6.63	4.61	3.78	3.32	3.02	2.80	2.64	2.51	2.41

$F_{.99}$ (use with $\alpha = .01$)

f_1 / f_2	10	12	15	20	24	30	40	60	120	∞
1	6056	6106	6157	6209	6235	6261	6287	6313	6339	6366
2	99.40	99.42	99.43	99.45	99.46	99.47	99.47	99.48	99.49	99.50
3	27.23	27.05	26.87	26.69	26.60	26.50	26.41	26.32	26.22	26.13
4	14.55	14.37	14.20	14.02	13.93	13.84	13.75	13.65	13.56	13.46
5	10.05	9.89	9.72	9.55	9.47	9.38	9.29	9.20	9.11	9.02
6	7.87	7.72	7.56	7.40	7.31	7.23	7.14	7.06	6.97	6.88
7	6.62	6.47	6.31	6.16	6.07	5.99	5.91	5.82	5.74	5.65
8	5.81	5.67	5.52	5.36	5.28	5.20	5.12	5.03	4.95	4.86
9	5.26	5.11	4.96	4.81	4.73	4.65	4.57	4.48	4.40	4.31
10	4.85	4.71	4.56	4.41	4.33	4.25	4.17	4.08	4.00	3.91
11	4.54	4.40	4.25	4.10	4.02	3.94	3.86	3.78	3.69	3.60
12	4.30	4.16	4.01	3.86	3.78	3.70	3.62	3.54	3.45	3.36
13	4.10	3.96	3.82	3.66	3.59	3.51	3.43	3.34	3.25	3.17
14	3.94	3.80	3.66	3.51	3.43	3.35	3.27	3.18	3.09	3.00
15	3.80	3.67	3.52	3.37	3.29	3.21	3.13	3.05	2.96	2.87
16	3.60	3.55	3.41	3.26	3.18	3.10	3.02	2.93	2.84	2.75
17	3.59	3.46	3.31	3.16	3.08	3.00	2.92	2.83	2.75	2.65
18	3.51	3.37	3.23	3.08	3.00	2.92	2.84	2.75	2.66	2.57
19	3.43	3.30	3.15	3.00	2.92	2.84	2.76	2.67	2.58	2.49
20	3.37	3.23	3.09	2.94	2.86	2.78	2.69	2.61	2.52	2.42
21	3.31	3.17	3.03	2.88	2.80	2.72	2.64	2.55	2.46	2.36
22	3.26	3.12	2.98	2.83	2.75	2.67	2.58	2.50	2.40	2.31
23	3.21	3.07	2.93	2.78	2.70	2.62	2.54	2.45	2.35	2.26
24	3.17	3.03	2.89	2.74	2.66	2.58	2.49	2.40	2.31	2.21
25	3.13	2.99	2.85	2.70	2.62	2.54	2.45	2.36	2.27	2.17
26	3.09	2.96	2.81	2.66	2.58	2.50	2.42	2.33	2.23	2.13
27	3.06	2.93	2.78	2.63	2.55	2.47	2.38	2.29	2.20	2.10
28	3.03	2.90	2.75	2.60	2.52	2.44	2.35	2.26	2.17	2.06
29	3.00	2.87	2.73	2.57	2.49	2.41	2.33	2.23	2.14	2.03
30	2.98	2.84	2.70	2.55	2.47	2.39	2.30	2.21	2.11	2.01
40	2.80	2.66	2.52	2.37	2.29	2.20	2.11	2.02	1.92	1.80
60	2.63	2.50	2.35	2.20	2.12	2.03	1.94	1.84	1.73	1.60
120	2.47	2.34	2.19	2.03	1.95	1.86	1.76	1.66	1.53	1.38
∞	2.32	2.18	2.04	1.88	1.79	1.70	1.59	1.47	1.32	1.00

Bibliography

Abramson, J. H. 1974. *Survey Methods in Community Medicine*. Edinburgh: Churchill Livingstone.

Armitage, P. 1971. *Statistical Methods in Medical Research*. Oxford: Blackwell Scientific.

Backstrom, C. H., and G. D. Hursh. 1963. *Survey Research*. Evanston, Ill.: Northwestern University Press.

Belloc, N. B. 1973. Relationship of health practices and mortality. *Preventive Medicine* 2:67–81.

Berkson, J. 1946. Limitations of the application of fourfold table analysis to hospital data. *Biometrics Bulletin* 2:47–53.

Billings, K., and D. Moursund. 1979. *Are You Computer Literate?* Beaverton, Ore.: Dilithium Press.

Brown, B. W., and M. Hollander. 1977. *Statistics: A Biomedical Introduction*. New York: Wiley.

Cole, P., and A. S. Morrison. 1980. Basic issues in population screening for cancer. *Journal of the National Cancer Institute* 64:1263–72.

Colton, T. 1974. *Statistics in Medicine*. Boston: Little, Brown.

Cutler, S. J., and F. Ederer. 1958. Maximum utilization of the life table method in analyzing survival. *Journal of Chronic Diseases* 8:699–713.

Dixon, W. J., and F. J. Massey. 1969. *Introduction to Statistical Analysis*. 3d ed. New York: McGraw-Hill.

Elveback, L. R., C. L. Guillier, and F. R. Keating. 1970. Health, normality, and the ghost of Gauss. *Journal of the American Medical Association* 211:69–75.

Flesch, R. 1974. *The Art of Readable Writing*. 25th anniversary ed. New York: Harper & Row.

Frenzel, L. E. 1978. *Getting Acquainted with Microcomputers*. Indianapolis: Bobbs-Merrill.

———. 1980. *The Howard W. Sams Crash Course in Microcomputers*. Indianapolis: Bobbs-Merrill.

Hammond, E. C. 1966. Smoking in relation to the death rates of one million men and women. *National Cancer Institute Monograph* 19:127–204.

Hill, A. B. 1963. Medical ethics and controlled trials. *British Medical Journal* 1:1043.

Huff, D. 1954. *How to Lie with Statistics*. New York: Norton.

Kuzma, J. W. 1967. A comparison of two life table methods. *Biometrics* 23:51–64.

———. 1970. Planning and management aspects of cooperative trials. *Journal of Clinical Pharmacology* 10:79–87

Kuzma, J. W., and W. J. Dixon. 1966. Evaluation of recurrence in gastric adenocarcinoma patients. *Cancer* 19:677–688.

Kuzma, J. W., and D. G. Kissinger. 1981. Patterns of alcohol and cigarette use in pregnancy. *Neurobehavioral Toxicology and Teratology* 3:211–221.

Kuzma, J. W., and R. J. Sokol. 1982. Maternal drinking behavior and decreased intrauterine growth. *Alcoholism: Clinical and Experimental Research* 6:396–401.

Lilienfeld, A. M., E. Pedersen, and J. E. Dowd. 1967. *Cancer Epidemiology: Methods of Study*. Baltimore: Johns Hopkins University Press.

MacMahon, D., and F. Pugh. 1970. *Epidemiology Principles and Methods.* Boston: Little, Brown.

MacMahon, B., and F. Pugh. 1970. *Epidemiology: Principles and Methods.* Boston: Little, Brown.

McMillen, M. M. 1979. Differential mortality by sex in fetal and neonatal deaths. *Science* 204:89–91.

McWilliams, P. A. 1982. *The Personal Computer Book.* Los Angeles: Prelude Press (distributed by Ballantine Books).

Mainland, D. 1963. *Elementary Medical Statistics.* 2d ed. Philadelphia: Saunders.

Medical Research Council. 1948. Streptomycin treatment of pulmonary tuberculosis. *British Medical Journal* 2:769.

Muir, C. S., and J. Nectoux. 1977. Role of the cancer registry. *National Cancer Institute Monograph* 47:3–6.

National Center for Health Statistics. *Monthly Vital Statistics Report.*

———. *Vital and Health Statistics Series.* Washington: Government Printing Office.

———. *Vital Statistics of the United States.* Vol. 1, *Natality*; vol. 2, *Mortality*; vol. 3, *Marriage and Divorce.* Washington: Government Printing Office.

———. 1976. *Vital Statistics of the United States,* 1972. HRA Publication no. 75-1101. Rockville, Md.

———. 1981. *User's Manual—The National Death Index.* Public Health Service Publication no. 81-1148. Hyattsville, Md.: U.S. Department of Health and Human Services, Public Health Service.

———. 1982. Advance report: Final mortality statistics, 1979. *Monthly Vital Statistics Report* 31(6), suppl. 4.

Nie, N. H., C. H. Hull, J. G. Jenkins, K. Steinbrenner, and D. H. Gent. 1975. *SPSS: Statistical Package for the Social Sciences.* 2d ed. New York: McGraw-Hill.

Paul, O. 1976. The multiple risk factor intervention trial (MRFIT). *Journal of the American Medical Association* 235:825–827.

Remington, R. D., and M. A. Schork. 1970. *Statistics with Applications to the Biological and Health Sciences.* Englewood Cliffs, N.J.: Prentice-Hall.

Rimm, A. A., A. J. Hartz, J. H. Kalbfleisch, A. J. Anderson, and R. G. Hoffmann. 1980. *Basic Biostatistics in Medicine and Epidemiology.* New York: Appleton-Century-Crofts.

Sackett, D. L. 1979. Bias in analytic research. *Journal of Chronic Diseases* 32:51–63.

Savage, E. R. 1981. *BASIC Programmer's Notebook.* Indianapolis: Bobbs-Merrill.

Scheaffer, R. L., W. Mendenhall, and L. Ott. 1979. *Elementary Survey Sampling.* 2d ed. Boston: Duxbury Press.

Sheen, A. P. 1982. *Breathing Life into Medical Writing—A Handbook*. St. Louis: Mosby.

Shyrock, H. S., and J. S. Siegel. 1973. *The Methods and Materials of Demography*. Washington: U.S. Bureau of the Census.

Simpson, W. S. 1957. A preliminary report on cigarette smoking and the incidence of prematurity. *American Journal of Obstetrics and Gynecology* 73:808–815.

Slonim, M. J. 1960. *Sampling—A Quick, Reliable Guide to Practical Statistics*. New York: Simon and Schuster.

Snedecor, G. W. 1956. *Statistical Methods*. Ames: Iowa State College Press.

Spencer, D. D. 1978. *Fundamentals of Digital Computers*. 2d ed. Indianapolis: Bobbs-Merrill.

Steel, R. G. D., and J. H. Torrie. 1980. *Principles and Procedures of Statistics*. 2d ed. New York: McGraw-Hill.

Stocks, P. 1944. The measurement of morbidity. *Proceedings of the Royal Society of Medicine* 37:593–608.

Tukey, J. W. 1977. *Exploratory Data Analysis*. Reading, Mass.: Addison-Wesley.

United Nations. Secretariat. Department of Economic and Social Affairs. Statistical Office. 1983. *Demographic Yearbook*. New York: United Nations Publishing Service.

U.S. Bureau of the Census. *Census of Population*. Washington: U.S. Government Printing Office.

———. *Statistical Abstract of the United States*. Washington: U.S. Government Printing Office.

U.S. Department of Health, Education and Welfare. 1965, 1971. *Health Consequences of Smoking: A Report to the Surgeon General*. Washington: Public Health Service, Health Services and Mental Health Administration.

———. 1979. *Smoking and Health: A Report to the Surgeon General*. Washington: Public Health Service, Office of Smoking and Health.

Veterans Administration Cooperative Study Group on Antihypertensive Agents. 1970. Effects of treatment on morbidity in hypertension: II, Results in patients with diastolic blood pressure averaging 90–114 mmHg. *Journal of the American Medical Association* 213:1143.

———. 1972. Effects of treatment on morbidity in hypertension: III, Influence of age, diastolic pressure, and prior cardiovascular disease; further analysis of side effects. *Circulation* 45:991.

Willis, J., and M. Miller. 1983. *Computers for Everybody*. Beaverton, Ore.: Dilithium Press.

Winslow, C. E. A., W. G. Smillie, J. A. Doull, and J. E. Gordon. 1952. *The History of American Epidemiology*. St. Louis: Mosby.

World Health Organization. 1977. *Manual of the International Statistical Classification of Diseases, Injuries, and Causes of Death*. Geneva.

Answers to Selected Exercises

Chapter 2

2.1 Simple random sample

2.2 Stratified random sampling

2.3 (a) Systematic sampling
(b) Yes, if the variable you are sampling has periodic variation.

2.4 (a) 7683 persons enrolled in the Honolulu Heart Study, 1969
(c) Statistic
(d) Parameter

Chapter 3

3.1 (a)

Education	qualitative
Weight	quantitative
Height	quantitative
Smoking	qualitative
Physical activity	qualitative
Blood glucose	quantitative
Serum cholesterol	quantitative
Systolic blood pressure	quantitative
Ponderal index	quantitative
Age	quantitative

(b)

Weight	continuous
Height	continuous
Blood glucose	continuous
Serum cholesterol	continuous
Systolic blood pressure	continuous
Ponderal index	continuous
Age	continuous

(c)

Education	bar chart *or* pie chart
Weight	frequency polygon or ogive
Height	frequency polygon or ogive
Smoking	bar chart or pie chart
Physical activity	bar chart or pie chart
Blood glucose	frequency polygon or ogive
Serum cholesterol	frequency polygon or ogive
Systolic blood pressure	frequency polygon or ogive
Ponderal index	frequency polygon or ogive
Age	frequency polygon or ogive

3.2 Diastolic blood pressure — quantitative continuous
Sex — qualitative
Diet status — qualitative

3.3 (a) Approximately symmetrical
(b) Distribution of smokers and nonsmokers would not be similar. Smokers' distribution would have a slight positive skew.

3.4 Extreme values are to the left in a negatively skewed distribution and to the right in a positively skewed one.

3.8 (a) Histogram
(b) Frequency polygon
(c) Pie chart
(d) Line graph

3.9 Stem and leaf display:

		Frequency
40–49	7 9	2
50–59	0 1 2 2 2 2 3 3 5 5 5 5 5 6 6 6 6 7 7 8 8 8 9 9 9 9 9 9 9 9	30
60–69	0 0 0 0 0 1 1 1 1 1 1 1 1 1 1 2 2 2 3 4 4 5 5 5 6 6 6 6 6 6 6 6 6 7 7 8 8 8 8 8 8	41
70–79	0 0 0 0 0 0 1 1 1 3 3 3 3 3 5 5 5 7 7 7 8	21
80–89	0 0 2 3 6	5
90–99	1	1
	Total	100

Chapter 4

4.1 Mean $= \dfrac{\Sigma x}{n} = \dfrac{24}{6} = 4$
Median $= 4$
Mode $= 5$
Range $= 8 - 1 = 7$
Variance $= \dfrac{\Sigma(x - \bar{x})^2}{n - 1} = \dfrac{32}{5} = 6.40$
Standard deviation $= \sqrt{\text{variance}} = 2.53$

4.3 Range $= 102 - 40 = 62$; median $= 72$; mode $= 70$

4.7 (a) $CV_H = \dfrac{100s}{\bar{x}} = \dfrac{100(5.60)}{161.75} = 3.46$
$CV_W = \dfrac{100s}{\bar{x}} = \dfrac{100(8.61)}{64.22} = 13.41$
(b) Weight, approximately four times larger

4.8 (a) $\bar{x} = \dfrac{13{,}010}{100} = 130.10$
$s^2 = \dfrac{1{,}737{,}124 - 1{,}692{,}601}{99} = 449.73 \quad s = 21.21$
(b) 108.89, 151.31

(c) 87.69, 172.51
(d) 66.48, 193.72
(e) 68.3% 95.4% 99.7%

4.10 Variance = $s^2 = (38.82)^2 = 1506.99$

4.14 (a) (i) 138,190,128,152,134,108,118,138,108,126,176,112,92,152,98, 112,120,140,94,150,144,156,140,150,162

(ii) 116,140,146,134,162,162,118,142,104,140,142,112,116,134,108, 114,154,128,116,140,122,122,172,128

$$\bar{x}_1 = \frac{\Sigma x}{n} = \frac{3338}{25} = 133.52$$

$$s_1 = \sqrt{\frac{\Sigma x^2 - (\Sigma x)^2/n}{n-1}} = \sqrt{\frac{460{,}748 - 445{,}688.76}{24}} = \sqrt{627.43} = 25.05$$

$$\bar{x}_2 = \frac{\Sigma x}{n} = \frac{3152}{24} = 131.33$$

$$s_2 = \sqrt{\frac{\Sigma x^2 - (\Sigma x)^2/n}{n-1}} = \sqrt{\frac{421{,}472 - 413{,}962.67}{23}} = \sqrt{326.49} = 18.07$$

(b) The first set has the larger standard deviation: 25.05 − 18.07 = 6.98.
(c) The first set of observations is more dispersed than the second.

Chapter 5

5.1 {TT, TH, HT, HH}
$P(0H) = (\frac{1}{2})(\frac{1}{2}) = \frac{1}{4}$
$P(1H) = (\frac{1}{2})(\frac{1}{2}) + (\frac{1}{2})(\frac{1}{2}) = \frac{1}{2}$
$P(2H) = (\frac{1}{2})(\frac{1}{2}) = \frac{1}{4}$

5.3 {TTT, TTH, THT, THH, HTT, HTH, HHT, HHH}
(a) $P(2H) = \frac{3}{8}$
(c) P(at most 2H) = $\frac{7}{8}$

5.4 {GGG, GGB, GBG, GBB, BGG, BGB, BBG, BBB}
(a) $P(2B + 1G) = \frac{3}{8}$
(c) $P(0G) = \frac{1}{8}$
(e) P(2B followed by 1G) = $\frac{1}{8}$. Note that (a) doesn't consider order.

5.7 (a) P(sum 8) = 5/36
(d) P(sum 7 and both dice < 4) = 0

5.8 (a) $P(O \text{ or } R) = \frac{10 + 15}{10 + 30 + 20 + 15} = \frac{25}{75} = \frac{1}{3}$

(c) $P(\text{not } B) = \frac{55}{75} = \frac{11}{15}$

(e) $P(R, W, \text{or } B) = \frac{60}{75} = \frac{4}{5}$

5.9 P(white mouse in 10 hours) = $\frac{7}{10}$; P(black mouse in 10 hours) = $\frac{9}{10}$

(a) $P(\text{both alive}) = \left(\frac{7}{10}\right)\left(\frac{9}{10}\right) = \frac{63}{100}$

(b) P(black alive and white dead) = $\left(\frac{9}{10}\right)\left(\frac{3}{10}\right) = \frac{27}{100}$

(d) P(at least one alive) = $\frac{7}{10} + \frac{9}{10} - \frac{63}{100} = \frac{97}{100}$

5.10 (a) P(vegetarian) = $\frac{18 + 22}{18 + 22 + 20 + 23} = \frac{40}{83}$

(c) P(male vegetarian) = $\frac{18}{83}$

5.11 (a) P(completed high school) = $\frac{19}{100}$

(c) P(physically inactive) = $\frac{49}{100}$

(e) P(serum cholesterol > 250; systolic blood pressure > 130) = $\frac{9}{100}$

5.12 5! = 120

5.13 $P(10,4) = \frac{10!}{(10-4)!} = \frac{3,628,800}{720} = 5040$

5.15 $C(9,5) = \frac{9!}{5!(9-5)!} = \frac{362,880}{(120)(24)} = 126$

5.16 (b) $C(6,4) = \frac{6!}{4!(6-4)!} = \frac{720}{24(2)} = 15$

P(n,r) > C(n,r) because order is considered

5.17 $C(10,4) = \frac{10}{4!(10-4)!} = \frac{3,628,800}{(24)(720)} = 210 = C(10,6)$

5.18 (a) P(3 out of 5) = $\frac{5!}{3!(5-3)!}(.5)^3(1-.5)^2 = \frac{120}{6(2)}(.5)^3(.5)^2$

$= .3125$

(c) P(at most 1) = P(0) + P(1) = $.03125 + \frac{5!}{1!(5-1)!}(.5)^1(.5)^4$

$= .03125 + .15625 = .1875$

$n = 20$; $p = .25$

5.19 (a) P(3) = .1339
(c) P(< 3) = 1 − P(≥ 3) = 1 − 9087 = .0913

5.20 $n = 10$, $p = .1$
(a) P(10) = 0
(c) P(≥ 3) = 1 − (.3487 + .3874 + .1937) = .0702

5.21 $n = 12$, $p = .25$
(a) P(4) = .1936
(c) P(≥ 4) = 1 − .6488 = .3512

5.22 10 males, 15 females; P(M smoke) = $\frac{1}{2}$, P(F smoke) = $\frac{1}{3}$
(a) [P(4 of 10 M smoke) = .2051 and
P(6 of 15 F smoke) = .1786] = (.2051)(.1786) = .0366
(c) [P(0 of 10 M smoke) = .0010 and
P(0 of 15 F smoke) = .0023] = (.0010)(.0023) = .0000

Chapter 6

6.1 (a) .4911
(c) 2(.4678) = .9356
(e) .4990

6.2 (a) .5 − .4582 = .0418
(c) .5 − .4946 = .0054
(e) 0

6.3 (a) 1.645
(c) ±1.96
(e) ±1.645

6.4 (a) 1.645
(c) 0

6.5 (a) For 40%, Z_1 will be ±1.282;
for 45%, Z_2 will be ±1.645.
(b) $x = \mu \pm Z\sigma = 130 \pm 1.282(17)$; x = (108.2, 151.8)

6.6 (a) $Z_1 = (x - \mu)/\sigma = (45 - 60)/10 = -1.5$
$Z_2 = (75 - 60)/10 = 1.5$; area = 2(.4332) = .8664 = 86.6%
(c) <50Z = (50 − 60)/10 = −1; area = .5 − .3413 = .1587 = 15.9%
(e) ≥75Z = (75 − 60)/10 = 1.5; area = .5 − .4332 = .0668 = 6.7%

6.8 Mean = 75, σ = 8; 90th percentile; Z = 1.28
1.28 = (x − 75)/8; x = (1.28)8 + 75 = 85.24 = 86%

6.9 Mean = 50, σ = 12
$P(x < 35) = (35 - 50)/12 = -1.25$; area = .5 − .3944 = .1056

6.10 $\bar{x} = 73, s^2 = 121$
(a) $P(80 < x < 100)$; $Z_1 = (80 - 73)/11 = .64$; $Z_2 = (100 - 73)/11 = 2.45$;
area = .4929 − .2389 = .254
(c) $P(x > 90)$; $Z = (90 - 73)/11 = 1.55$; area = .5 − .4394 = .0606

6.12 $\bar{x} = 217, s^2 = 1507$
(a) $P(150 < x < 250)$; $Z_1 = (150 - 217)/38.82 = -1.73$, $A_1 = .4582$;
$Z_2 = (250 - 217)/38.82 = .85$, $A_2 = .3023$; area = .4582 + .3023 = .7605
(c) $P(x < 150)$; $Z = -1.726$; area = .5 − .4582 = .0418

Chapter 7

7.1 n = 36, μ = 130, σ = 17
Follows an approximately normal distribution with a mean equal to the population mean and a standard deviation of $\sigma/\sqrt{n}$

7.2 n = 25, μ = 60, σ = 10
(a) $P(57 < \bar{x} < 63)$; $Z_1 = (57 - 60)/(10/5) = -1.5$, A = 2(.4332);
$Z_2 = (63 - 60)/2 = 1.5$, A = .8664 = 86.6%
(c) $P(\bar{x} > 64)$; $Z = (64 - 60)/2 = 2$; A = .5 − .4772 = .0228 = 2.3%

7.3 (a) The areas are equal. The area of Exercise 7.2 is between 57 and 63. The area of Exercise 6.6 is between 45 and 75. In Exercise 7.2 the measure of variation is much smaller.
(b) The area to the right of 75 is larger in Exercise 6.6, because the measure of variation is larger there.

7.4 $n = 25, \mu = 60, \sigma = 10$; 95th percentile

$$1.645 = \frac{\bar{x} - 60}{10/\sqrt{n}} = \frac{\bar{x} - 60}{2}; \bar{x} = 2(1.645) + 60 = 63.29$$

7.5 $\mu = 50, \sigma = 12$

(a) $SE(\bar{x}) = 12/\sqrt{16} = 3$

(c) $SE(\bar{x})$ decreases when n increases.

7.6 $\mu = 71, \sigma = 8, n = 15$

(a) $P(\bar{x} \geq 77)$; $Z = (77 - 71)/(8/\sqrt{15}) = 2.905$; $A = .0019$

(b) $P(65 < \bar{x} < 75)$

$$Z = \frac{65 - 71}{8/\sqrt{15}} = -2.905 \qquad A = .9720$$

$$Z = \frac{75 - 71}{8/\sqrt{15}} = 1.936$$

7.7 $\mu = 52.5; \sigma = 4.5; P(\bar{x} > 56)$

(a) $n = 10$; $Z = (56 - 52.5)/(4.5/\sqrt{10}) = 2.460$; $A = .0069$

7.8 $\mu = 3360, \sigma = 490$

(a) $Z_1 = (2300 - 3360)/490 = -2.1633$,
$Z_2 = (4300 - 3360)/490 = 1.9184$; $A = .9572$

(c) $Z = (5000 - 3360)/490 = 3.3469$; $A = <.001$

7.9 (b) $Z_1 = (3100 - 3360)/(490/\sqrt{49}) = -3.7143$, $A \simeq 1.0$;
$Z_2 = (3600 - 3360)/(490/\sqrt{49}) = 3.4286$

(c) $Z = (2500 - 3360)/(490/\sqrt{49}) = -12.2857$, $A = 0$

Chapter 8

8.1 $.64 - .51 \pm (1.96)(.17)\sqrt{(1/30) + (1/27)}$
$.04 < \mu_1 - \mu_2 < .22$

8.3 $\mu = 200$

$\bar{x} = 225, \sigma = 16.67, n = 49, z = 1.96$

(a) 95% CI of $\mu = 225 \pm (1.96)(16.67/\sqrt{49})$
$220.33 < \mu < 229.67$

(b) $n = [(1.96)(16.67)]^2/10^2 = 10.67 \approx 11$

8.4

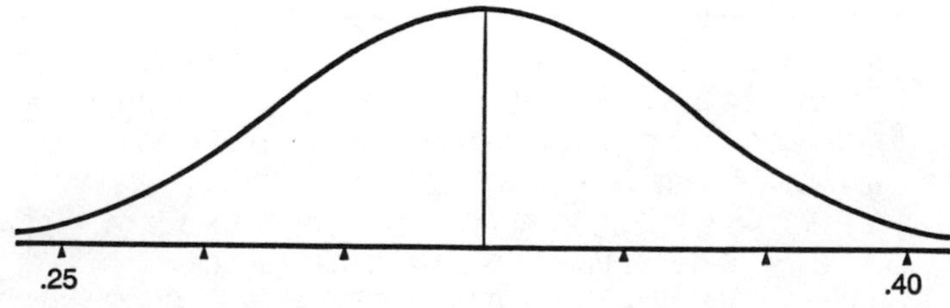

(a) $\bar{x} = .33$

$.25 = \bar{x} - 3.00\,s$

$= .33 - 3.00\,s$

$s = .03$

(b) The 99% confidence interval formula for μ is
99% CI for $\mu = \bar{x} \pm ts/\sqrt{n}$
$.33 \pm t(.03)/\sqrt{n}$
Exact values for CI can be determined for a known value of n.

8.7

	Mean	s	n	
Male	74.9	12.0	38	$s_p^2 = 131.51$
Female	71.8	11.0	45	

$$3.10 \pm 2.58(11.47)\sqrt{\frac{1}{38} + \frac{1}{45}}$$

$$-3.42 < \mu_1 - \mu_2 < 9.62$$

8.8 $\bar{x}_1 = 163.33 \qquad s_1 = 25.07$
$\bar{x}_2 = 179.90 \qquad s_2 = 33.87$

$$s_p = \sqrt{\frac{(25.07)^2(53) + (33.87)^2(50)}{54 + 51 - 2}} = 29.67$$

$$16.57 \pm (2.576)(29.67)\sqrt{\frac{1}{54} + \frac{1}{51}}$$

$$1.65 < \mu_1 - \mu_2 < 31.49$$

Chapter 9

9.1 (a) −1.645 or 1.645
(c) −3.012 and 3.012
(e) −1.96 and 1.96

9.2 (a) Z test in (a) and (d)
(b) t test in (b), (c), and (e)

9.3 (a) H_0: $\mu \leq 30$, H_1: $\mu > 30$
(d) H_0: $\mu \geq 31.5$, H_1: $\mu < 31.5$
(e) H_0: $\mu = 16$, H_1: $\mu \neq 16$

9.4 (a) −1.96 and 1.96
(c) −2.576 and 2.576
(e) −2.602

9.6 (a) Fail to reject H_0.
(c) Reject H_0.
(e) Fail to reject H_0.

9.7 $\mu = 85$, $n = 25$, $\bar{x} = 80.94$
$Z(.05) = -1.645$; $t(.05, n-1 = 24)$; H_0: $\mu \geq 85$, H_1: $\mu < 85$

(a) $Z = \dfrac{80.94 - 85}{11.6/\sqrt{25}} = -1.750$ Reject H_0 and conclude that the boys were indeed underfed.

(b) $t = \dfrac{80.94 - 85}{12.3/\sqrt{25}} = -1.645$ Fail to reject H_0 since $t = -1.645$ does not fall beyond the critical value $t = -1.711$.

9.9 Exercise 8.2: $Z = \dfrac{16 - 17}{2/\sqrt{25}} = -2.50$ $\quad p = 2(.0062) = .0124$

Exercise 8.3: $Z = \dfrac{225 - 200}{16.67/\sqrt{49}} = 10.50$ $\quad p = .0000$

Exercise 9.7a: $Z = -1.750$ $\quad p = .0401$

Exercise 9.8: $t = 4.72$ $\quad p < 2(.005) = .01$

Exercise 9.17: $t = \dfrac{73 - 70}{11.6/\sqrt{83}} = 2.36$ $\quad p < .01$

9.11 (a) $s_p = 11.55$; $\alpha = .05$; H_0: $\mu_v = \mu_{nv}$, H_1: $\mu_v \neq \mu_{nv}$

$$t = \frac{73.5 - 72.9}{11.55\sqrt{(1/40) + (1/43)}} = .236$$

Fail to reject H_0 and state the evidence was insufficient to indicate a difference in mean blood pressures between the two groups.

9.13 $\alpha = .05$; H_0: $\mu = 15$, H_1: $\mu \neq 15$ $\quad z = (16 - 15)/(2/\sqrt{25}) = 2.50$
Two-tailed test: $z \pm 1.96$ Reject H_0 and conclude that the mean hemoglobin level is significantly different (higher) in this sample from that of the population mean.

9.15 (a) paired t test $\quad$ (b) $\bar{x}_d = 275 - 260.6 = 14.4$
$t(.99, 9) = 3.25$ $\quad$ H_0: mean difference between labs $= 0$
H_1: mean difference $\neq 0$

$$s_d = \sqrt{\frac{2486 - (144)^2/10}{9}} = 6.77$$

$$t = \frac{14.4 - 0}{6.77/\sqrt{10}} = 6.72$$

Reject H_0 and conclude that there is a significant difference between means of the two laboratories.

(c) $t = (275 - 260.6)/20.62\sqrt{1/10 + 1/10} = 1.56$

9.17 $t = (73 - 70)/(11.6/\sqrt{83}) = 2.356$
H_0: $\mu \leq 70$, H_1: $\mu > 70$ $\quad$ $t(.01, 82, \text{one-tailed}) = 2.33$
Reject H_0 in favor of H_1 and conclude that the mean blood pressure of this group is significantly higher than 70.

9.19 (a) $s_p = 29.67$
$t = (163.33 - 179.90)/29.67\sqrt{(1/54) + (1/51)} = -2.860$
$t(.05, 103, \text{one-tailed}) = -1.65$ $\quad$ H_0: $\mu_v - \mu_{nv} \geq 0$, H_1: $\mu_v - \mu_{nv} < 0$
Reject H_0 in favor of H_1 and conclude that the mean cholesterol level of vegetarians is significantly lower than that of nonvegetarians.

Chapter 10

10.1 (a) H_0: $\mu_1 = \mu_2 = \mu_3$ (mean number of children is same for all groups)

(b)

Source of variation	SS	df	MS	F ratio
Between	381.67	2	190.84	26.88
Within	191.80	27	7.10	$F_{.95}(2,27) = 3.35$
Total	573.47	29		

(c) Reject H_0 and conclude that the need for family planning counsel differs by the number of children per family.

10.3

Source of variation	SS	df	MS	F ratio
Between	8,296.62	2	4,148.31	23.95
Within	3,118.33	18	173.24	$F_{.95}(2,18) = 3.55$
Total	11,414.95	20		

Reject H_0: $\mu_1 = \mu_2 = \mu_3$ and conclude that the mean ages of the three communities are different.

Chapter 11

11.1 (a) p_1 (none) = 25/100 = .25
p_2 (primary) = 32/100 = .32
p_3 (intermediate) = 24/100 = .24
$p_4 + p_5$ (high school and technical school) = 19/100 = .19
(c) p_1 (mostly sitting) = .49; p_2 (moderate) = .51; p_3 (much) = 0

11.2 $\mu = np = 7683(.37) = 2842.71$
$\sigma = \sqrt{npq} = \sqrt{7683(.37)(.63)} = 42.32$

11.3 H_0: $p_H = .31$
H_1: $p_H \neq .31$
$\alpha = .05$
Critical region: $Z > 1.96$, $Z < -1.96$

$$Z = \frac{\hat{p}_H - p}{\sqrt{pq/n}} = \frac{.37 - .31}{\sqrt{(.31)(.69)/100}} = 1.30$$

Fail to reject H_0 and conclude that the evidence is insufficient to indicate that the proportion of smokers in Honolulu is significantly different from that in the United States in general.

11.5 $p_1 = 4/7 = .57;\ p_2 = 7/21 = .33$

$$p' = \frac{4 + 7}{7 + 21} = .39$$

$$SE(\hat{p}_1 - \hat{p}_2) = \sqrt{\frac{(.39)(.61)}{7} + \frac{(.39)(.61)}{21}} = .213$$

H_0: $p_1 - p_2 = 0$
H_1: $p_1 - p_2 \neq 0$
$\alpha = .05$

$$Z = \frac{.57 - .33}{.213} = 1.127$$

$Z(.025) = \pm 1.96$

Fail to reject H_0. There is no difference in the proportion of smokers between the two groups.

11.6 90% CI for $p_1 - p_2 = \hat{p}_1 - \hat{p}_2 \pm 1.645\sqrt{\frac{(.57)(.43)}{7} + \frac{(.33)(.67)}{21}}$

$$= .24 \pm .35$$
$$= -.11 < \hat{p}_1 - \hat{p}_2 < .59$$

11.8 $\hat{p} = 29/99 = .293$

99% CI for $p = .293 \pm 2.576\sqrt{\frac{(.293)(.707)}{99}}$

$$= .293 \pm .118$$
$$= .175 < p < .411$$

11.10 $\hat{p}_1 = \frac{55}{219} = .251;\ \hat{p}_2 = \frac{117}{822} = .142$

$\alpha = .01$

$$p' = \frac{55 + 117}{219 + 822} = .165;\ q' = .835$$

$$SE(p_1 - p_2) = \sqrt{\frac{(.165)(.835)}{219} + \frac{(.165)(.835)}{822}} = .028$$

H_0: $p_1 - p_2 = 0$

$$Z = \frac{.251 - .142}{.028} = 3.893$$ Critical region is ± 2.576 (for $\alpha = .01$)

Reject H_0 and conclude that there was a significantly higher proportion of those who started smoking at an earlier age among "abusers" than among "nonusers."

11.12 (a) 99% CI for 11.10

$$p_1 - p_2 = \hat{p}_1 - \hat{p}_2 \pm 2.576\sqrt{\frac{(.251)(.749)}{219} + \frac{(.142)(.858)}{822}}$$
$$= .109 \pm .082$$
$$= .027 < p_1 - p_2 < .191$$

Chapter 12

12.1 (a)

	Smokers		Nonsmokers	
	Observed	Expected	Observed	Expected
None	9	9.25	16	15.75
Primary	15	11.84	17	20.16
Intermediate	12	8.88	12	15.10
Senior high	1	3.33	8	5.67
Technical school	0	3.7	10	6.3

H_0: There is no association between smoking and educational level.
$\alpha = .05$
$\chi^2 = 11.54$
$\chi^2_{.95}(\text{df} = 4) = 9.49$
Reject H_0.

(b)

	Smokers		Nonsmokers	
	Observed	Expected	Observed	Expected
None	9	9.25	16	15.75
Primary	15	11.84	17	20.16
Intermediate	12	8.88	12	15.10
Senior high and technical school	1	7.03	18	11.97

$\alpha = .05$
$\chi^2 = 11.1$[illegible]
$\chi^2_{.95}(\text{df} = 3) = 7.81$
Reject H_0 and conclude that smoking is dependent on one's educational level—namely, smoking is less frequent among the more highly educated.

12.3 (a)

	Egg consumption							
	0		<1		2–4		Daily	
	O	*E*	*O*	*E*	*O*	*E*	*O*	*E*
Low	5	5.36	13	13.66	8	9.91	4	1.07
Medium	4	6.7[illegible]	20	17.30	14	12.55	0	1.36
High	11	7.86	18	20.04	15	14.54	0	1.57

H_0: There is no association between egg consumption and age at menarche.
$\alpha = .05$
$\chi^2 = 14.59$
$\chi^2_{.95}(\text{df} = 6) = 12.59$
Reject H_0 and conclude that age at menarche is dependent on one's level of egg consumption.

(b)

	Egg consumption					
	0		<1		2–7	
	O	E	O	E	O	E
Low	5	5.36	13	13.00	12	10.98
Medium	4	6.79	20	17.30	14	13.91
High	11	7.86	18	20.04	15	16.11

H_0: There is no association between egg consumption and age at menarche.
$\alpha = .05$
$\chi^2 = 3.26$
$\chi^2_{.95}(\text{df} = 4) = 9.49$
Fail to reject H_0: The data do not refute the H_0 of *no* association between age at menarche and egg consumption.

12.4 (a)

	Smoking		No smoking		
	O	E	O	E	Total
Hypertension group	4	2.75	3	4.25	7
Control group	7	8.25	14	12.75	21
Total	11		17		28

H_0: $p_1 = p_2$ (there is no difference in the proportion of smokers in the two groups).
$\alpha = .05$
$\chi^2 = 1.25$
$\chi^2_{.95}(\text{df} = 1) = 3.84$
Fail to reject H_0: The data do not refute the H_0 of no association.

12.5

Age interval	Heartbeat O	Heartbeat E	O − E	$\frac{(O-E)^2}{E}$
25–34	18	43.12	−25.12	14.63
35–44	33	38.56	−5.56	0.80
45–54	54	37.17	16.83	7.62
55–64	48	30.42	17.58	10.16
≥65	35	38.72	−3.72	0.36
	188			33.57

$$E_1 = \frac{140{,}195(188)}{611{,}152} = 43.13$$

H_0: The age distribution of the heartbeat group is the same as that of the SMSA.
$\alpha = .05$
$\chi^2 = 33.58$ and $\chi^2_{.95}(\text{df} = 4) = 9.49$

Reject H_0: The heartbeat age distribution is significantly different from the SMSA age distribution.

Chapter 13

13.1 (a) Range −1 to 1
(b) The sign tells the direction of the slope.
(c) It tells the strength of the linear relationship.
(d) It tells how good the prediction is likely to be.
(e) Yes, they would have the same sign. No, they would not have the same magnitude.

13.2 (a) $r = \dfrac{3{,}371{,}580 - (15{,}214)(21{,}696)/100}{\sqrt{2{,}611{,}160 - (15{,}214)^2/100} \cdot \sqrt{4{,}856{,}320 - (21{,}696)^2/100}}$

$= .336$

13.3 (a) Plot of systolic blood pressure in row 3 (R3) versus cadmium level in row 1 (R1):

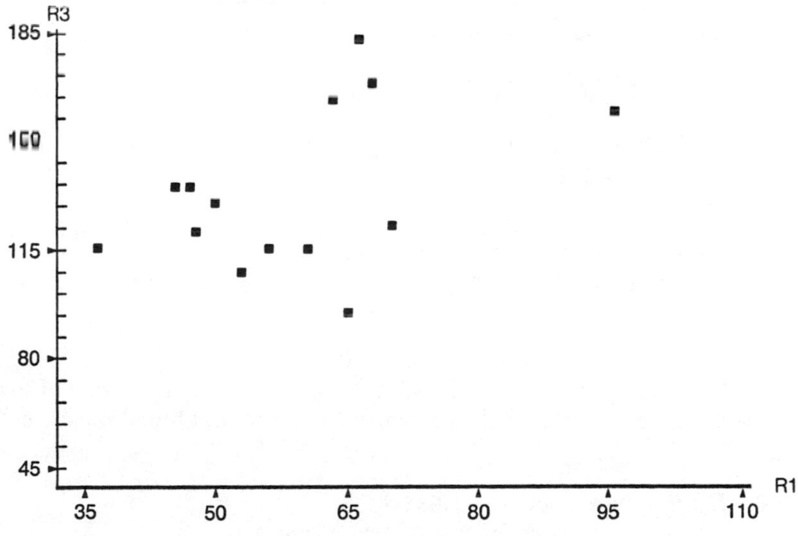

13.3 (b) The plot does not support the notion that there is a strong linear relationship between the two variables.
(c) Correlation of R1 and R3 = 0.439.

(d) Plot of zinc level in row 2 (R2) versus cadmium level in row 1 (R1):

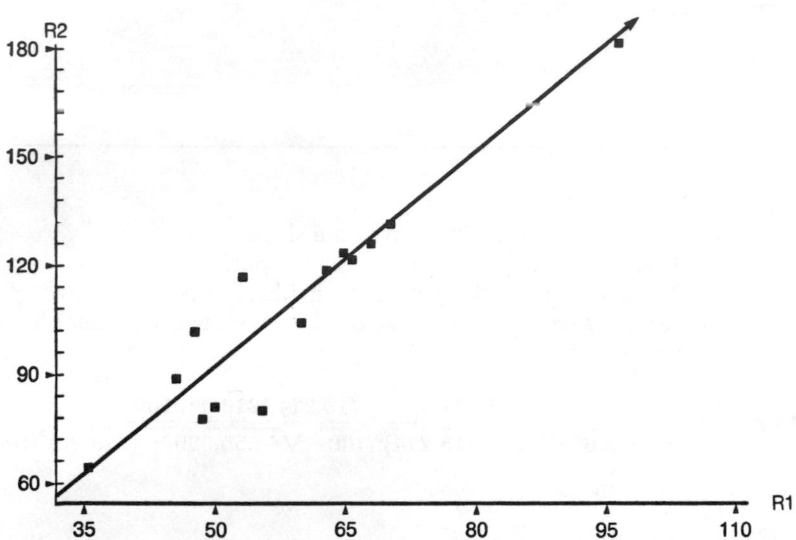

Correlation of R1 and R2 = .931.

(e) Yes, since it appears to follow a straight line.

(f) $b = \dfrac{94{,}517 - (823)(1516)/14}{51{,}169 - [(823)^2]/14} = 1.936$

$a = 108.286 - (1.936)(58.786)$
$= -5.523$
$\hat{y} = 1.936x - 5.523$

(g) $\hat{y} = 1.936(80) - 5.523 = 149.36$

(h) No, since this is not possible to assess with this method.

13.5 (a) $\alpha = .05$; $r = .447$; $n = 14$; $-.10 < \rho < .77$
(b) Since $\rho = 0$ is included in the confidence interval, we fail to reject the H_0 of no relationship between cadmium and blood pressure.

13.6 H_0: $\beta = 0$; $\alpha = .05$; $b = 1.936$

$\text{SE}(b) = \sqrt{\dfrac{232.363}{46{,}364.357}} = .071; t = \dfrac{1.936 - 0}{.071} = 27.3$

Reject H_0 and conclude that the population regression coefficient is significantly different from zero.

Chapter 14

14.1

Breastfed			Not breastfed		
No.	Age	Rank	No.	Age	Rank
1	14	10	1	9	4
2	15	11	2	10	5.5
3	12	7.5	3	8	3
4	13	9	4	6	1.5
5	19	12	5	10	5.5
			6	12	7.5
			7	6	1.5
			8	20	13
	$W_1 = 49.5$			$W_2 = 41.5$	
	$\bar{R}_1 = 9.90$			$\bar{R}_2 = 5.2$	

(a) H_0: Breastfed babies have more cavities than, or the same number of cavities as, nonbreastfed babies.
(b) H_1: Breastfed babies have fewer cavities than nonbreastfed babies.

$W_e = 35 \quad \sigma_W^2 = 46.67; \sigma_W = 6.83 \quad Z = \frac{W_1 - W_e}{\sigma_W} = \frac{49.5 - 35}{6.83} = 2.12$

One-tailed test: $Z(.05) = 1.64$

Reject H_0 in favor of H_1 and conclude that breastfed babies have fewer cavities.

14.2 (a) Vegetarians: $W_1 = 295$; $\bar{R}_1 = 16.4$; $n_1 = 18$

Nonvegetarians: $W_2 = 400$; $\bar{R}_2 = 21.5$; $n_2 = 19$

$W_e = \frac{18(18 + 19 + 1)}{2} = 342; \sigma_w = 32.9$

$Z = (295 - 342)/32.9 = -1.43$

Since $Z = 1.43$ is less than $Z(\alpha = .05) = 1.96$, we conclude there is no significant difference in diastolic blood pressure between the two groups.

14.3 (a) H_0: The number of cavities for town A is the same as for town B.
(b) H_1: The number of cavities for the two towns is different.
(c)

Town A			Town B		
Person	# Cavities	Rank	Person	# Cavities	Rank
1	0	1	1	3	15
2	1	4	2	2	9
3	3	15	3	2	9
4	1	4	4	3	15
5	1	4	5	4	19.5
6	2	9	6	3	15
7	1	4	7	2	9
8	2	9	8	3	15
9	3	15	9	4	19.5
10	1	4	10	3	15
		$W_1 = 69$			$W_2 = 41$
		$R_1 = 6.9$			$R_2 = 14.1$

$W_e = 105$, $\sigma_w = 13.2$

Since $z = -2.73$, which is less than -1.96, reject H_0

$\Sigma r_d = 55 \qquad \Sigma r_{d(+)} = W_1 = 51.5$
$W_e = 27.5 \qquad \Sigma r_{d(-)} = W_2 = 3.5$

$$Z = \frac{51.5 - 27.5}{\sqrt{(20 + 1)27.5/6}}$$

Since $Z = 2.45$ is greater than 1.96, we reject H_0 in favor of H_1 and conclude that the two towns have different cavity levels; that is, the level is higher in the town with unfluoridated water.

14.5

	Inspector (1)	Inspector (2)	Inspector (1) Rank	Inspector (2) Rank
	Column: C1	C2	C11	C22
Row	Count: 11	11	11	11
1	2.	1.	3.5	1.5
2	3.	3.	6.5	7.0
3	2.	3.	3.5	7.0
4	3.	2.	6.5	4.0
5	1.	2.	1.5	4.0
6	4.	5.	9.5	11.0
7	5.	4.	11.0	9.5
8	3.	2.	6.5	4.0
9	1.	1.	1.5	1.5
10	3.	4.	6.5	9.5
11	4.	3.	9.5	7.0

Correlation of C11 and C22 = .736

$$t = \frac{.736\sqrt{9}}{\sqrt{1 - (.736)^2}}$$
$$= 3.262$$

Two-tailed test: $t(.975, 9) = 2.26$

(a) H_0: There is no association between the cleanliness rankings of the two inspectors.

(b) H_1: There is an association between the cleanliness rankings of the two inspectors.

$\alpha = .05$

Since $t = 3.262$ is greater than $t(.975, 9) = 2.26$, we reject H_0 and conclude that there is a high correlation between the cleanliness rankings of the two inspectors.

Chapter 15

Note: Data are from *Statistical Abstract of the United States* for 1984.

15.1 1970: 205.1 million
1980: 227.7 million
1990: 246 million (lowest projection)

15.3 (a) 227,000

15.5

	Alaska	Kansas
Birthrate	23.7/1000	17.2/1000
Death rate	4.3/1000	9.3/1000

15.6 (1) Diseases of heart; (2) Malignant neoplasms; (3) Cerebrovascular diseases; (4) Accidents; and (5) Chronic obstructive pulmonary diseases

15.7 1950: whites, 61.1 per 1000; nonwhites, 221.6 per 1000 (excludes Alaska and Hawaii)

15.9

	Deaths		
	Total	Infant	Neonatal
Riverside	5404	106	145
San Bernardino	6180	152	208

15.10 (a) Alaska, 23.7 per 1000 population; Arizona, 18.4 per 1000 population
(b) The birthrate in Alaska is higher because of the higher proportion of the population in the child-bearing age group.

Chapter 16

16.1

Age interval	l_x	d_x	$_nL_x$	T_x	$\hat{e}_x$
70–75	62,481	12,640	281,437	755,828	12.10
75–80	49,841	14,175	214,476	474,391	9.52
80–85	35,666	13,714	142,674	259,915	7.29

16.4 (a) $_1q_0 = \frac{_1d_0}{l_0} = \frac{1902}{100{,}000} = .01902$

(c) $_5q_0 = \frac{_5d_0}{l_0} = \frac{1902 + 314}{100{,}000} = .02216$

16.5 (b) $_{10}q_{35} = \frac{_{10}d_{35}}{l_{35}} = \frac{1155 + 1720}{94{,}657} = .03037$

16.6 (a) $_{45}p_{20} = \frac{l_{65}}{l_{20}} = \frac{72{,}324}{96{,}848} = .7468$

16.7 (a) At birth, $\hat{e} = 71.02$.
(c) At 35 years, $\hat{e} = 39.24$.

Author Reference Index

Armitage 1971, 128, 155, 175

Belloc 1973, 4
Berkson 1946, 225
Brown & Hollander 1977, 182, 184, 186

Colton 1974, 9, 227

Dixon & Massey 1969, 186

Elveback, Guillier & Keating 1970, 66

Flesch 1974, 224

Hammond 1966, 31
Hill 1963, 9
Huff 1954, 3

Kuzma 1970, 9
Kuzma 1967, 215
Kuzma & Dixon [illegible], 208
Kuzma & Kissinger 1981, 146, 148
Kuzma & Sokol 1982, 163

Lilienfeld, Pedersen & Dowd 1967, 205

MacMahon et al. 1981, 153
MacMahon & Pugh 1970, 8
Mainland 1963, 2
Medical Research Council 1948, 9
Morbidity and Mortality Weekly Reports, 192
Muir & Nectoux 1977, 193

National Center for Health Statistics 1982, 34
National Center for Health Statistics 1981, 192
National Center for Health Statistics 1977, 203

Owen 1962, 85

Paul 1976, 4

Remington & Schork 1970, 205
Rimm et al. 1980, 155

Sackett 1979, 225
Scheaffer & Mendenhall 1979, 15
Sheon 1982, 224
Shyrock & Siegel 1973, 207, 213
Simpson 1957, 3
Smoking and Health, Surgeon General's Report 1979, 4
Snedecor 1979, 128
Snedecor 1973, 128
Statistical Abstract of the United States, 191
Steel and Torrie 1980, 128
Stocks 1944, 226
Surgeon General's Report 1965, 132, 136
Surgeon General's Report 1971, 168

Tukey 1977, 29

United Nations 1983, 194

Veterans Administration 1972, 5
Veterans Administration 1970, 5
Vital and Health Statistics, 193
Vital Statistics of the United States, 192
Vital Statistics Report, 192

Winslow et al. 1952, 192
World Health Organization 1977, 223

Subject Index

Abscissa, 27
Absolute values, 39
Acceptance region, 105
Addition rule, 52
Adjusted rates, 194, 202, 205
Age-specific death rate, 195
Alpha (α) error, 111–113
Alternative hypothesis, 104
Analysis of variance (ANOVA), 121–129
  application of, 126–128
  assumptions, 126
  calculations, 123–126
  function of, 122
  rationale for, 122–123
  table, 127
Analytical surveys, 8
Answers to problems, 251
Arithmetic mean, 37
Array, 24
Average, 38

Bar chart, 30
Before-and-after experiment, 97–98
Berksonian bias, 225
Beta (β) error, 111–113
Bias
  definition, 7
  dropout, 226
  interviewer, 222
  lead-time, 226
  memory, 226
  observer, 225
  participant, 226
  response, 225
  sampling, 223, 225
  selection, 225
Bimodal distribution, 28
Binomial distribution, 58, 61, 132–139
  approximation of, to normal distribution, 133
  confidence intervals for p, 137–139
  mean of, 132
  proportion, 132
  standard deviation of, 133
  term, 58
  test of significance, 134–136
Birth certificate, 191
Birth rate, crude, 200
Bit, 231
Bivariate data, 161
BMD, 232
Byte, 231

Case-control study, 6
Case-fatality proportion, 202
Cause-and-effect relationship, 159
Census, 3
Central limit theorem, 81
Central processing unit (CPU), 230
Central tendency, 37
Chi-square (χ^2)
  homogeneity test, 148
  table, 145
  test, 142, 145, 151
  test of difference between two proportions, 150
  test of goodness of fit, 151
Classification of data, 24–26
Clinical trial, 8–10
Clinical limits, 66
Coding, 223
Coefficient of variation, 42
Cohort studies, 7
Combinations of n objects taken r at a time, 56
Compiler, 231
Concurrent control group, 9
Confidence interval, 91
  for difference of $p_1 - p_2$, 138
  for p, 137
  for ρ (rho), 167
Contingency table, 142
  for regression coefficient, 175
  2 × 2, 152
Continuous variables, 24
Control group, 9
Convenience sampling, 14
Correlation coefficient, 161, 164–169
  confidence belts for, 167
  perfect, 164
Counting rules, 54
Critical region, 104
Critical values, 123
Cumulative frequency polygon, 29

Cumulative percentage, 26
Cumulative relative frequency, 26

Data
  analysis of, 224, 227
  categorical, 142
  collection of, 223, 227
  enumeration, 142
  frequency, 142
  qualitative, 142
  quantitative, 132
Death certificate, 191
Death rate, 195, 196
Decennial census, 190
Degrees of freedom (d.f.)
  ANOVA, 127
  before-and-after experiments, 97–98
  chi-square, 144
  correlation, 166
  F-distribution, 123
  paired *t*, 98
  pooled *t*, 94
  regression, 175
  single *t*, 84
Dependent variable, 161
Descriptive statistics, 3
Dichotomous variables, 58
Direct method of adjustment, 203
Discrete variables, 24
Distribution
  bell-shaped, 67
  bimodal, 28
  binomial, 58, 132–139
  Gaussian, 67
  normal, 66
  Poisson, 134
  probability, 56
  rectangular, 28
  skewed, 28
  standard normal, 69
  symmetrical, 28
Distribution-free methods, 179, 180
Distribution of sample means, 79
Double blind, 9
Double notation, 124

Errors
  systematic, 7
  type I, 111–113
  type II, 111–113
Estimation
  confidence intervals, 91–97
  confidence limits, 92
  correlation coefficient, 161–164
  difference between means, 94–95
  difference between two proportions, 138
  mean, 90
  point, 90
  proportion, 137
  regression line, 171
  standard deviation, 83
Evaluation of a research report, 224
Events
  equally likely, 49
  independent, 51
  mutually exclusive, 51–53
Expected frequency (E), 142
Experiments, 5
  planning and designing, 97–98

F-distribution, 122, 123
F-statistic (test), 125
F-table, 244
Factorial notation, 55
Fertility measures, 200, 201
Fetal death ratio, 199
Five year survival rate, 215
Fourfold table, 152
Frequency distribution, 24, 25
Frequency polygon, 28
Frequency table
  class boundaries, 26
  class frequency, 25
  class intervals, 24
  class limits, 25

Gaussian distribution, 67
General fertility rate, 201
GIGO syndrome, 230
Gradient, 170
Graphic presentations, 26–34
Grouped data, 42–44
  means, 43
  variance, 43

Hardware, computer, 230
Health survey, 219
Histogram, 27
Honolulu Heart Study, 18, 21–28, 30–31, 42–43, 79–80, 86, 96–97, 105–108, 111–13, 233–238
Hypothesis tests
  ANOVA, 121–129
  binomial proportion, 134
  correlation coefficient, 166
  goodness of fit, 151
  homogeneity, 148
  means
    one, σ known, 106, 107
    one, σ unknown, 109, 110
    two (difference between dependent), 115
    two (difference between independent), 113

Hypothesis tests *continued*
  nonparametric, 180–186
  proportions
    one, 134
    two, 135, 150
  relationship of, to confidence intervals, 115
  signed rank test, 186
  slope of regression line, 174
  Spearman rank correlation coefficient, 184–186
  2 × 2 contingency, 152
  Wilcoxon rank-sum test, 181
  Wilcoxon signed-rank test, 184

Incidence rate, 201
Independent observations, 155
Independent samples, 93, 113
Independent trials, 58
Independent variable, 161
Indirect method of adjustment, 205
Infant mortality rate, 198
Inferences, types. *See* Estimation; Hypothesis tests
Inferential statistics, 3
Intercept (β_0), 171
Interviews, 222

Kruskal-Wallis test, 184

Least-squares method, 171
Level of confidence, 91, 92
Level of significance, 104
Life expectation, 211
Life tables
  abridged, 208
  cohort, 208
  complete, 210
  current, 208
  follow-up, 214
Line of best fit, 163
Linear correlation coefficient, 161
Lost to follow-up, 214, 215
Lower subscript, 150

Maternal mortality ratio, 198
Median, 37, 38
Mean, 37
Mean deviation, 39
Mean square (MS), 127
Measures of central tendency, 37
Measures of variation (dispersion), 39–42
Microcomputers, 238, 239
Mode, 37, 38
Morbidity, 201
Mortality data, 192
Mu (μ), 44, 45
Multiple-range test, 129
Multiple Risk Factor Intervention Trial (MRFIT), 4
Multiple tests, 128
Multiplication rule, 51
Mutually exclusive events, 51, 53

National Health Survey, 193
Neonatal mortality proportion, 199
Nominal numeral, 21
Nonparametric tests, 179–180
Normal deviate, 69
Normal distribution, 66
Normal limits, 66
Null hypothesis, 104
Numbers, sum of 1 through *n*, 180

Objectives of a study, 221
Observed frequencies, 142
Odds ratio, 153
Ogive, 29
One-tail test, 108
Ordinal numeral, 21
Ordinate, 27
Outcome variable, 6
Output, computerized data, 237–238
Outliers, 167

p-value, 104
Paired data (before and after experiment), 97–98
Parameter, 13
Parametric methods, 179
Pearson's product-moment r, 164
Peer review, 224
Percentile, defined, 29
Perinatal mortality proportion, 200
Permutations, 55
Person-years, 211
Phi (ϕ) coefficient, 154
Pie chart, 32
Placebo, 5, 9
Planning a health survey, 219–224
Point estimate, 90
Poisson distribution, 134
Pooled sample variance, 94
Population
  mean, 45
  parameters, 13
  target, 221
  variance, 45
Population at risk, 195
Power of a statistical test, 112
Prediction equation, 161
Pretest, 223
Prevalence proportion, 202
Probability
  a posteriori, 93
  addition rule, 52

definition, 49
distribution, 56
multiplication rule, 51
Professional Activity Study, 193
Program, computer, 230
Proportion, 194
Proportional mortality, 197
Prospective studies, 7

Qualitative data, 132
Qualitative variables, 24
Quantitative data, 132
Quantitative variables, 24
Questionnaire, 222

Random allocation, 9
Random number table, 15
Random sample, 16
Random sampling, 14
Random variable, 57, 161
Range, 39
Rank correlation coefficient, 184
Rank-order tests, 180–186
Rates
adjusted, 194
crude, 194, 195
specific, 194–197
Ratio, 194
Ratio scale, 21
Record, computer, 233
Rectangular distribution, 28
Registry, chronic disease, 193
Regression, 161
coefficient, 170
line, 163, 170–175
point ($\bar{x}$, $\bar{y}$), 172
slope (gradient), 170
Rejection region, 104
Relative deviate, 69
Relative frequency, 25
Relative odds, 153
Relative risk, 153
Research report, 224
Residual, 163, 171
Retrospective study, 6
Rho (ρ), 166, 168

Sample size determination, 99, 100
Sample statistics, 43
Samples, 13
cluster, 15
convenience, 14
independent, 93, 113
large (size), 13
random, 14, 16
representative, 18
stratified, 14
systematic, 14
Sampling
convenience, 14
distribution, 78, 80
frame, 14
stratified, 14
systematic, 14
SAS, 232
Scatter diagram, 162, 163
Short-cut formula (variance), 43
Sigma (σ), lower case, 45
Sigma (Σ), upper case. *See inside cover*
Significance level, 104
Single blind, 9
Skewed distribution, 28
Slope (β_1), 170
Software, computer, 230, 231
Solutions to problems, 251
Spearman correlation coefficient, 185
Spearman rank-order correlation coefficient, 184
SPSS, 232
Square root, 41
Standard deviation
calculation, 41, 43, 45
definition, 40
pooled estimate, 94
Standard error
of the difference, 93
of the difference between proportions, 136
of the estimate, 174
of the mean, 81
Standard Metropolitan Statistical Areas (SMSAs), 190
Standard normal distribution, [illegible]
Stationary population, 211
Statistic, 13
Statistically significant, 110
Statistics, 2
Stem-and-leaf display, 30
Stimulus variable, 6
Student's *t* distribution, 84
Subscript notation
F, 125
t, 84
χ^2, 150
"Success," 58–60
Sum of squares, 125
Summation notation (Σ). *See inside cover*
Surgeon General's Reports, 4, 132, 136, 168
Surveys, 5
analytical, 8
descriptive, 8
planning of, 10, 219–224
Symmetrical distribution, 28
Systematic sampling, 14

Tables
  binomial probability, 241–243
  χ^2, 145
  F, 244–247
  random numbers, 15
  t, 85
  Z, 70
Tables, guidelines for constructing, 24, 25
Tally, 25
Target population, 221
Test of significance, 106. *See also* Hypothesis tests
Test statistic, 104
Time-sharing, 232
Treatment group, 9
Tree diagram, 50
2 × 2 contingency table, 152
Two-tail test, 108
Type I error, 111–113
Type II error, 111–113

Universe. See Population
U.S. standard million, 204

Variables, 221
  continuous, 24
  dependent, 161
  discrete, 24
  independent, 161
  outcome, 161
  random, 57
Variance, pooled sample, 94
Variation, measures of
  defined, 40
  formula, 41, 45
  short-cut formula, 43
  sources, 41
Venn diagram, 53
Verification, data, 234–235
Veterans Administration Cooperative Study, 5
Vital events, 190
Vital statistics, 190

Wilcoxon rank-sum test, 180
Wilcoxon signed-rank test, 182
Within-group variance, 123

Yates continuity correction, 152
y-axis intercept (β_0), 171

Z standard score, 69, 83, 106

normal curve - Z score pg 70 two tailed

t dist. pg 85 one tailed in <u>this</u> book

χ^2 (chi square) 145 "automatically given a 2 tailed test"